Atlas of Minimally Invasive Surgery in Esophageal Carcinoma

Shailesh Puntambekar
Miguel A. Cuesta

Atlas of Minimally Invasive Surgery in Esophageal Carcinoma

Springer

Dr. Shailesh Puntambekar
Galaxy Laparoscopic Institute
Pune-411004
India

Dr. Miguel A. Cuesta
Vrije Universiteit Medical Center
1007 MB Amsterdam
The Netherlands

ISBN 978-1-4471-6008-3 ISBN 978-1-84882-768-4 (eBook)
DOI 10.1007/978-1-84882-768-4
Springer Dordrecht Heidelberg London New York

Additional material to this book can be downloaded from http://extra.springer.com.

Printed on acid-free paper.

Springer is part of Springer Science+Business Media (www.springer.com)

Foreword

Esophageal cancer remains both a life-threatening disease and an everyday challenge for both patients and surgeons. Controversies regarding its management are prevalent, creating confusion and uncertainties. Preoperative mortality and morbidity, limited overall and disease-free survival, and dismal prognosis make decision making regarding the choice of management difficult.

Prof. Puntambekar is an enthusiastic surgeon, full of energy and inspiration. This young colleague offers contemporary possibilities for management of esophageal carcinoma. Prof. Cuesta is an experienced surgeon working in Europe. These two authors have compiled their work in this atlas and enrich the reader with experience encompassing two different continents. This book is an update of novel surgical techniques of combined thoracoscopic and laparoscopic approach in minimally invasive management of esophageal carcinoma.

Prof. Puntambekar's outstanding experience and expertise in this field is fully illustrated in this book in a step-by-step description of the operative procedures. This book should be regarded as a landmark for the surgical management of esophageal carcinoma.

The book is distinctive and the technical steps are original, reflecting a deep knowledge of the regional anatomy and a unique ability of visual and operative orientation.

I read the book with care and admiration and would like to ensure every potential reader that not only is this book one of its kind on the international front but it also opens up new discussions and possibilities for the management of esophageal cancer with minimal morbidity. The approach is practical, easy to comprehend, and replicate. The oncological and operative concepts are well elucidated.

The contributions of Prof. Puntambekar and Prof. Cuesta are outstanding and applicable in everyday clinical and surgical practice. This innovative and original work will remain a precious heritage in the surgical management of esophageal carcinoma.

Prof. N. J. Lygidakis

Preface

The role of minimal invasive surgery (MIS) in esophageal cancer is slowly but surely being established. We started MIS in 2004. Starting with transhiatal esophagectomy, we ventured into thoracoscopy later in 2005. We had been performing open surgery for esophageal cancer for almost 12 years before embarking on the laparoscopic version. But with MIS, we realized that though the hospitalization time did not change, the overall morbidity decreased considerably. Avoiding thoracotomy was probably solely responsible in bringing down the lung complications. The magnification allowed a better and cleaner visualization of the structures. Surgeons performing open thoracotomy do realize the depth in which one has to perform the surgery, especially the supra-azygous dissection. Thoracoscopy allowed an easy access to these regions.

We started performing laparoscopy keeping in mind the open surgical steps in esophagectomy, the bottom line being that the basic surgical procedure must remain the same, only that the modality changed from open to laparoscopy. Hence, the procedures described here are a duplication of the open surgical steps. Thus, thoracoscopy was also started in lateral position since, as surgeons we were more accustomed to the anatomy in lateral position.

After gaining considerable experience in MIS in esophageal cancers, we realized the need for detailing the surgical steps. Any surgeon wishing to adapt MIS in esophageal surgery should have a readymade atlas which can describe the steps. The steps should be clear, precise, and duplicable. This atlas is an attempt to describe the surgeries in a stepwise fashion.

The first chapters give an overview of role of surgery in esophageal cancer. We are indebted to Prof. Praful Desai for his invaluable contribution to this book. He is my guru and mentor. But more than that, this thought process comes from a stalwart having 40 years of experience in esophageal surgery! He started doing esophageal surgery at the time when very few surgeons dared to venture into this territory, owing to the high morbidity and mortality involved. He has to his credit the experience of performing more than 1000 esophageal resections and who better than him can understand this surgery! Coming from the era of open surgery and great open surgeons, he has witnessed the emergence of this new technique and endorsed it with an open mind. His thoughts and views serve as a balance between open and laparoscopic surgery in esophageal cancer.

The thoracoscopy is described in two different positions so that the reader can have the unbiased option of choosing any option to suit the needs. Prof. Cuesta has described the procedure in prone position, while we describe the same in lateral position. Two approaches with different positions will provide a complete anatomical picture to the reader. Prof. Cuesta has a huge experience of esophageal cancers and his contribution to this book remains invaluable. He has also described a different technique for Laparoscopic Transhiatal esophagectomy.

Change is a constant and vital feature of any scientific technique, and this book would not have been complete without discussing the future in MIS. We have included the chapter on Robotic surgery for this very reason. As more and more centers get equipped with the facility of Robotics, this surgery may be done more commonly.

Dr. Geetanjali Agarwal, a laparoscopist and cancer surgeon, is my associate who has taken a great effort in compiling the world literature on MIS. She is a part of our operating team, and shares our surgical experience.

Dr. Ravi Sathe is a senior laparoscopist and surgeon. He is my associate and team member. He is a technocrat and has in-depth knowledge of the laparoscopic instruments and staplers. His chapter gives a detailed account and working knowledge of the staplers. This will help one to decide and choose the right type of staplers for a given surgery.

This book would not have been possible without the dedicated and painstaking efforts of my colleague, Dr. Anjali Patil, who is a consultant laparoscopist and surgeon in our institute. She is also a visiting surgeon to Athens, Greece. The recording of surgeries, selecting, and compiling of the material is a monumental task. It is thanks to her that we could accomplish our goal.

Dr. Neeraj Rayate, Dr. Rajan Jaggad, and Dr. Saurabh Joshi are all my associates and accomplished laparoscopists and surgeons. Together they went through a collection of multiple patient recordings to shoot more than 5000 pictures. These had to be sorted and compiled. After going through the photographs, many had to be discarded and replaced by new ones. The final photographs were changed more than 20 times, and every time I changed them, these young surgeons were again at their task, enthusiastically compiling the legends with new ones. I cannot thank all these colleagues enough and am grateful to them for their tireless support and enthusiasm. Every small effort and every nut in a car is equally important in their own place to the final product! I thank them all for everything.

I would like to thank my wife and my daughters for their unconditional help, support, and inspiration.

Last, but not the least, the most important people behind the creation of this book are all my patients without whom the book would not have happened! They have taught me compassion, courage, and humility. I thank them with all my heart!

We have made a sincere effort to encompass the different techniques and aspects of MIS in esophageal cancers in this atlas. We do realize that there may be many more techniques and many more experts performing these surgeries. Our views and technique are our own and in no way do we wish to be dogmatic. We sincerely believe that this atlas will be used as a first step toward adapting MIS in esophageal cancers. One can develop and add individual variations and techniques later.

Every step taken in the right direction brings you closer to your goal, and we would consider our goals achieved if we can urge and motivate more and more surgeons to follow this path!

Shailesh Puntambekar
Pune, India

Miguel A. Cuesta
Amsterdam, The Netherlands

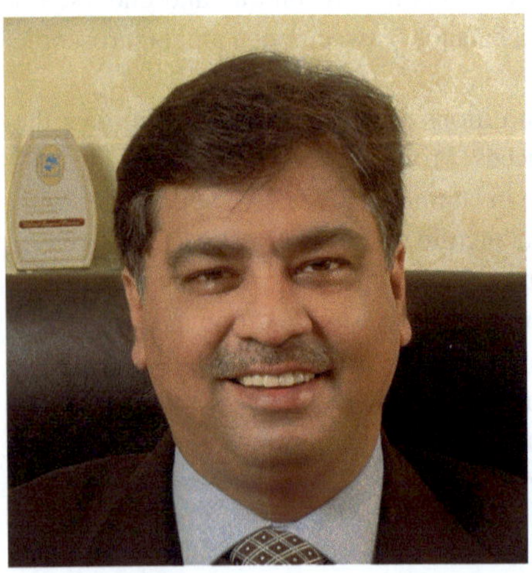

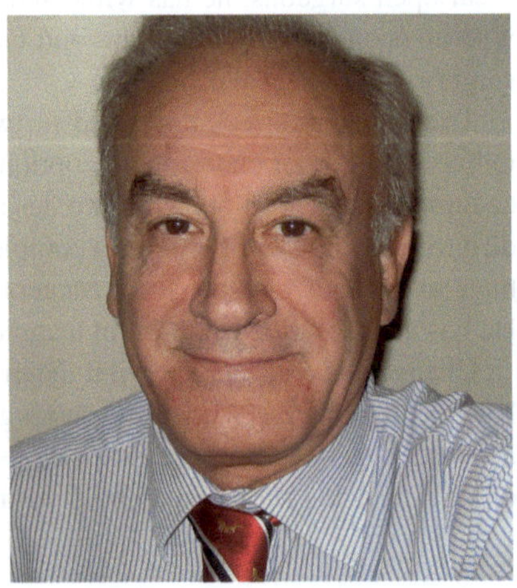

Contents

Contributors

Geetanjali A. Agarwal, MBBS, MS Galaxy Laparoscopy Institute, Pune, Maharashtra, India

Surya S. A. Y. Biere, MD Department of Surgery, VU Medical Center, Amsterdam, The Netherlands

Judith Boone, MD, PhD Department of Surgery, University Medical Center Utrecht, Utrecht, The Netherlands

Miguel A. Cuesta, MD, PhD Department of Surgery, VU Medical Center, Amsterdam, The Netherlands

Praful B. Desai, MS Department of Oncosurgery, Bombay Hospital and Research Centre, Mumbai, Maharashtra, India

Bob H. M. Heijnen, MD Department of Surgery, VU Medical Center, Amsterdam, The Netherlands

Rajan B. Jagad, MD Department of Gastrointestinal and Laparoscopic Surgery, Haria L. G. Rotary Hospital, Vapi, Gujarat, India

Saurabh N. Joshi, MBBS, MS Galaxy Laparoscopy Institute, Pune, Maharashtra, India

Wolter Oosterhuis, MD, PhD Department of Surgery, VU Medical Center, Amsterdam, The Netherlands

Anjali M. Patil, MS Department of Advanced Laparoscopic Surgery, Galaxy Laparoscopy Institute, Pune, Maharashtra, India

Shailesh Puntambekar, MS Galaxy Laparoscopy Institute, Pune, Maharashtra, India

Neeraj V. Rayate, MS, DNB Department of Advanced Laparoscopic Surgery, Galaxy Laparoscopy Institute, Pune, Maharashtra, India

Ravindra M. Sathe, MBBS, DA (Anesthesia), MS (Surgery) Department of Minimal Access Surgery, Galaxy Laparoscopy Institute, Pune, Maharashtra, India

Joris J. B. Scheepers, MD Department of Surgery, Erasmus Medical Center, Rotterdam, The Netherlands

Donald L. van der Peet, MD, PhD Department of Surgery, VU Medical Center, Amsterdam, The Netherlands

Richard van Hillegersberg, MD, PhD Department of Surgery, University Medical Center Utrecht, Utrecht, The Netherlands

1

Surgery for Cancer of the Esophagus "The Continuing Evolution"

Praful B. Desai

Introduction and History

Ever since Torek [1] reported the first successful total esophagectomy, there has been a continuing evolution and appraisal of many different surgical techniques and approaches which are now practiced in the surgical management of this difficult cancer. Unavoidably, a lot has changed in our overall therapeutic approach based on our knowledge of imaging techniques, preoperative assessment, the efficacy of chemotherapy (CT) and radiotherapy (RT) which, when necessary, can be appropriately incorporated in the treatment planning based on the clinical setting of a given patient.

It is important to realize, however, that surgery has remained steadfast in the management of esophageal cancer when the disease is loco-regional and is amenable to a complete surgical clearance. Surgery of esophageal cancer is probably one of the most demanding and challenging procedure for the surgeon and the patient alike – with a significant morbidity and mortality, particularly in inappropriately selected patients. The approach and the extent of surgery undertaken, therefore, vary widely based on a surgeon's experience, expertise, bias, and comfort zone.

Newer technology of minimally invasive surgery (MIS.) for cancer of the esophagus is making slow and steady inroads into traditional open surgery and probably will be used with increasing frequency in the future as experience and expertise steadily increase [2, 3].

The first half of the last century saw standardization of various surgical approaches, that is, the left thoraco-abdominal and the Ivor Lewis/Tanner approach with effective clearance of lymphatic drainage in the abdomen (left gastric/celiac/hepatic/paraesophageal and mediastinal nodes).

Various authors like Adams [4], Garlock, Sweet [5], Ellis, and many others contributed a great deal – McOwen's and Makayamas three stage approaches helped to standardize total esophagectomy and cervical anastomosis. The transhiatal approach (Orringer) [6–8] in the 1970s was mainly devised to avoid intrathoracic anastomosis which had a high anastomotic disruption rate at that time.

The extent of surgery (total or subtotal esophagectomy), the site of anastomosis (cervical or intrathoracic), and two- or three-field lymph node dissections continue to be debated, though large experiences have now been collated by many authors.

The advent of MIS in the late 1980s & 1990s has slowly seen acceptance at the present time, after adequate experience in the new millennium. The fact that so many different approaches and techniques exist indicates that no one procedure or technique can be applied to all patients. It would also be correct to state that one procedure cannot be labeled as superior to another, despite numerous good studies and comparisons of the procedures seen in the literature.

This is particularly so because carcinoma of the esophagus is a heterogeneous disease treated across the globe by a large number of institutions and surgeons of varying infrastructure, surgical expertise and experience.

It is, therefore, prudent to select a procedure which appears to be suitable for a given patient based on a given clinical setting to serve his best interests. Individualization of surgical procedure therefore should be based on the patients' medical status, the type and extent of the lesion, and the possibility of considering nonsurgical treatment as well as the use of neo-adjuvant or adjuvant therapies. Factors mentioned above should therefore finally decide the most appropriate surgical approach in a given patient.

Preoperative Evaluation

The single most important factor for a successful surgical outcome in cancer esophagus is case selection. It cannot be overemphasized that the morbidity which results after inappropriate surgery (R_2 resections, severe postoperative complications) is often worse than the existing disease itself and severely impacts negatively on the quality of life issues. This is apart from hospital costs and the necessity to be confined. We would leave patients infinitely worse after unnecessary explorations for a nonresectable disease or leaving behind disease (R_2 resections). Appropriate preoperative evaluation, therefore, must pay attention to:

i. Overall assessment (many are smokers, alcohol addictives, poor nutritional states, cardiopulmonary, hepatic, and renal function evaluations, routine urine, blood chemistry, etc.)
ii. Endoscopic assessment (to identify skip-lesions and morphology or the type of growth either cicatrizing and obstructive or proliferative or nonobstructive)
iii. Imaging procedures

Apart from routine procedures like CXR and esophagogram, a CT-scan is mandatory. Endoscopic ultrasound (EUS) and PET-CT are optional but should be strongly considered when the lesion appears to be a borderline case for a surgical approach. In published literature [9], in nearly 25%, the treatment approaches may change after PET-CT or EUS studies. The PET positivity should be confirmed by histology before rejecting a patient from a surgical approach.

Despite very efficient current chemotherapyradiotherapy (CT/RT), surgery remains the treatment of choice in a loco-regionally confined cancer of the esophagus (except in carcinoma of the cervical esophagus and high Supra-aortic lesions at the thoracic inlet – which are poor subjects for surgery). A lesion more than 6–7 cm in its vertical extent (if localized) should be downstaged by Neo-adjuvant chemotherapy and then assessed for surgery.

Globally there is an increase in the incidence of Barrets' esophagus, dysplasia, and adenocarcinoma of the lower esophagus. The principles of surgical treatment have remained the same, that is, removing the primary lesion with a good proximal margin of at least 5–7 cm (to avoid skip lesions) and clearance of regional lymph nodes.

Variations of this approach by always doing a total esophagectomy and two- or three-field dissections are open to continued discussions and debates – which will not end. Different procedures yielding the same or better results with minimal morbidity still holds the sway, depending on the site of the lesion, the experience, the expertise, and the comfort zone of the surgeon.

In a recent review [10] of 517 esophagectomies from Mayo clinic, 392 were Ivor Lewis, 57 total esophagectomy, and 68 transhiatal esophagectomy (TTE). The report documents that lymph node retrieval is better in open transthoracic approach than transhiatal.

Similar reports have been reported in literature by Holscher et al. [11] There is no doubt that more adequate retrieval of nodes is possible by a TTE (transthoracic esophagectomy) than by THE. In lesions of the lower third and cardio-esophageal junction a TTE (Ivor Lewis) is often preferable and is currently more frequently performed globally except probably in Japan, and those surgeons who always prefer THE. The currently low anastomotic leakage rate of 2–4% has taken the sting and the danger out of intrathoracic anastomosis.

Standard surgical approaches

Site of lesion			Surgical approaches
Adenocarcinoma, squamous Ca	C.O.Jn.lower esophagus cardia	⟶	Left thoraco abdominal (TTE) Ivor-Lewis/Tanner (TTE) Transhiatal (THE)
Squamous Ca, adenocarcinoma (rare)	Mid 1/3 lesion	⟶	High Ivor. Lewis/Tanner (TTE) Three stage total esophagectomy (TTE) Transhiatal esophagectomy (THE)
Cervical Supra aortic Thoracic inlet		⟶	Poor candidates for surgery CT/RT/Stenting etc. are better options

This recent well-documented study from a major institution (Mayo clinic) clearly indicates that any emphatic and definitive statement about a particular method in clinical medicine indicates a personal bias, dogma, and inability to view the subject in a balanced manner. The concept of total esophagectomy and cervical anastomosis basically evolved to avoid an intrathoracic anastomotic disruption and its inherent morbidity and mortality. Actually, in all the series, cervical anastomotic disruption and subsequent morbidity are considerably higher than the intrathoracic anastomosis. With experience and proper case selection, the incidence of anastomotic leaks (intra thoracic) by high-volume surgeons and hospitals ranges between 3 and 5%. With aggressive management, most of these patients can be salvaged and the mortality is between 2 and 3%.

The surgery of cancer is indeed the surgery of the lymph nodes. The old adage of *"remove the growth, the growth as a whole and the growing ends of the growth (lymph nodes)"* has stood the test of time for a successful outcome. The concept of "Sentinal Nodes" has not yet been studied in esophageal cancer and till such time that we have data, reliance on appropriate lymph node clearance will remain the "Sine-qua-non" for surgery for esophageal cancer.

The chaotic and profuse lymphatic drainage of an organ extending over three anatomic regions is a major issue in the surgical treatment of esophageal cancer.

In an advanced esophageal carcinoma ($T_{3,4}$ $N_{1,2}$), it is likely that lymph nodes away from the site may be involved (say cervical nodes from a lower esophageal carcinoma); however, these are hardly the cases that one would plan for a surgical therapy. For a routinely resectable case ($T_{1,2,3}$ $N_{0,1}$) – the incidence of node metastasis at a faraway site is around 10% or less. This is, therefore, not a strong reason to subject the other 90% to a total esophagectomy and a three-field dissection at all times keeping in mind the morbidity, complications and long-term survival results, which has not shown a significantly increased survival in this group subjected to such a major procedure.

It, therefore, stands to reason that a good loco-regional dissection (two-field – abdomen and thoracic up to paratracheal region) in cancer of the lower 1/3, c.o.jn (cardio-esophageal junction) and cardia lesions is a sound surgical approach. Intrathoracic anastomosis at the level of the azygos vein or just proximal always provides a good and safe proximal margin of more than 5 cm.

Lesions of the mid-1/3, when a good proximal margin is not available, should have a total esophagectomy with cervical anastomosis and pick up of cervical nodes in its lower reaches.

For the same reasons, routine sacrifice of the thoracic duct and the entire azygos vein are not routinely indicated unless the lesion is very bulky, is locally advanced, and has a large nodal burden in the medastinum. Such lesions are not surgically rewarding and with proper preoperative evaluation could be treated with nonsurgical modalities like CT/RT/stenting etc. to control the symptoms and relieve dysphagia.

Personal experiences in two-field loco-regional dissections reveal that the opinions expressed by the author here are justified [12].

Total esophagectomy and three-field dissections are justified in a lesion of the mid 1/3 where proximal margin is inadequate and indeed the neck has to be entered and the lower cervical nodes can be dissected with ease.

Lesions of the cervical esophagus and those at the thoracic inlet and supra-aortic esophagus yield uniformly poor results with surgery and are best treated by CT/RT/stenting as needed.

Complications in Surgery for Cancer of the Esophagus

Prevention

Adequate preoperative assessment should be initiated by a thorough clinical examination, endoscopic examination and CT scan. The EUS and PET/CT are optional but may be indicated in borderline operability cases. Nutritional status, blood chemistry (proteins, albumin levels, etc.) are of vital importance before doing the case selection for surgery. The existing comorbidities should be carefully assessed and rectified before subjecting a patient to surgery with particular emphasis to cardiopulmonary and renal function evaluation.

If a patient is otherwise fit and appropriately selected, the postoperative recovery is generally smooth and uneventful.

Routine Complications After Any Major Surgery

Esophageal surgery entails severe surgical and anesthetic stress because of the age (generally above 50 years), combined abdomino-thoracic and often, as needed, cervical approaches. Routine postoperative anesthetic care in the ICU is preferable for the first 2 or 3 days. Cardiopulmonary evaluation is a major issue during this time. Effective physiotherapy will prevent consolidation and pneumonic changes, and proper attention at surgery will avoid wound infections and other routine complications.

Specific Complications

Anastomatic disruption is a major complication which requires vigilant postoperative care to detect it early so as to ensure a quick therapeutic response. With experience, this complication should not exceed 5–8% and with proper care most of these patients can be salvaged.

In more than 90% of cases, the disruption is due to a technical miss by the surgeon. Rarely, low levels of nutrition, allowing the gastric conduit to distend/dilate due to delayed gastric emptying could be one of the reasons.

Necrosis at the anastomosis mostly occurs because of the gastric conduit ischemia due to poor vascularity and tension at the anastomotic site or less than secure anastomosis.

Adequate thoracic drainage is crucial to keep the lungs fully expanded.Routine drainage of the posterior (retro-gastric) mediastinum by a negative vacuum suction tube will reveal abnormal discharges (saliva, infected, necrotic material) indicating a leak at a very early stage. Most large thoracic drains do not show any evidence of abnormal discharge as the drains are at the periphery near the chest wall and the infective discharges often localized in the anterior or posterior mediastinum.

A *major leak*, however, produces an emergency situation with hydro-pneumothorax, tachypnea, and tachycardia, and a shock-like state which calls for an emergency exploration. Rapid evacuation of the infected discharges, appropriate drainages, and disengaging the anastomosis with a cervical esophagostomy and a feeding gastrostomy by returning the gastric conduit to the abdomen are necessary. Colonic reconstruction at a later date will have to be considered after the patient recovers from this severe complication. Majority of these patients will recover if early intervention is undertaken.

Minor leaks will heal (if adequate drainage, lung expansion, and proper nutrition are in place). There is no indication for intervention.

A doubtful or questionable leak when suspected should be confirmed by an oral contrast study.

(a) Anastomosis

The single most important and vital step in surgery for cancer of the esophagus is the anastomosis to restore the continuity of the GI tract. There is no doubt that a stomach fashioned into a tube which snugly lies in the posterior mediastinum is the ideal conduit. Colon may be the next choice, particularly for reconstruction after a major anastomotic breakdown.

It has been proven many times over; by hard data that incidence of anastomotic disruptions is inversely proportional with high-volume surgeons and institutions where esophageal surgery is common. It is difficult to define "high volume"; however, around 50 resections a year could be comfortably labeled as high volume [13].

It is important to emphasize that anastomotic disruptions are *not* due to the type of a suture material used, or whether the anastomosis is hand-sewn or stapled. As long as the esophageal and stomach ends are vascular and the anastomosis is devoid of tension, it will heal rapidly.

Oral feeds (clear liquids) can be started as early as on the third postoperative morning if the course is uneventful and stable.

(b) Delayed Complications

Long-term consequences like anastomotic strictures, delayed gastric emptying (DGE) and acid gastric reflux can occur following these procedures.

Esophageal surgery often has negative impact on the quality of life (QOL) issues even if the surgery has been smooth and recovery expeditious; it has to be emphasized that a R_2 resection (leaving behind macroscopic disease) and/or a complicated recovery will leave the patient in a suboptimal condition, from which recovery is long and protracted.

The DGE and consequent gastro-esophageal reflux are a source of significant distress which may continue for months or even longer. The only way to prevent this is to ensure a good pyloric function by a liberal pyloro-myotomy. Pyloro-plasty often produces very free regurgitation and consequent reflux which may lead to anastomotic strictures. Erythromycin may help to relieve symptoms marginally. Most strictures within the first six months are a result of this reflux and should be treated conservatively. The DGE/reflux/anastomotic strictures are thus a summation of cause and effect reflects consequent to the surgical procedure which severely alters the anatomy and physiology of the upper G.I. tract.

Apart from the reasons stated earlier, debate has ranged about the suture material and the incidence of strictures. Many studies have shown that "incidence of strictures" is almost similar with hand-sewn or stapled anastomosis. Some reviews indicate a greater incidence with staples (foreign body); however, none of the studies are statistically significant – however, it stands to reason that absorbable polyglactin or polydioxanone sutures 3.0 or 4.0 would be an ideal suture material to minimize the incidence of strictures due to unabsorbable sutures.

(c) Type of Anastomosis

Anastomotic disruptions has nothing to do with the type of anastomosis, whether continuous or interrupted, as long as the ends are vascular; however, the author prefers only a few – 4 or 5 – (too many sutures are a source of stenosis) interrupted one layer through and through sutures with special attention at the corners, which should be inverted by the serosa of the stomach and the muscle layer of the esophagus. A few inverting sutures of esophageal muscle and stomach serosa will ensure a safe anastomosis. End-to-end or end-to-side, with a flap or without one, a vascular tension-free anastomosis will unite. The author prefers an end-to-end anastomosis which avoids creation of a stump. In its final analysis, the best anastomosis depends on the comfort zone of the surgeon.

Summary of Fundamental Facts for Esophageal Cancer Surgery

- Surgery, when the disease is loco-regional, (except cervical and thoracic inlet lesions) is the current standard of care for esophageal Squamous cell carcinoma and adenocarcinoma. This includes lesions of the c.o.jn and cardia.

- Preferably and ideally, the surgical procedure should be attempted by high-volume surgeons and institutions with adequate infrastructure and expertise, as the morbidity and mortality with low-volume surgeons/hospitals are significantly higher. Those interested should pursue the learning curve [14].
- A lesion at the cardia, c.o.jn, and extreme lower esophagus cancer can be adequately dealt with by a left-sided abdomino-thoracic approach; with a high intrathoracic anastomosis between the pulmonary vein and the aortic arch.
- Lesions of the lower esophagus and low mid esophagus can be adequately managed by an Ivor Lewis-Tanner approach with a high right-sided intrathoracic anastomosis at the level of the aortic arch – with a two-field lymph node clearance. The nodes retrieved are significantly more by this approach.
- Alternatively in patients with poor cardiopulmonary status, a THE could be considered if the disease is localized to the esophageal wall ($T_{1,2,3}$) and does not have a large tumor or nodal burden.
- Total esophagectomy should be considered for mid 1/3 and higher lesions above aortic arch where the three-field cervical node clearance could be added.
- The MIS is gathering popularity and with experience the procedure will gain increasing acceptance – long-term results and oncologic outcomes still require solid documentation.
- The learning curve for esophageal surgery – traditional or thoracoscopic is long and arduous and should be cultivated at a large center with experienced surgeons.
- Case selections for surgery should be based on a good preoperative assessment with precise imaging techniques.
- Neo-adjuvant or adjuvant therapies should be appropriately combined with surgery where indicated – this will positively impact on the QOL and also survival.
- Nonsurgical candidate (advanced disease; poor medical condition with comorbidities) should have the benefit of CT/RT/stenting/dilatations/ as indicated to provide and achieve good palliation for dysphagia.
- It will be a long while before CT/RT can replace surgery as the therapy of choice for loco-regional carcinoma of the esophagus.
- Complications will occur, but can be effectively controlled with high postoperative vigilance and aggressive therapy as indicated. The overall postoperative mortality should be below 5% and in a good center with experience, it should be around 2–3%.
- Surgery for carcinoma esophagus is challenging and demanding; *"The bigger (surgery), the better"* does not hold true in surgical oncology. It is better to individualize a surgical approach for a given patient out of so many choices now available. This must depend on the experience, expertise, and the comfort zone of the surgeon. He should do what he knows best.
- In surgical oncology, "Technique is the Prince, Selection is the Queen, Biology is the King" [15].

The Future

Throughout the last millennium and the present years, appropriate surgery for esophageal cancer has remained deeply entrenched as the most curative therapy ensuring a good quality of life (relief of dysphagia), prolonged control, and a few cures.

Chemotherapy is continually improving with better and newer molecules as is sophistication in RT techniques. Majority of patients present late and surgery is often not feasible when CT and RT should be appropriately utilized. Studies on neoadjuvant CT and/or RT are continuing and should be utilized to downstage the disease before surgery (if feasible) can be attempted. Most meta-analyses have not shown increase in overall survival, though some have shown beneficial results [16]. Most patients are nutritionally low and combined aggressive therapies will require the highest level of supportive care, often unavailable at many centers. These factors have to be taken into consideration before planning treatment.

Recent studies on targeted (biological) therapies along with CT show some minor incremental benefits of a few months; however, the cost and toxicity are significant and the therapy should be attempted within the ambit of clinical trials.

Further studies and research, in the gene profile expressions of this cancer, planning targeted or tailored therapies still remain a distant dream.

Prevention is paramount but difficult to achieve. This is the best way to the future.

This article is predominantly a summary of surgical approach and has aimed to avoid too many statistics and data, which are easily available in the literature.

Results and Conclusions

Based on our experiences the authors believe that intrathoracic anastomosis in the left side or the right side of the chest, is a time-tested surgical procedure which effectively control cancers of the lower reaches of the esophagus (within 5 cm above the diaphragm), cardia and c.o.jn. – The surgical procedure is safe, quick, and lends itself to a good clearance of the primary lesion and nodal metastasis. It should remain in the armamentarium of all surgeons involved in the treatment of these cancers. *Total esophgectomy is not always necessary for this group of cancers except in those who are unfit for a thoractomy due to medical conditions, when a transhiatal total esophagectomy could be considered.*

The author feels that total esophagectomy is not always necessary for all patients with esophageal cancer. Lesions in the lower reaches can be effectively dealt with by a subtotal esophagectomy with intrathoracic anastomosis and THE may be resorted when patient has cardiopulmonary dysfunction. Every patient should be individualized for a particular therapy based on the clinical setting.

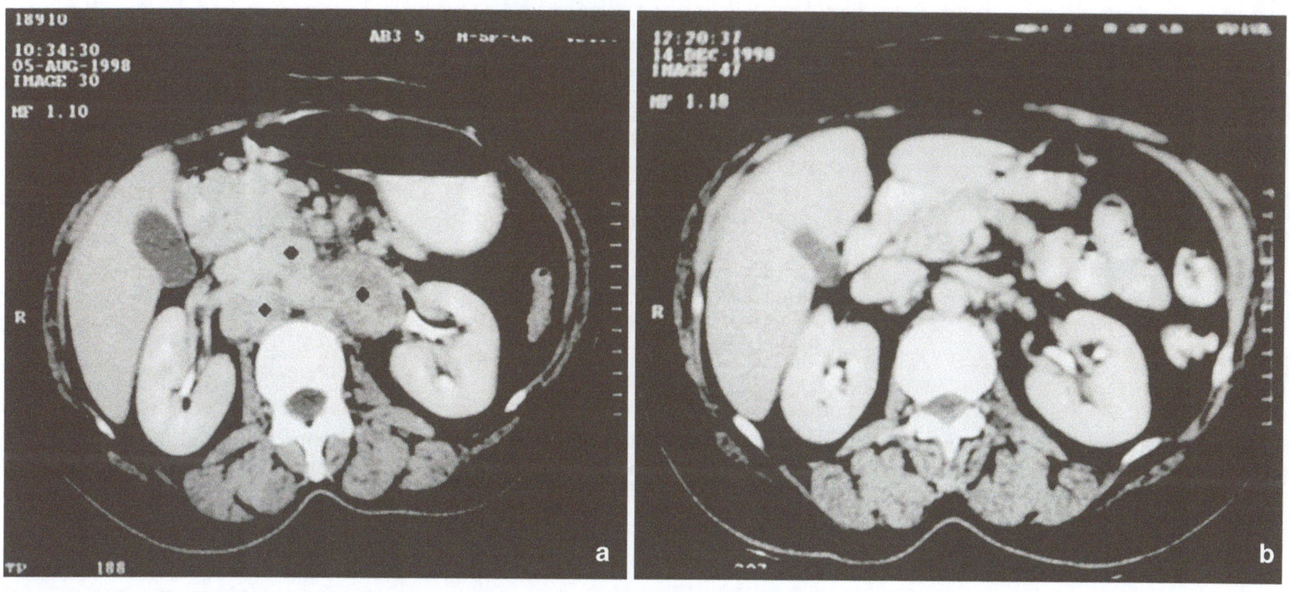

Fig. 1.1 (**a, b**) Locally advanced nodal burden (para-aortic nodes – *black dots*) can be effectively reduced by neo-adjuvant chemotherapy as shown in this slide from a primary lesion of cardio-esophageal cancer. The patient subsequently underwent a successful resection of the lesion

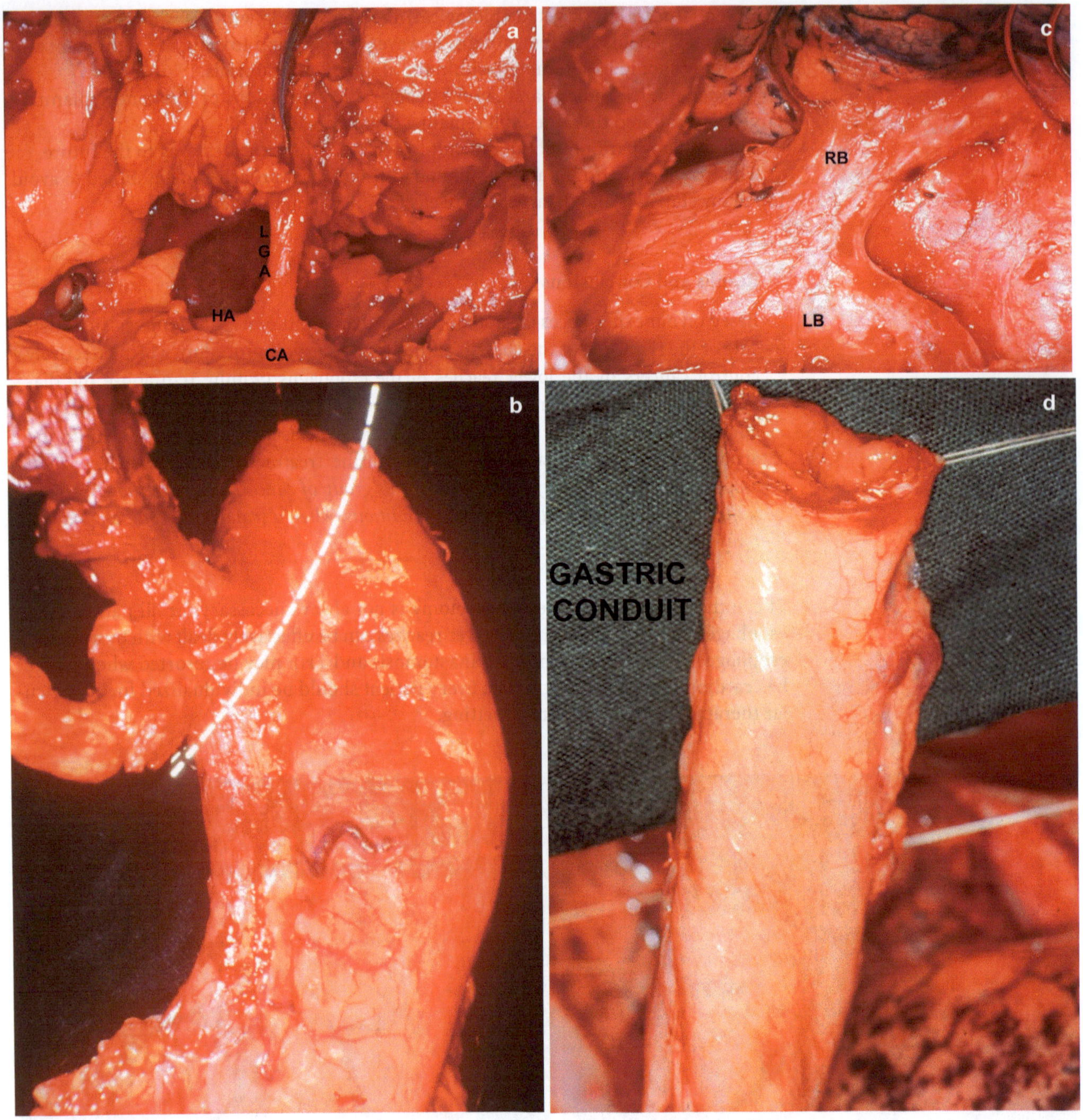

Fig. 1.2 Operative photographs showing nodal clearance at the coeliac axis (**a**), lesser curvature of the stomach (**b**), and the carinal region (**c**) in the mediastinum. A vascular gastric conduit (**d**) is prepared which can snugly fit in the posterior mediastinum

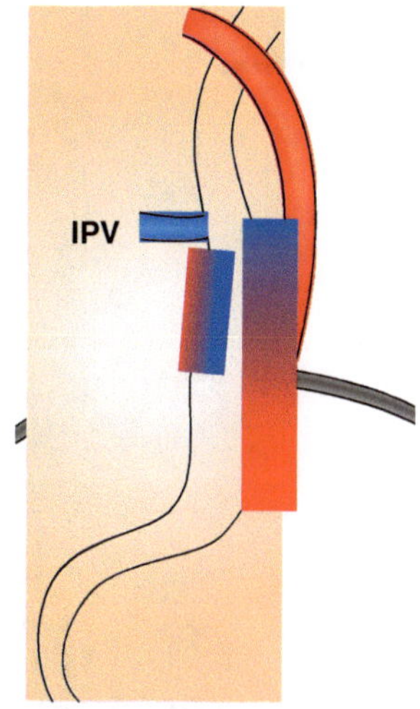

Fig. 1.3 A diagrammatic representation of an area of excision for a lesion at the cardia, lower esophagus and c.o.jn. The nodal dissection can proceed proximally in the mediastinum as needed. Intrathoracic anastomosis could be done on the right side (Ivor-Lewis) or in the left thorax always aiming for a good proximal margin of 5–7 cm

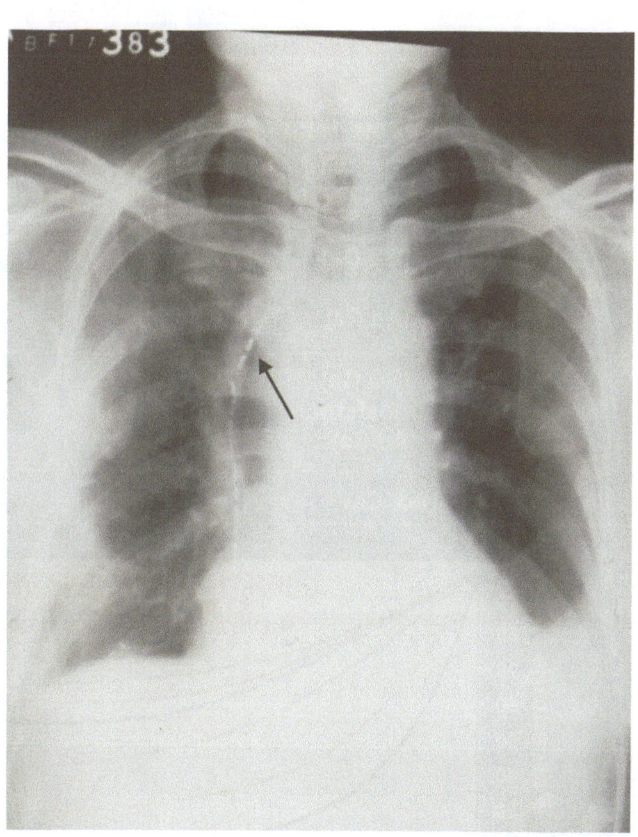

Fig. 1.4 The stomach conduit is seen here lying snugly in the mediastinum with the anastomosis (*arrow*) above the arch of the aorta in the right chest

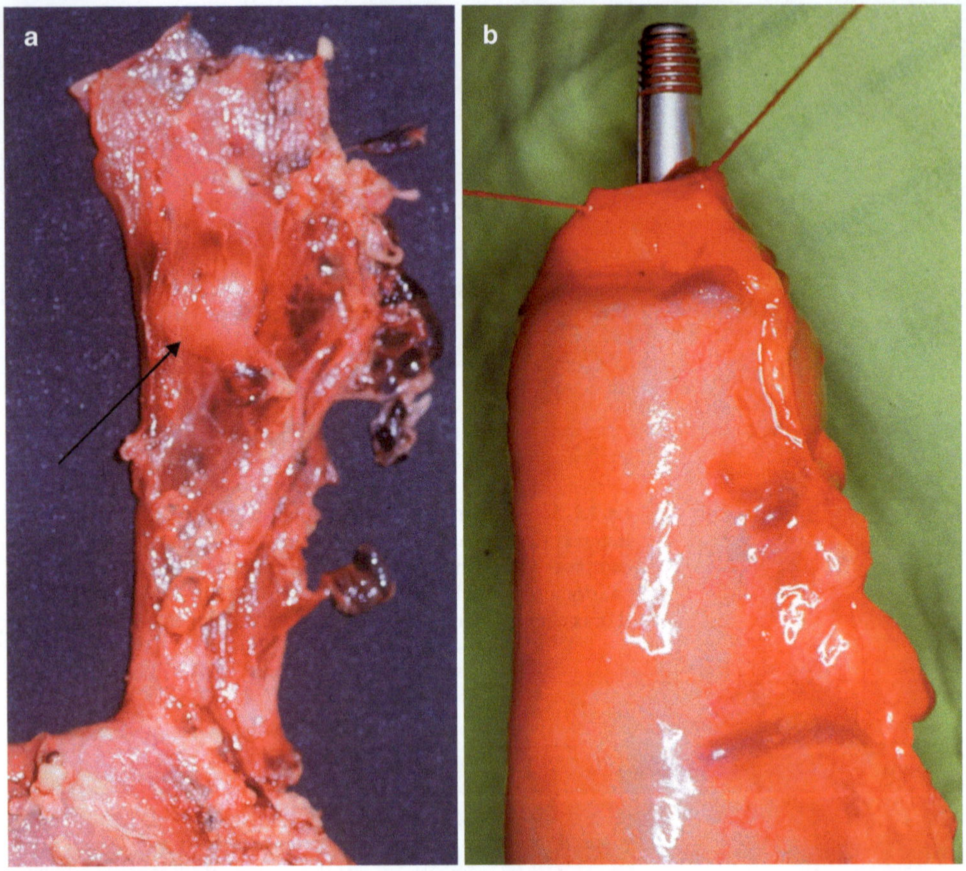

Fig. 1.5 (**a**) Specimen of total esophagectomy shows en-mass excision of the tumor (arrow) pleura and lymph nodes. (**b**) Gastric tube conduit being readied for stapled anastomosis. Note the normal vascularity of the conduit

Left Thoracic Abd. Approach for Cancers of the Cardia, C.O. JN and lower Esophagus

Total 330 Resections (1990 – 2002)

No.		Site	%
186	→ 69 (SQ Ca) → 19 (Ad.Ca)	Lower Esoph.	56
46	→ 21 (SQ Ca) → 8 (Indeterm.) → 17 (Ad.Ca)	C.OJN	14
98	(Ad. Ca)	Fundus	30

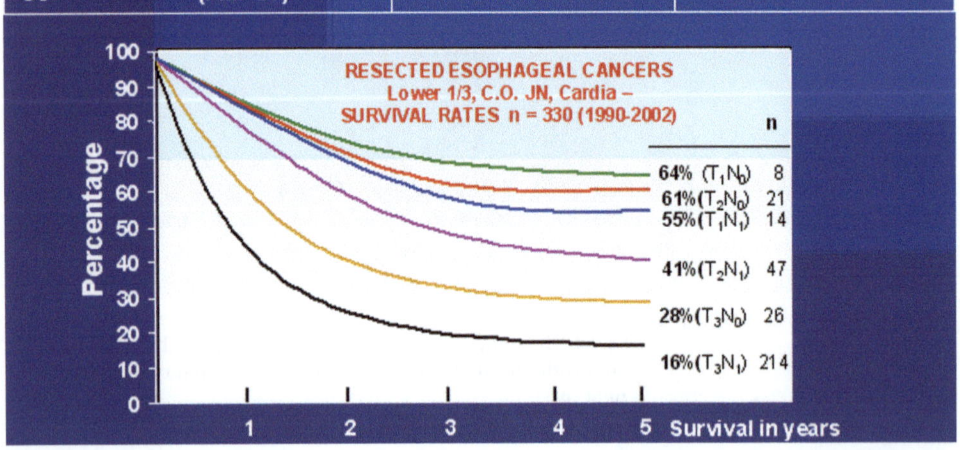

Fig. 1.6 Results of 330 esophageal resections over a period of 12 years at the Tata Memorial Hospital (TMH), Bombay Hospital, and Breach Candy Hospital. All intrathoracic anastomosis (right or left)

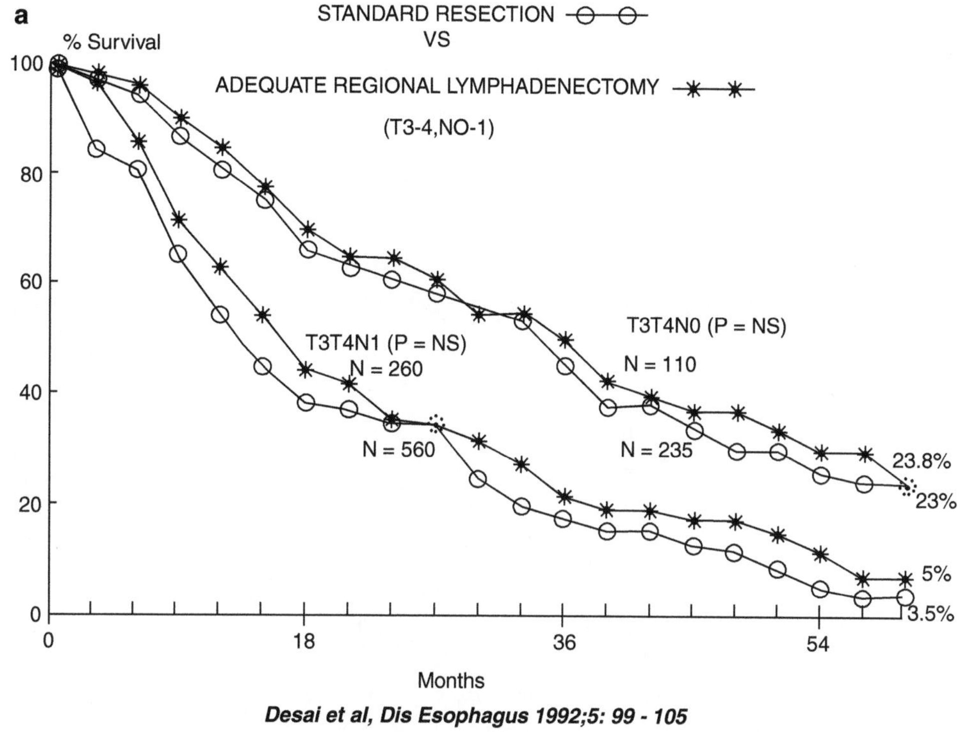

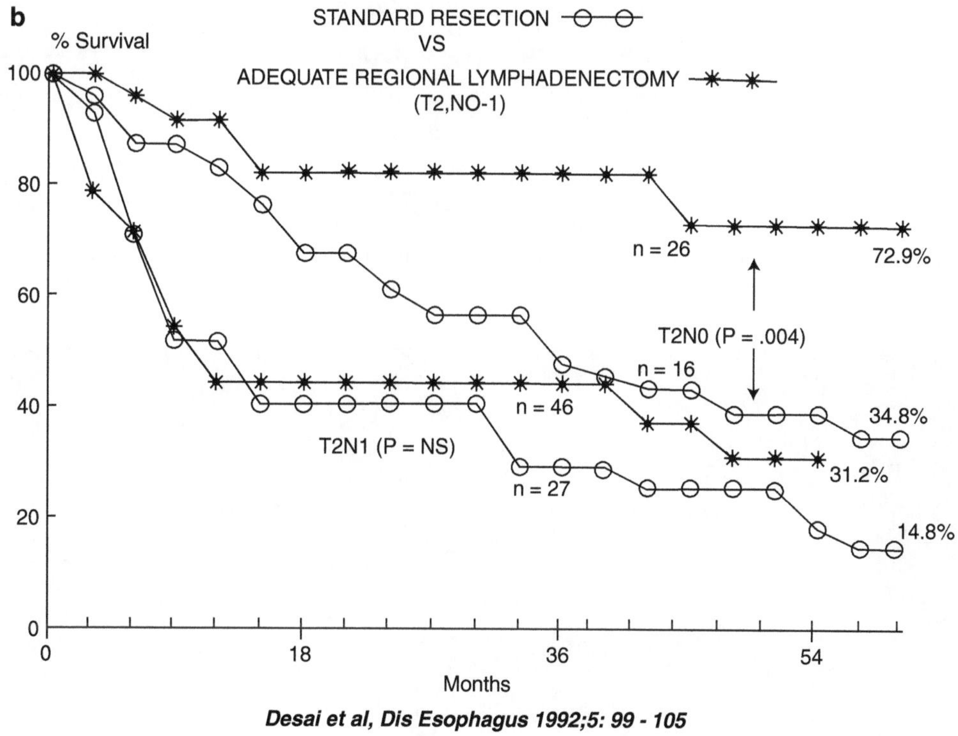

Fig. 1.7 (a, b) Excellent responses of neo-adjuvant chemotherapy to proliferative lesions. No evidence of viable tumor on histology of the operative specimen. Adequate regional two-field (abdomen and mediastinum). Lymphadenectomy gives better results when the lesions are T1, T2, and N1 with limited number of nodal involvement

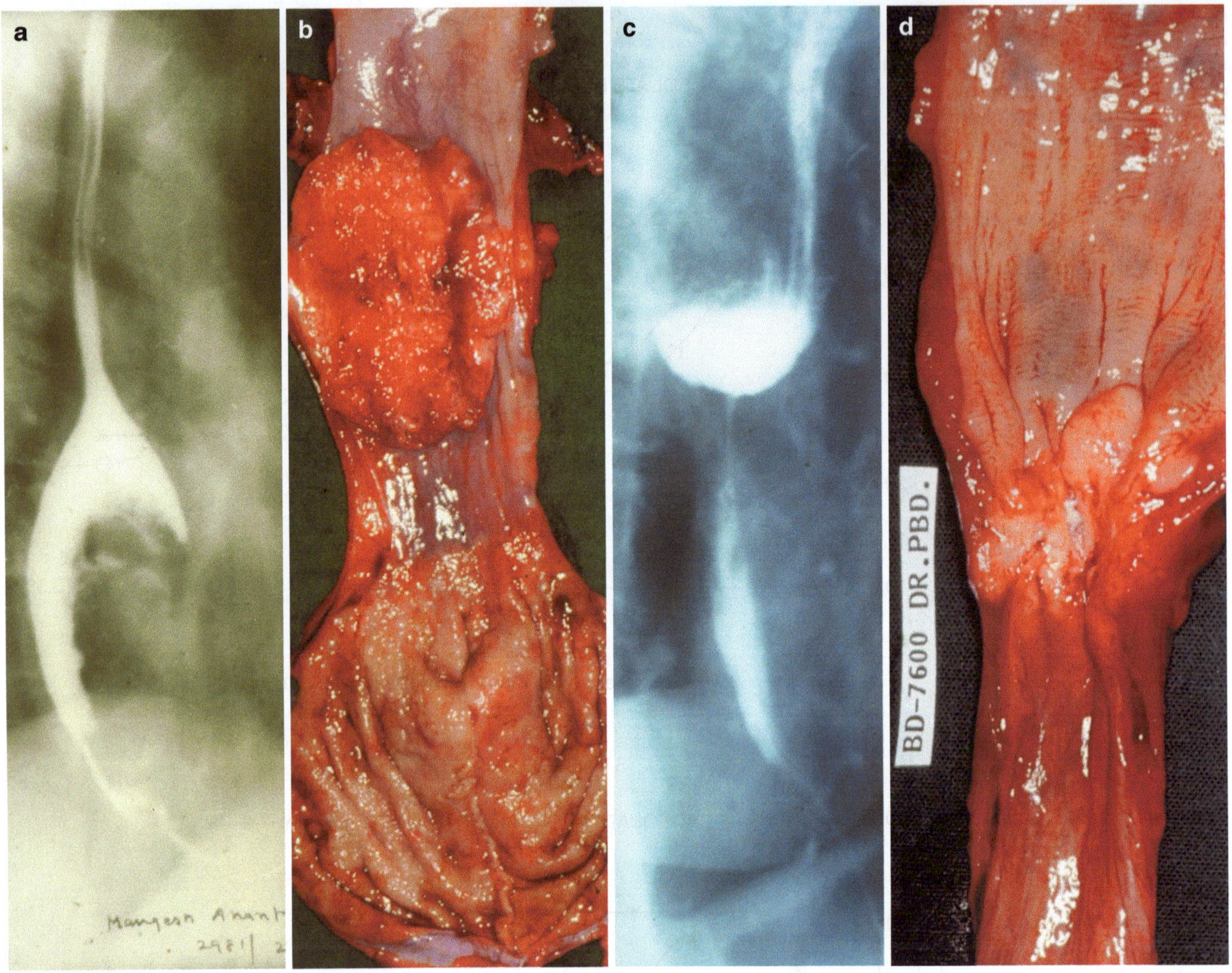

Fig. 1.8 Esophagograms and specimens of a predominantly proliferative lesion (**a, b**) and obstructive, cicatrising lesion (**c, d**). The former responds very effectively with neo-adjuvant chemotherapy unlike the obstructing lesions which respond poorly

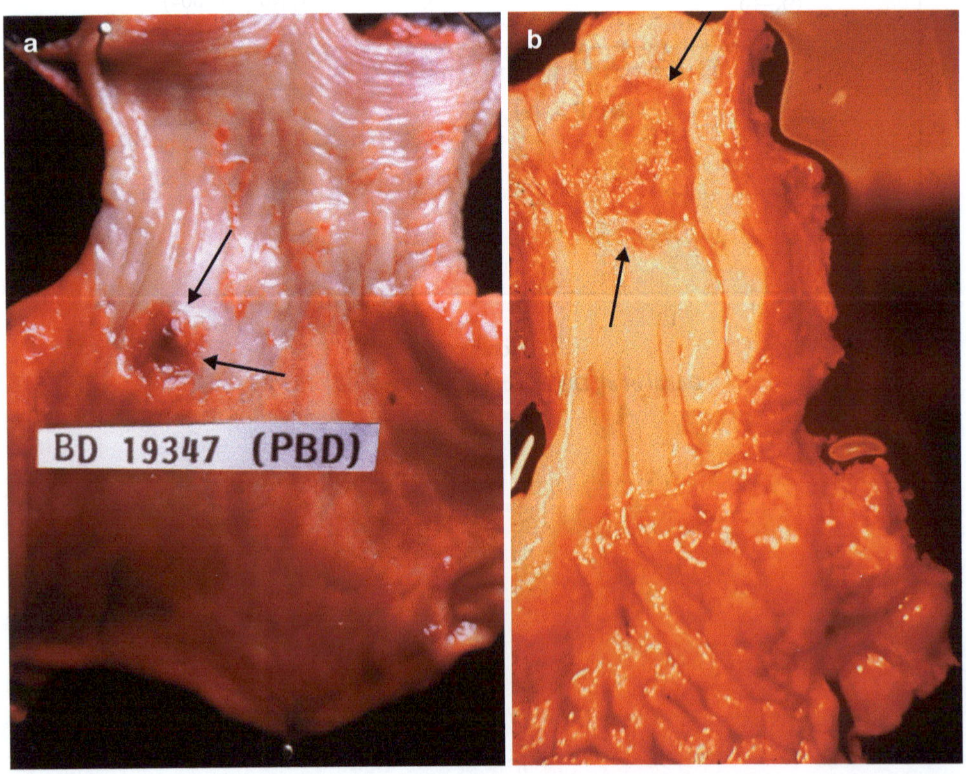

Fig. 1.9 (**a, b**) Excellent responses of neo-adjuvant chemotherapy to proliferative lesions (indicated by arrows). No evdence of viable tumor on histology of the operative specimen

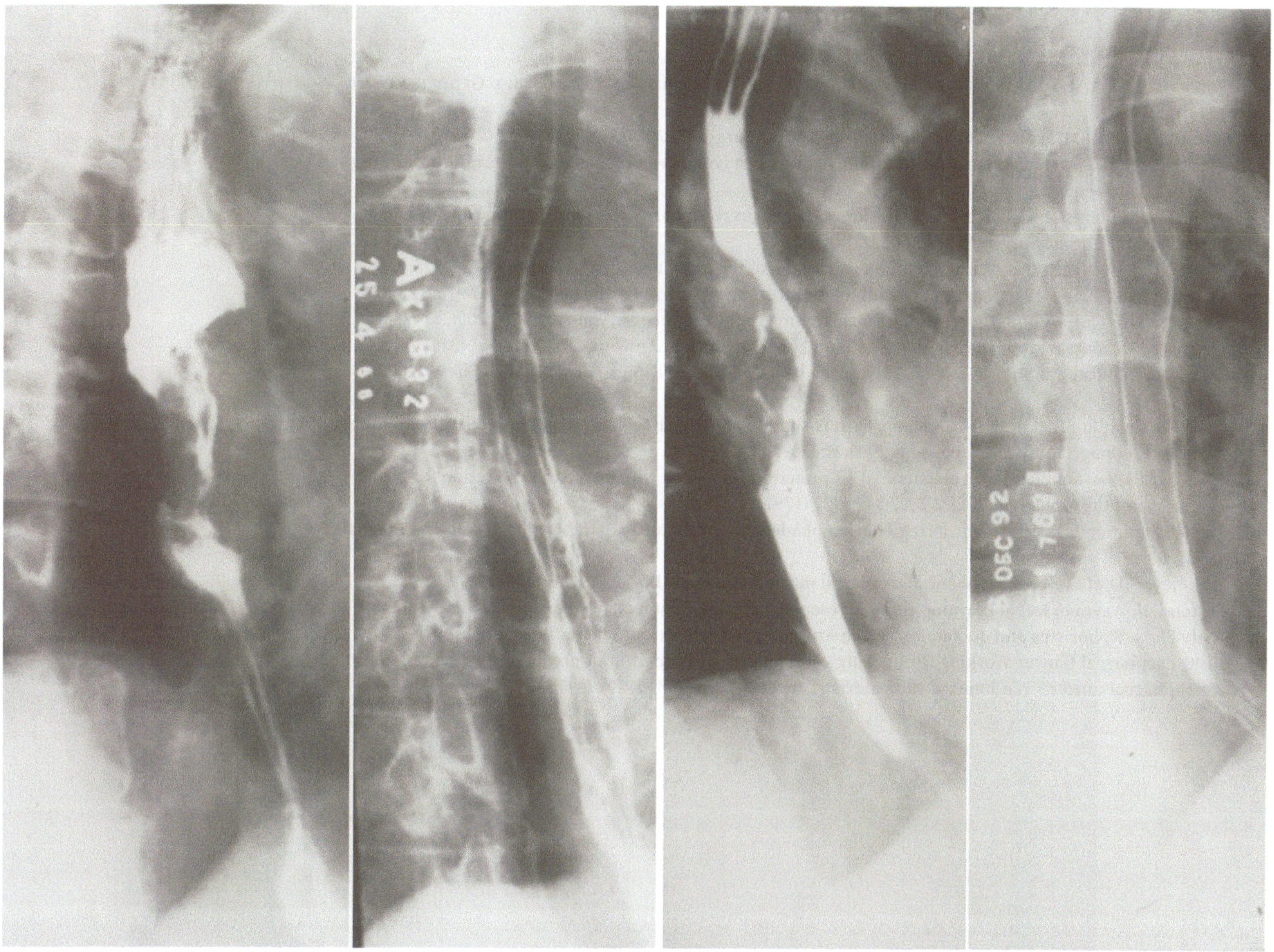

Fig. 1.10 Two different patients with locally advanced lesions of the middle esophagus showing good responses with chemo-radiotherapy producing excellent response with prolonged palliation extending from 8 months to 4 years

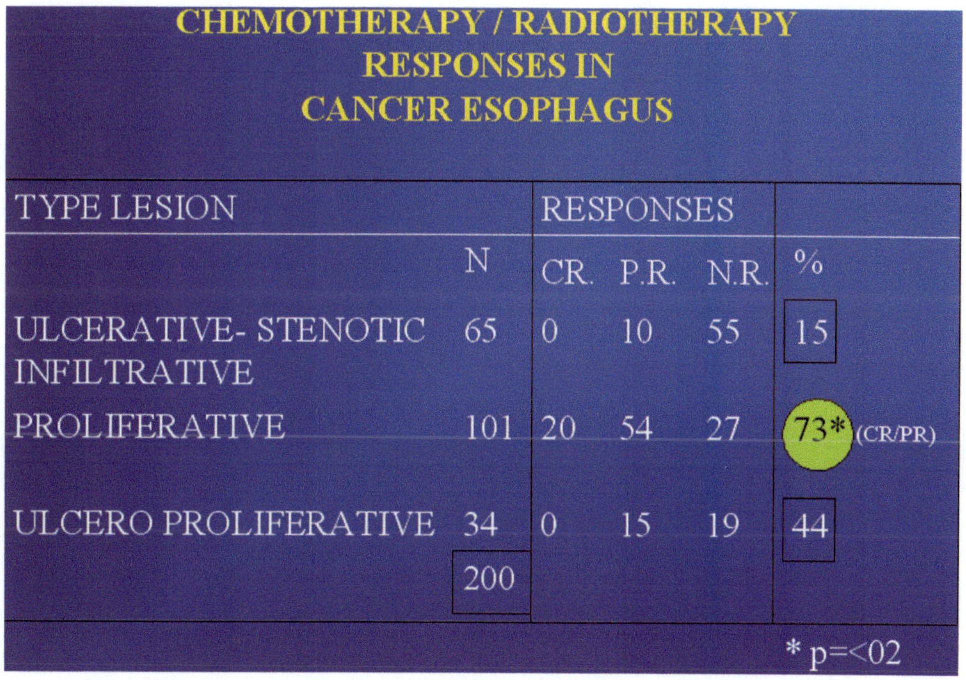

CHEMOTHERAPY / RADIOTHERAPY
RESPONSES IN
CANCER ESOPHAGUS

TYPE LESION	N	RESPONSES CR.	P.R.	N.R.	%
ULCERATIVE- STENOTIC INFILTRATIVE	65	0	10	55	15
PROLIFERATIVE	101	20	54	27	73* (CR/PR)
ULCERO PROLIFERATIVE	34	0	15	19	44
	200				

* p=<02

Fig. 1.11 Data of responses of chemo-radiotherapy in obstructive and proliferative lesions

References

1. Torek F. The first successful case of resection of the esophagus for cancer. Surg Gynecol Obstet 1913;16:614–617.
2. Luketich JD, et al MIS for cancer esophagus. Ann Thorac Surg 2000;70:906–911.
3. Bizakis C, et al Initial experiences with minimally invasive Ivor-Lewis esophagectomy. Ann Thorac Surg 2006;82(2):402–406.
4. Adams WE, Phemister IB. Carcinoma of the lower esophagus report of a successful resection and esophagogastrostomy. J Thorac Surg 1938;7:621–632.
5. Sweet RH. Late results of surgical treatment carcinoma of the esophagus. JAMA 1954;155:422–425.
6. Orringer MB, Sloan H. Esophagectomy without thoracotomy. J Thorsc Cardiovasc Surg 1978;76:643–654.
7. Orringer MB. THE without thoracotomy for carcinoma of the esophagus. Ann Surg 1984;200:282–288.
8. Orringer MB, Marshal B. THE changing trends and lessons learned. Ann Surg 2007;246:363–374.
9. Rice TW. Clinical staging of esophageal cancer by CT, EUS, PET. Surg Clin N Am (Chest) 2000;10: 471–485.
10. Wolf CS, Castillo SF, et al Ivor-Lewis approach is superior to transhiatal approach in retrieval of lymph nodes at esophagectomy. Dis Esophagus 2008;21:328–333.
11. Holscher JB, Van Sandick JW, et al Extended TT resection compared with limited TH resection for adenocarcinoma of the esophagus. NEJM 2002;347:1705–1791.
12. Desai P, Deshpande R, et al Adequate regional lymphadenectomy in cancer of the esophagus. Dis Esophagus 1992;5:99–105.
13. Birkmeyer JD, et al Hospital volume and surgical mortality in US. NEJM 2002;346:1128–1137.
14. Sutton DN, Wayman J, et al Learning curve for esophageal cancer surgery. Br J Surg 1998;85:399–402.
15. Cady Blake. Aphorisms and quotations for the surgeon, editor by Moshe Schein. Tfm, Shrewsbury.
16. MRC Esophageal Cancer Working Group. Surgical resection with or without preoperative chemotherapy in esophageal cancer – randomized clinical trial. Lancet 2002;359(9319):1727–1733.

2

Minimally Invasive Surgery in Esophageal Cancer: World Literature

Geetanjali A. Agarwal

Introduction

Esophageal cancer is the sixth leading cause of cancer death with median survival of 11 months. Controversies about management are prevalent.

Czerny first successfully resected a cancer of cervical esophagus in 1877. Surgical resection became the primary form of therapy for local and loco-regional disease because of its superior and more durable quality of swallowing, as compared with nonoperative modalities. Short-term outcome of surgical resection improved between 1970 and 1993 because of changes in perioperative and surgical management. Long-term survival too improved due to earlier detection of tumors.

Goals and Approaches

Traditionally, esophagectomy has been performed either by a thoracoabdominal, transhiatal, or transthoracic approach. However, all these methods have an acknowledged high intraoperative and postoperative morbidity. Goldminc et al. in 1993 conducted a prospective randomized trial of 67 patients undergoing esophagectomy by either a transhiatal approach or right-sided thoracotomy. They concluded that long-term survival was unaffected by the type of operation performed or the addition of preoperative chemotherapy or radiotherapy. In general, the choice of operative approach depends on the tumor location, stage of disease, the fitness of the patient, and the experience of the surgical team. Proponents of transhiatal route argue that it avoids a thoracotomy and the attendant respiratory complications. Those favoring thoracotomy emphasize the ability to clear the tumor and involved lymph nodes and the relative safety of the procedures, if other mediastinal structures are adherent.

The aim of surgical treatment defined is as below:

1. Complete resection of all disease
2. Lymph node sampling
3. Resection of regional lymph node
4. Replacement of the esophagus with appropriate conduit

Regardless of the surgical procedure used, avoidance or at least minimizing complications and rapid return to preoperative status are obvious surgical goals.

MIS

Minimally access surgery has revolutionized many areas of surgery since its introduction in late 1980s. The common denominator in minimal access surgery is to perform the same operation as in the open approach but through a smaller incision. This reduces the

Table 2.1 Laparoscopic transhiatal esophagectomy

Author	No	Conversion	Mean op time (min)	Mean blood loss	Mortality	Morbidity	Mean hospital stay (days)	Mean number of lymph nodes
De Paula et al.	12	1 (8.3)	256		0	5	7.6	NA
Swanstrom et al.	9	0	390	290	0	4	6.4	NA
Avital et al.	22	1 (4.5)	380	220	1 (4.5)	4	8	14.3
Puntambekar et al.	98	0	155	250	5 (5.5)	10	8	10

Table 2.2 Laparoscopic transthoracic esophagectomy

Author	No	Conversion	Mean op time	Mean blood loss	Mortality	Morbidity	Hospital stay	Mean number of lymph nodes
Martin et al.	36	2	190–360	Upto 1,500	2 (5.5%)	15	8–61	-
Nguyen et al.	46	2	210–520	Upto 1,000	4.3%	12	4–60	10.3
Puntambekar et al.	108	2	180	Upto 500	2 (3.7%)	5	5–20	15

operative trauma without compromising the principles of the surgical operation. Laparoscopic cholecystectomy and fundoplication are accepted as gold standards. However, application of laparoscopy in esophagectomy has been slow because of associated complexities, decreased tactile control, possibly increasing the risk of injuring adjacent vital structures, compromised margins, inadequate lymph node retrieval, and tumor dissemination including portsite metastasis. But with the potential to reduce trauma, using these methods may reduce high morbidity and mortality associated with these procedures. The laparoscopic approach also holds the advantage in those cases in which radiological evidence of operability is equivocal, avoiding a major laparotomy and delay in further palliative management.

The various minimally access surgical techniques to esophagectomy use either thoracoscopy, laparoscopy, or a combination of both techniques.

Transhiatal approach was initially described by Denk in 1913 and later popularized by Orringer. The side effect of transhiatal approach was blunt mediastinal dissection, resulting in intraoperative bleeding and recurrent laryngeal nerve injury. De Paula et al. (1995) were the first to demonstrate the feasibility of laparoscopic transhiatal esophagectomy in a series of 12 patients. Shmuel Avital et al. in 2005 published a retrospective analysis of 22 patients undergoing THE (Table 2.1). Simon Law et al. (2005) retrospectively analyzed 29 patients and mentioned the advantages of magnified dissection in laparoscopic THE, especially of gastroesophageal junction. The pressure of pneumoperitoneum aids the dissection of the esophagus and ensures a wide dissection. Concerns about adequate nodal dissection were raised.

Torek (1913) performed the first successful transthoracic esophageal resection. Right thoracotomy and abdominal approach was described by Lewis in 1946. Tanner in 1947 described the Ivor Lewis procedure. In 1998 Luketich and colleagues described the combined thoracoscopic and laparoscopic approach overcoming the disadvantage of laparoscopic transhiatal approach mainly difficulty in mobilizing the middle third esophagus. Smithers et al. (2001) reported their experience with 162 patients who underwent thoracoscopic esophageal mobilization in prone position. Martin et al. (2005) promoted the prone position as the deflated lung lies forward out of the operating field and requires no extra port for a lung retractor (Table 2.2). Smithers et al. (2001) reported their experience with 162 patients who underwent laparoscopic TTE in prone position; the median survival time was 29 months which was similar to the same group's experience with an open Ivor Lewis technique. Nguyen et al. (2000) described a technique similar in principle to the technique described by Swanson and colleagues (2001), which consisted of an initial right thoracotomy for complete dissection of the esophagus followed by a laparotomy for mobilization of the gastric conduit and a cervical anastomosis. Nguyen used thoracoscopy instead of thoracotomy and laparoscopy instead of laparotomy. The advantages of thoracoscopy include improved visualization with better hemostasis, and the ability to evaluate proximal and middle-third tumor for possible extension to other mediastinal structures.

Use of hand-assisted laparoscopic and thoracoscopic surgery in radical esophagectomy with three-field lymphadenectomy for thoracic esophageal cancer was described by Suzuki et al. in 2005. But thoracoscopic esophagectomy fell into disrepute because of longer operative time, increasing morbidity hence defying its advantages.

Thus the choice for a particular minimally access approach to esophagectomy was based on the location of tumor, its extension, and radiological lymph node enlargement.

One of the major and common drawbacks of minimally access esophagectomy was the longer operative time and need for extensive surgical experience.

The learning curve as well as the time taken to complete these procedures can be reduced by standardization of steps, thus preventing repetition, which is the aim of this atlas. Luketich et al. recently (2003) reported the largest series to date of minimally invasive esophagectomies. They reported their experience in 222 patients operated during a 6-year period with a combined laparoscopic and thoracoscopic approach. They reported a 7.5 h median operative time which decreased to 4.5 h after the 29th procedure.

Ours is a high-volume laparoscopic oncosurgical unit. We perform laparoscopic THE and laparoscopic transthoracic esophagectomy, depending on the location of the tumor and patient status. We use stomach as a conduit. We do not perform any drainage procedure. Cervical anastomosis is done in two layers end-to-side hand sewn.

We compared our results retrospectively with other studies.

Selected Readings

1. Cuscheiri A. Thoracoscopic subtotal esophagetomy. Endosc Surg Allied Technol 1994;2:21–25.
2. De Paula et al Transhiatal approach for esophagectomy. In: Toouli J, Gossot D, Hunter JG, eds. Endosurgery. New York: Churchill Livingstone, 1996:293–299.
3. Luketich JD, et al Laparoscopic transhiatal esophagectomy for Barrets esophagus with high grade dysplasia. J Soc Laparoendosc Surg 1988;2:75–77.
4. Goldminc M, et al Oesophagectomy by a transhiatal approach or thoracotomy: a prospective randomized trial. Br J Surg 1993;80:367–370.
5. Nguyen NT, et al Thoracoscopic and laparoscopic esophagectomy for benign and malignant disease: lessons learned from 46 consecutive procedures. J Am Coll Surg 2003;197:902–913.
6. Orringer MB, et al Transhiatal esophagectomy: clinical experience and refinements. Ann Surg 1999;230:392–403.
7. Pisani P, et al Estimates of the worldwide mortality from 25 cancers in 1990. Int J Cancer 1999;83:18–29.
8. Putnam JB, et al Comparison of three techniques of esophagectomy within a residency training program. Ann Thorac Surg 1994;57:319–325.
9. Shmuel Avital MD, et al Laparoscopic transhiatal esophagectomy for esophageal cancer. Am J Surg 2005;190:69–74.
10. Simon Bann et al. Laparoscopic Transhiatal Surgery of the Esophagus JSLS 2005 Oct-Dec 9 (4) 376-81
11. Swanstron LL, et al Laparoscopic total esophagectomy. Arch Surg 1997;132:943–949.
12. Suzuki Y, et al Hand – assisted laparoscopic and thoracoscopic surgery (HALTS) in radical esophagectomy with three fi eld lymphadenectomy for thoracic esophageal cancer. EJSO 2005;31:1166–1174.

3

Staplers in Gastro-Esophageal Cancer Surgery

Ravindra M. Sathe

Introduction

As progress was made in laparoscopic instrumentation, the need to anastomose various gastrointestinal structures became evident. The answer to this problem was laparoscopic suturing and staplers. From the beginning of the practice of surgery, there has been concern about the amount of time required and the extent of tissue trauma associated with closure of the intestine and to perform gastrointestinal anastomoses with certain confidence. The primary goals were the restoration of function, to obtain effective hemostasis, the reduction of tissue trauma, and the prevention of postoperative morbidity, including infection and sepsis.

History

In 1908 a Hungarian surgeon, Professor Humer Hütl, demonstrated the first mechanical device using staples. This device, designed for use in distal gastrectomy, was widely acclaimed, although it was heavy and the assembly of its many parts was difficult and time-consuming. The design incorporated three principles that are still used in modern internal stapling devices – B-shaped configuration of closed staples, placement of staples in double-staggered rows, and use of fine wire as the staple material. In 1924, Petz Aladar, another Hungarian surgeon, developed the "Von Petz" instrument.

In 1934, Dr. Friedrich of Germany introduced the first stapling instrument to feature a replaceable, preloaded staple cartridge. This allowed for the multiple use of the instrument in the same surgical procedure.

The USSR began the first systematic program to develop stapling instruments. The first instrument designed in 1951was for vascular surgery. Since then, many other devices have been developed, each intended for a specific stapling application (e.g., bronchus, gastrointestinal tract, sclera, etc.), using a specific staple shape, size, and pattern. During a procedure, the surgeon selected the appropriate type of instrument for each application.

In 1978, Ethicon introduced the first preassembled disposable device – the PROXIMATE disposable skin stapler. Other types of disposable instruments soon followed, including, in 1980, the intraluminal stapler (ILS).

Advantages of Stapling

1. Clinical experience has shown that stapling of internal organs is faster than traditional suturing technique, hence reducing operating time. Furthermore, stapling can

reduce tissue trauma by minimizing tissue handling. In addition, the availability of stapling instruments has fostered the development of procedures that were difficult with traditional techniques because of limited access.

2. Many studies have shown that stapled tissue and anastomoses heal as reliably and rapidly as sutured anastomoses.

3. Effective and safe use of mechanical stapling devices depends upon good basic surgical technique, including clean, atraumatic dissection and careful hemostasis, attention to tissue condition and blood supply, and creation of tension-free anastomoses.

Various Types of Staplers

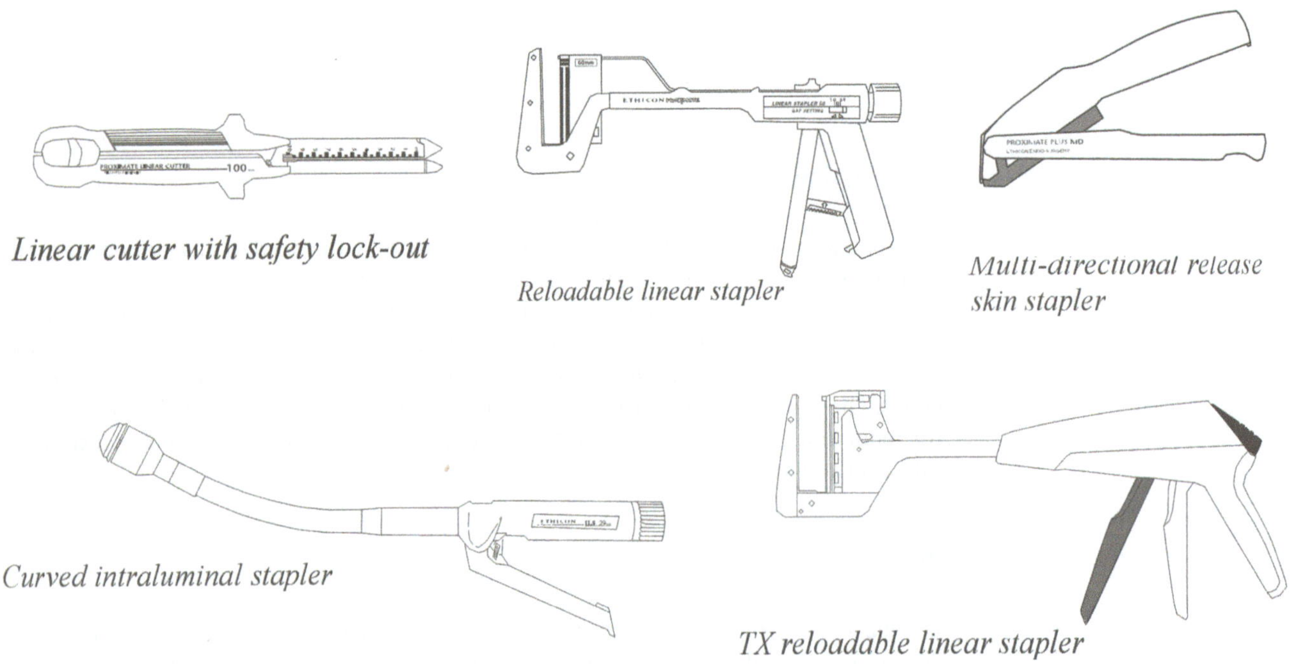

Fig. 3.1 Various types of staplers

Staple Configuration

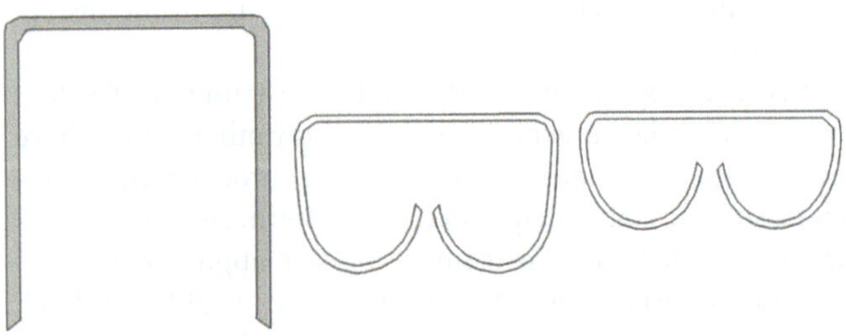

Fig. 3.2 Open and closed shapes of the staples used to approximate internal tissues

Internal Staplers

Internal staplers join tissues with B-shaped staples of fine metal wire (Fig. 3.2). As the instrument is fired, the open legs of the staple are driven through the tissue and formed into a B shape in a corresponding anvil indentation in the "anvil" jaw.

Linear Staplers

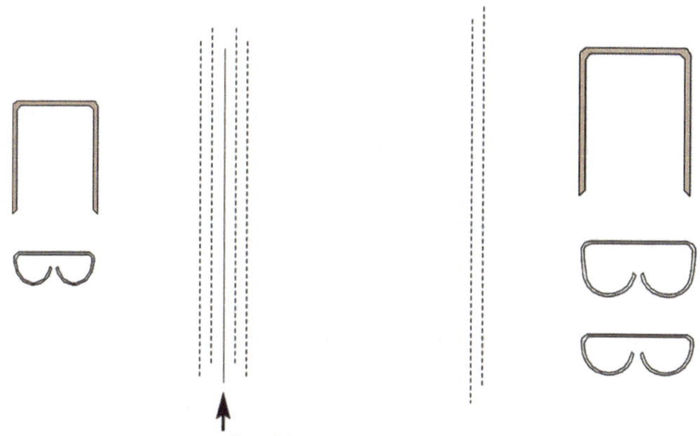

Fig. 3.3 Typical staple and staple line configuration of linear stapler-cutter

As the name suggests, a linear device places staples in one or two double-staggered rows (Fig. 3.3). It may have U- or V-shaped jaws, or separate forks.

Linear staplers with parallel closing jaws usually place one double-staggered row of staples, and do not contain a knife.

Forked staplers typically place two double-staggered rows of staples, and usually (but not necessarily) contain a knife that transects the tissue between the two double rows. They are known as linear cutters.

The flexible or articulating linear staplers are another variation. They have flexible or articulating components between the body and jaws that allow positioning versatility. This provides better access to otherwise difficult operative sites.

Linear Stapler Applications

Linear staplers are commonly used to close internal organs prior to transaction, and to close the common opening or enterotomy after the creation of an anastomosis with a linear cutter or an ILA. Since the linear cutter transects as it staples, this device is commonly used to transect organs, and to create side-to-side and functional end-to-end anastomosis.

The PROXIMATE Linear Cutter with Safety Lock-Out

(a) Indications

The PROXIMATE Linear Cutter with Safety Lock-Out is a linear stapler and has application in gastrointestinal, gynecologic, thoracic, and pediatric surgery for transection, resection, and/or creation of anastomoses.

(b) Contraindications

1. The instrument with blue reload should not be used on any tissue that requires excessive force to compress to 1.5 mm or on any tissue that compresses easily to below 1.5 mm.
2. The instrument with green reload should not be used on any tissue that requires excessive force to compress to 2.0 mm or on any tissue that compresses easily to below 2.0 mm.
3. The instrument should not be used on ischemic or necrotic tissue.

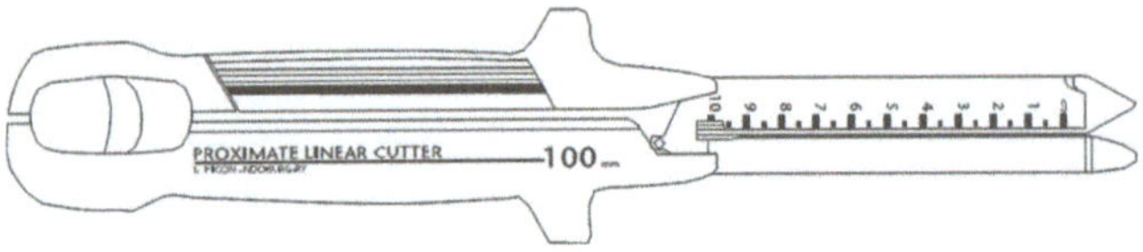

Fig. 3.4 The PROXIMATE linear cutter with safety lock-out

The PROXIMATE Linear Cutter with Safety Lock-Out delivers two double-staggered rows of staples while simultaneously dividing the tissue between rows.

Using the Linear Stapler

1. The instruments may be reloaded during a single procedure. Do not reload the instrument more than seven times for a maximum of eight firings per instrument (Fig. 3.4).

2. Separate the instrument halves by completely disengaging the alignment/locking lever.

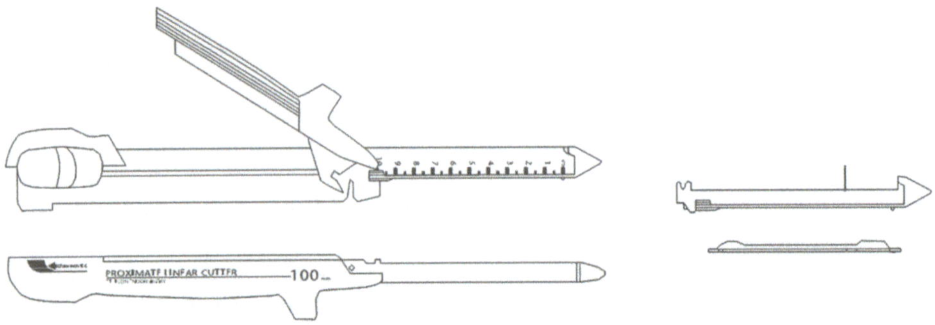

Fig. 3.5 The PROXIMATE linear cutter with safety lock-out parts

3. Grasp the edge of the staple retaining cap and lift straight up from the reload. Discard the staple retaining cap (Fig. 3.5).
4. Place the instrument across the tissue for transection (Fig. 3.6) or into the lumen to form an anastomosis (Fig. 3.7).

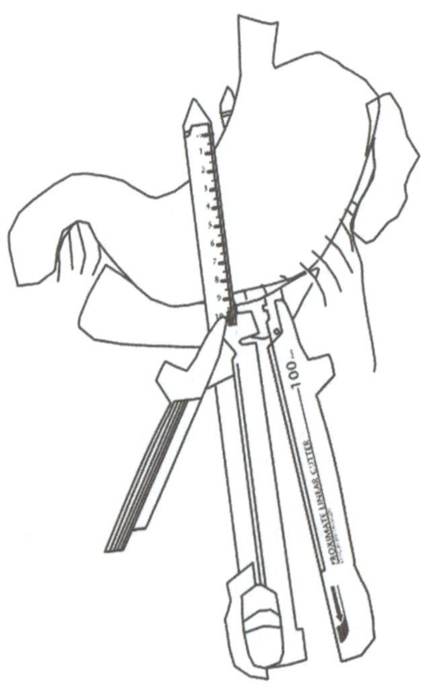

Fig. 3.6 The instrument is placed across the tissue for transection

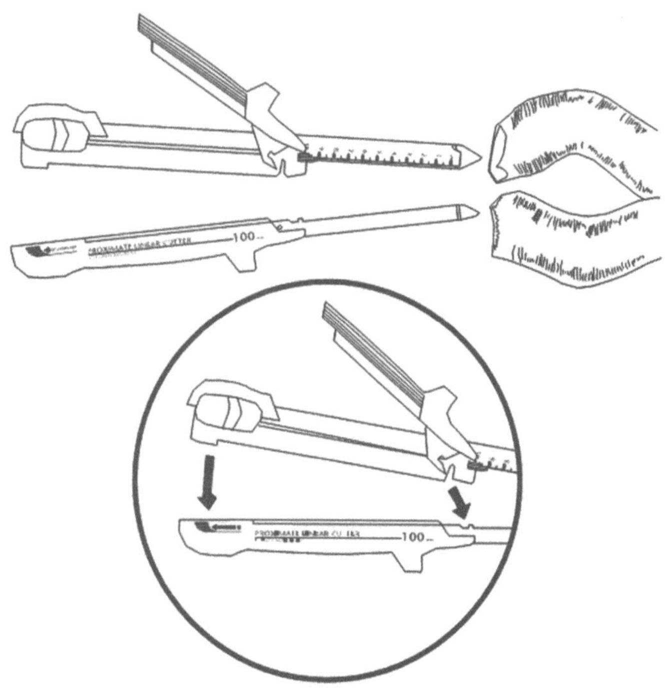

Fig. 3.7 The instrument is placed into the lumen to form an anastomosis

5. With the alignment/locking lever in the completely opened position, join the instrument halves together by aligning from either front, centre, or back of the instrument (Fig. 3.7).

6. To adjust tissue on the forks before firing, move the alignment/locking lever to the intermediate position. This allows manoeuvring of the tissue while the instrument halves are joined. Before firing, ensure that the instrument halves are aligned.

7. Close the alignment/locking lever completely when the tissue is properly in place. The tissue-retaining button helps secure the tissue in the proper position.

8. To fire the linear cutter, place the thumb on the firing knob and two fingers on the shoulders of the linear cutter, as if holding a syringe. Fire the instrument by pushing the firing knob completely forward. If the instrument size requires the use of two hands, an alternate method is to hold the instrument body firmly with one hand, and push the firing knob completely forward with the other hand. Care must be taken to clear the path of the firing knob.

9. Completely return the firing knob to the original "Return Knob Here" position and ensure a click is heard.

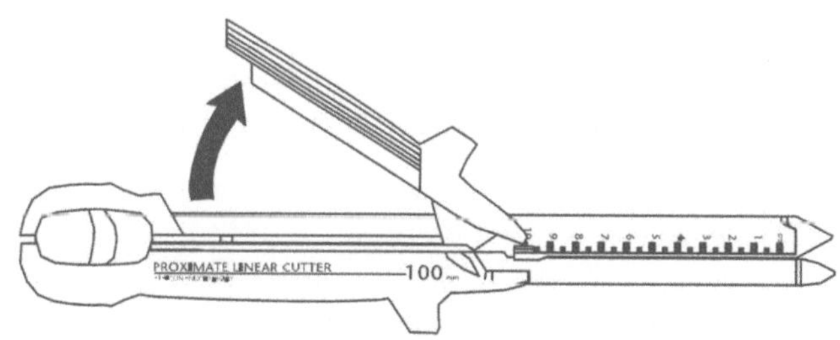

Fig. 3.8 The instrument halves are separated by opening the alignment/locking lever

10. Separate the instrument halves by opening the alignment/locking lever, and removing the instrument (Fig. 3.8). Caution: Examine the staple lines for proper staple closure.

Intraluminal staplers

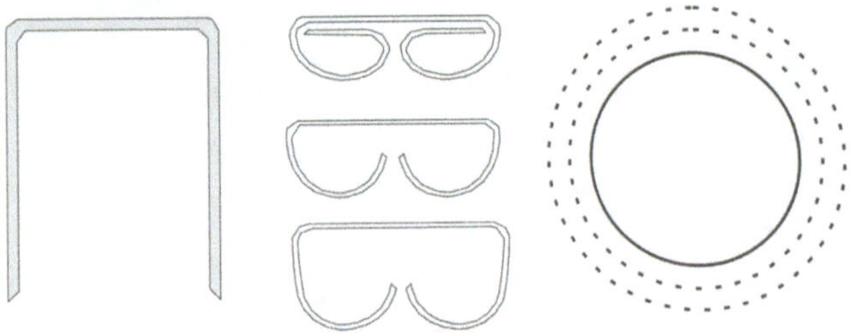

Fig. 3.9 Typical staple and staple line configuration of intraluminal (circular) staplers

This intraluminal type of instrument places staples in a double-staggered row but in a circular configuration (Fig. 3.9); this is why they are also known as circular staplers. As the instrument is fired, the staples are driven through the tissue; simultaneously, a circular knife cuts a uniform stoma in the joined tissue. Intraluminal staplers (ILS) are used to create anastomoses between hollow viscera.

The head of the ILS (Fig. 3.10) is inserted into the lumina of the organs to be joined through an enterotomy or, for low anterior resections, through the dilated anus. ILSs are available with various head diameters, permitting matching of instrument size to organ lumen.

PROXIMATE® ILS Curved Intraluminal Stapler

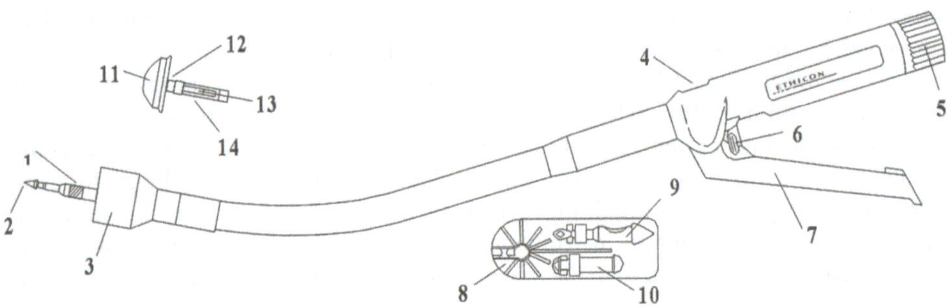

Fig. 3.10 Curved intraluminal stapler

(a) Indications

The PROXIMATE ILS curved intraluminal staplers have applications throughout the alimentary tract for end-to-end, end-to-side, and side-to-side anastomoses.

(b) Contraindications

Do not use where the combined tissue thickness is less than 1.0 mm or greater than 2.5 mm or where the internal diameter of the structure is less than 21 mm.

(c) Using the ILS

1. To remove the spacer tab, open the instrument by turning the adjusting knob counterclockwise two revolutions (Fig. 3.11.).

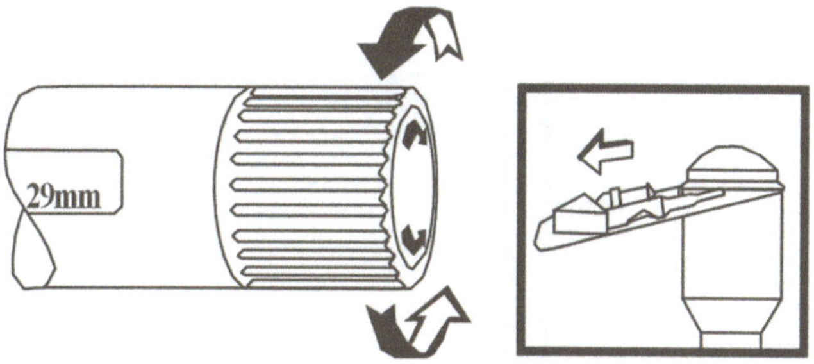

Fig. 3.11 Releasing the anvil

2. Place purse-string sutures (Fig. 3.12a) in the organs to be anastomosed. Based on surgeon experience and judgment, a closed- lumen technique (double- or triple-stapling technique (Fig. 3.12b)) may be employed as an alternative to a purse-string technique.

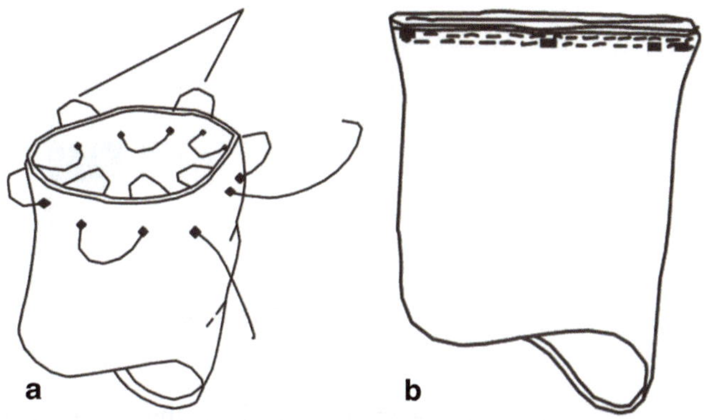

Fig. 3.12 (a) Purse-string suture and (b) stapled end with linear stapler

3. Insert the detachable head assembly into the lumen and secure the purse-string onto the anvil shaft above the tying notch (Fig. 3.13).

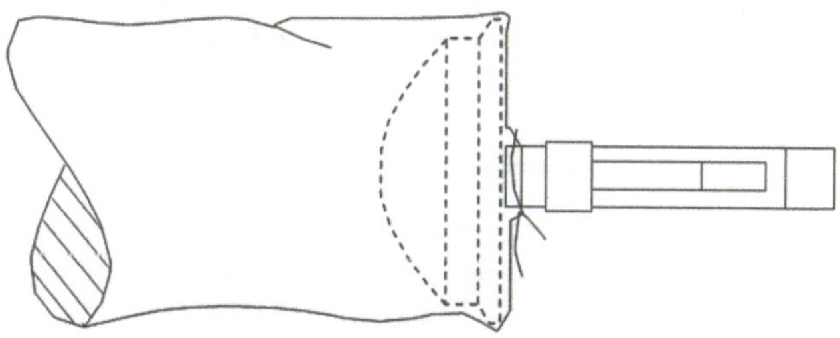

Fig. 3.13 Tying the purse-string onto the anvil shaft at proximal end of anastomosis

4. For a double-stapling technique, open the instrument using the adjusting knob until the orange tying area is visible. Remove the detachable head assembly to expose the trocar. Retract the trocar by rotating the adjusting knob clockwise until a stop is reached. Check trocar to verify that it is fully retracted before proceeding.

5. Insert the instrument up to the closed lumen with the detachable head assembly removed and the trocar fully retracted. Fully extend the trocar and pierce tissue by rotating the adjusting knob counterclockwise. Push the tissue down until the orange tying area is visible (Fig. 3.14).
Caution: Keep the trocar visible at all times to prevent personal injury or inadvertent trauma to adjacent structures.

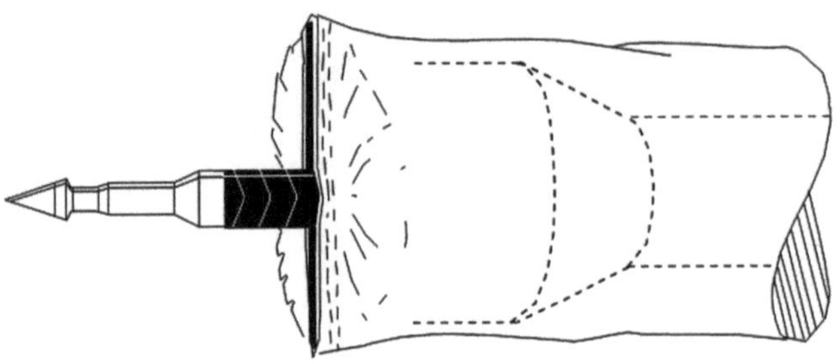

Fig. 3.14 Perforating the distal stump with the trocar till orange tying area is visible

6. Reattach the detachable head assembly by sliding the anvil shaft over the trocar and pushing until the detachable head assembly snaps into its fully seated position (Fig. 3.15).
Caution: Do not clamp across or grip on the locking springs when attempting to reattach the detachable head assembly.

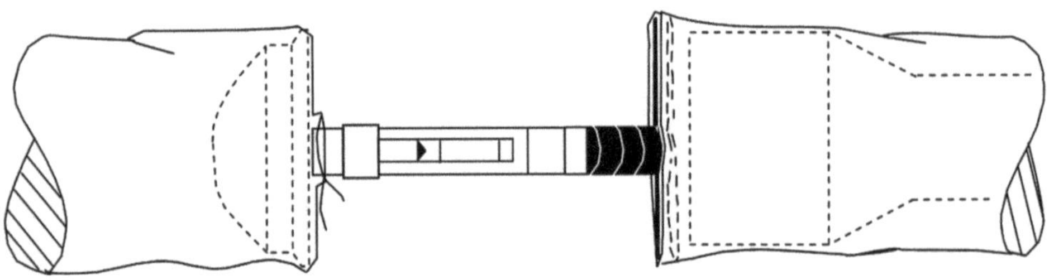

Fig. 3.15 Locking the stapler

7. While closing the instrument, keep the organ segments in proper orientation (Fig. 3.16). Inspect to ensure extraneous tissue is excluded. Turn the adjusting knob clockwise to close the instrument. As the final adjusting revolution is approached, the orange indicator (A) moves into the green range (B) of the gap setting scale. If the tissue segments to be anastomosed appear unusually thick or thin, the surgeon should adjust the instrument until, in his/her judgment, the tissue is adequately compressed or properly anastomosed. This is providing the orange indicator falls fully within the green range of the gap setting scale. This allows the surgeon to place staples at the height required for desired tissue compression (Figs 3.16 and 3.17).

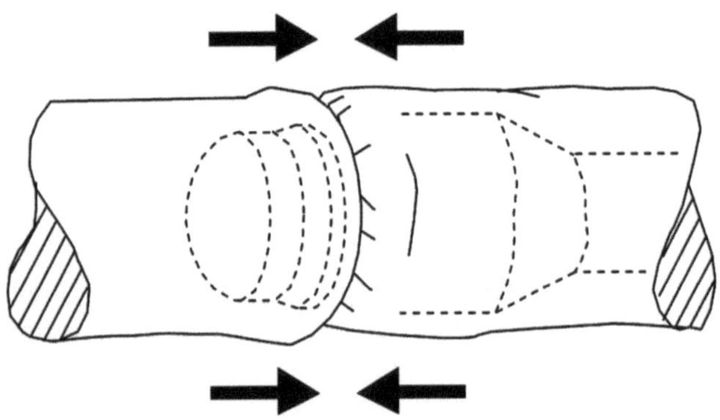

Fig. 3.16 Closing the stapler

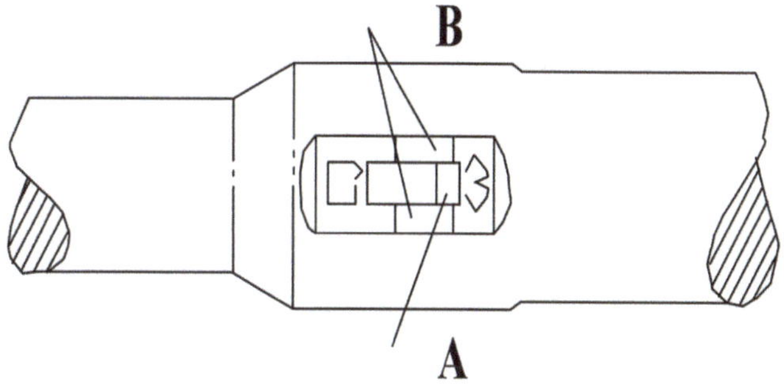

Fig. 3.17 Green (B) and orange (A) indicators on the handle showing adequate approximation

(d) Pre-Fire CheckList

- Orange indicator is fully within green range.
- Head assembly is securely attached.

To fire the instrument, draw the red safety lock back, toward the adjusting knob until it seats into the body of the instrument. If the red safety latch cannot be released, the instrument is not in the safe firing range. Once released, squeeze the firing handle with a firm, steady pressure. The surgeon will feel reduced trigger pressure and hear a "crunch" as the instrument completes the firing cycle. After firing, release the firing handle, allowing it to return to its original position, and re-engage the safety (Fig. 3.18).

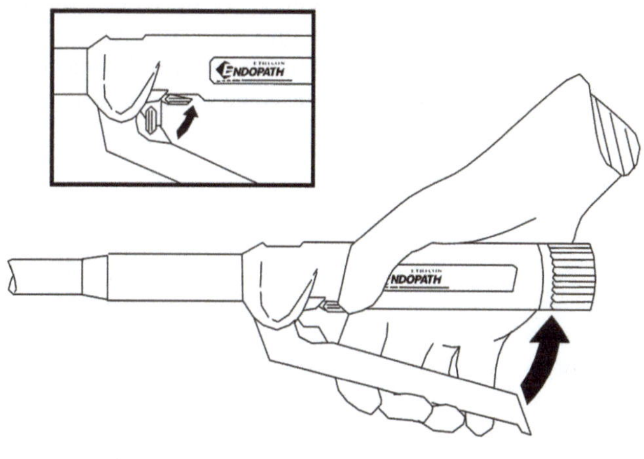

Fig. 3.18 Firing the instrument

8. Open the instrument by turning the adjusting knob counterclockwise, as indicated on the end of the knob. For easy removal, open the instrument only one-half to three-fourths revolutions (Fig. 3.19).

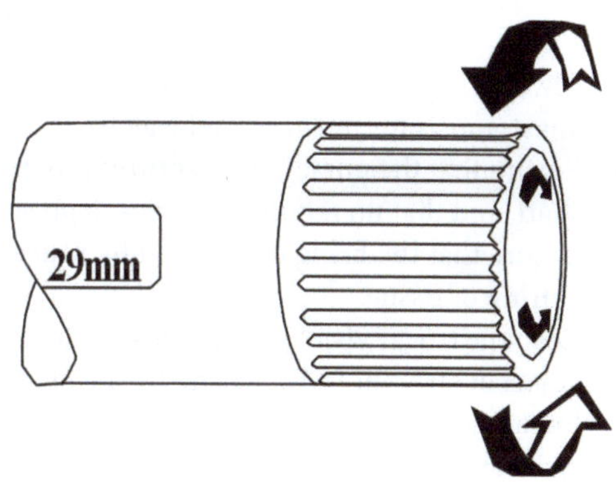

Fig. 3.19 Turning knob counterclockwise

9. To assure the anvil is free from tissue, rotate the instrument 90° in both directions. To withdraw the open instrument, gently apply rearward traction while simultaneously rotating (Fig. 3.20).

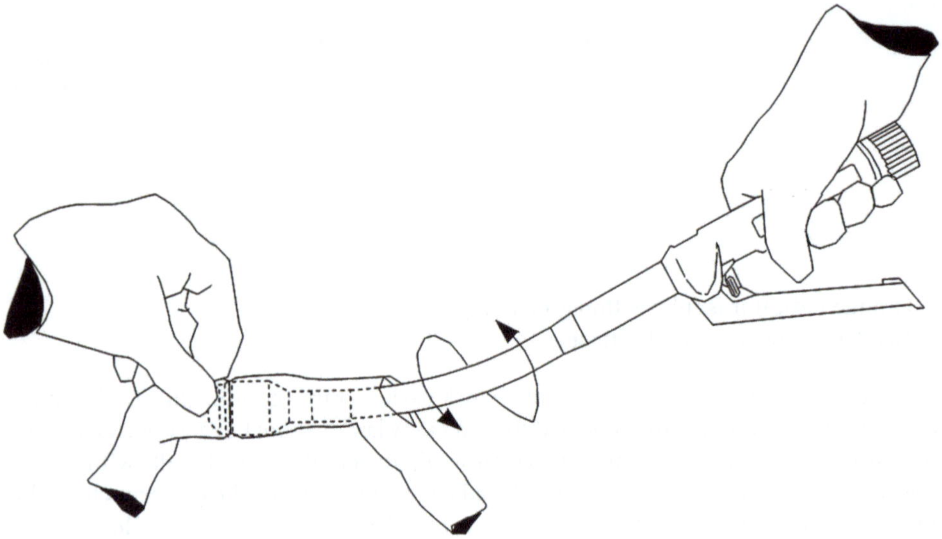

Fig. 3.20 Withdrawing the instrument

10. To inspect the donuts, remove the detachable head assembly, washer (if present), and donuts from within the circular knife. Examine the integrity of the donuts. Donuts should be intact and include all tissue layers. If donuts are not complete, the anastomosis should be carefully checked for leakage and appropriate repairs made (Fig. 3.21).

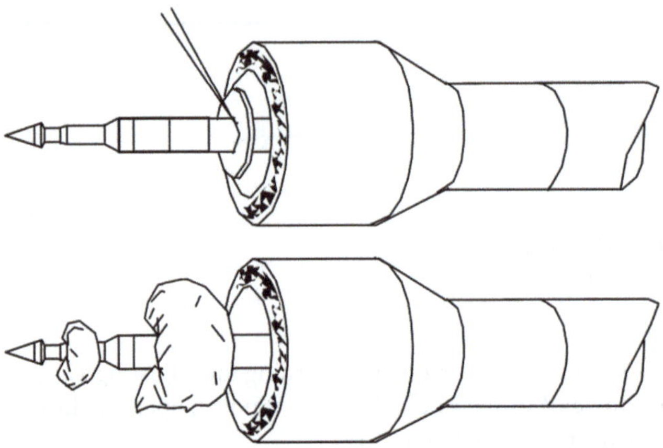

Fig. 3.21 Removing and checking the donuts

Important Points to Be Noted During Stapling

- Always inspect the anastomotic staple line for hemostasis, and check the completed anastomosis for integrity and leakage.
- Ensure that the purse-string sutures are tied snugly against the anvil shaft and trocar shaft, and that no redundant tissue is present.
- Ensure that the firing handle is fully squeezed to ensure proper staple formation and cutting of tissue.
- Keep the trocar visible at all times to prevent personal injury or inadvertent trauma to adjacent structures. Squeezing the firing handle will expose the knife.
- Engage the red safety latch prior to removing washer and donuts from within the circular knife.

Linear Stapler-Cutter for Laparoscopic Use

These instruments are designed for laparoscopic use; hence, the shafts are long and jaws are flexible. They allow you to select a color coded cartridge according to tissue thickness (see Fig. 3.23). The commonly used instruments are Endo GIA ETS45, and Echelon 60 stapler. ETS45

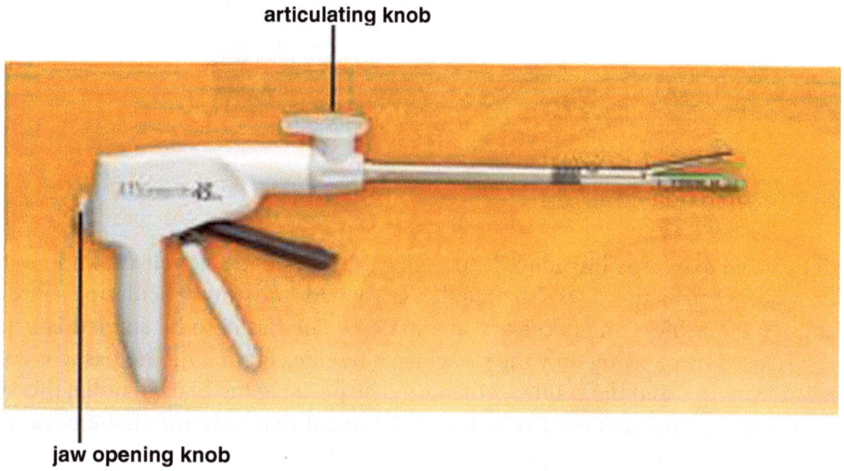

Fig. 3.22 Articulating linear stapler cutter: *Endo GIA ETS45*

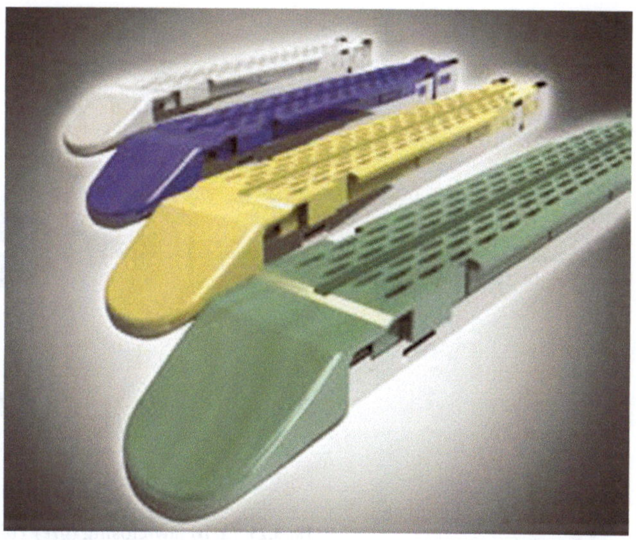

Fig. 3.23 Color-coded cartridges

This stapler cutter has a staple length of 40 mm. It staples two staggered rows of staples and cuts in between. It has two black marks on the jaw, which help the surgeon to decide the length of tissue to be stapled. The shaft is rotatable as well as articulating. This stapler is commonly used for linear stapling of the esophagus, or for the lesser curve of the stomach during esophageal surgery.

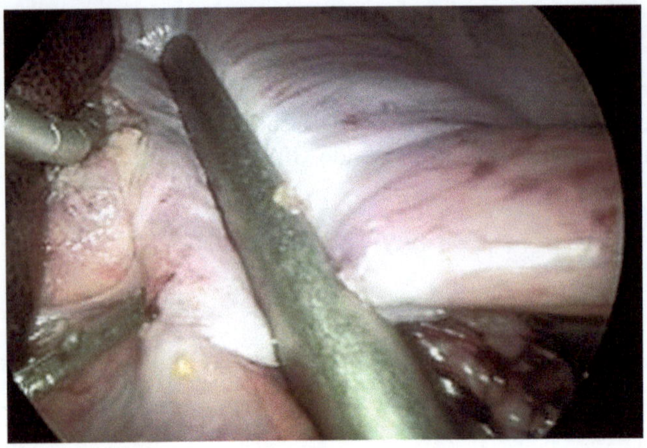

Fig. 3.24 Intracorporeal stapler application

Procedure

The closed stapler is introduced through a 12-mm port. The release knob at the end is pressed to open the jaws. The stapler is rotated and the articulating (flexion) knob adjusted to achieve the necessary angulations. The tissue to be stapled is held and the jaws closed by pressing only the jaw-closing handle (Fig. 3.25). The tissue is compressed for at least 15 s, and the stapler is then fired by pressing the black handle; this simultaneously staples and cuts the tissue. It is to be noted that only the tissue between the two black lines on the jaw is stapled and cut (Fig. 3.26).

Too fast stapling, too thick tissue, milking of excessive tissue into the jaws beyond the black indicators, and stapling across staple lines can result in poor or unsafe staple lines. Choosing the right type of stapler is hence very important.

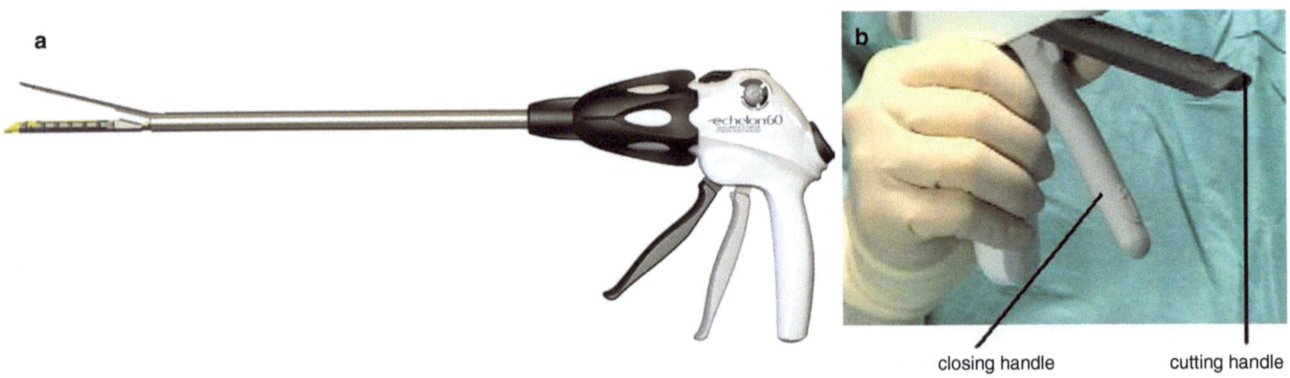

Fig. 3.25 (a, b) Jaw-closing (*grey color*) and stapler-firing (*black*) handles

Fig. 3.26 Two black indicators on the jaw: only the tissue between the two black lines on the jaw is stapled and cut

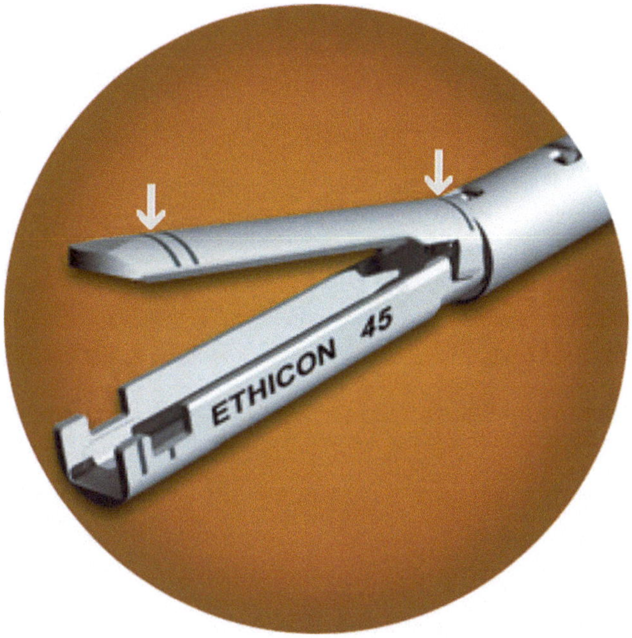

Echelon 60

The Echelon 60 delivers optimal hemostasis and mechanical strength. It has a wide jaw aperture and provides a 60 mm staple line. Since it fires two extra rows of staple lines, it improves the reliability as compared to the older staplers.

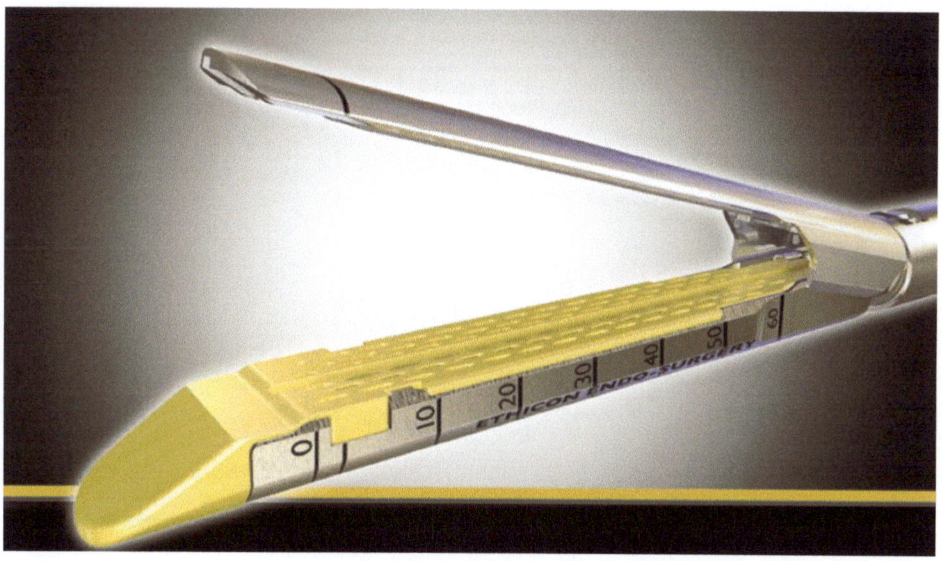

Fig. 3.27 The Echelon 60 with 6 rows of staples

It is inserted through a 12-mm port. It fires 6-rows of staples and cuts in-between. It is particularly useful in thick tissue. It is available in a wide range of cartridges – white, blue, gold, and green – and is applied as per the tissue thickness. We find the Gold stapler to be especially reliable and are extensively using it during gastrointestinal stapling and anastomosis.

4

Thoracoscopic and Laparoscopic Esophagectomy with Two-Field Nodal Clearance

Shailesh Puntambekar, Anjali M. Patil, Neeraj V. Rayate, and Saurabh N. Joshi

Introduction

The objectives of surgical management in carcinoma esophagus are

- A complete resection of the esophagus
- Adequate lymph node clearance
- Replacement of the esophagus by a suitable conduit
- Minimum morbidity

The salient features of the technique of combined thoracoscopic and laparoscopic esophagectomy with anastomosis in the neck described in this chapter are:

1. Thoracoscopic esophageal mobilization with lymphadenectomy, including the paratracheal, subcarinal, parabronchial and paraesophageal nodes.
2. Laparoscopic stomach mobilization with regional lymphadenectomy, including the lymph nodes along the lesser curvature of the stomach, the coeliac axis and the para-aortic nodes.
3. Specimen delivery through a small epigastric incision, and extracorporeal formation of stomach tube.
4. Intrathoracic placement of stomach tube and esophagogastric anastomosis in the neck.
5. Feeding jejunostomy in all patients.

Patient Selection

The choice of surgical procedure depends on

- Location and histology of tumor
- The stage of the disease
- Patient's general condition
- The pulmonary function tests

Indications of Thoracoscopic and Laparoscopic Esophagectomy

1. Cancers of the middle third of the esophagus
2. Cancers of the lower middle third of the esophagus

Contraindications

1. Cancers of the middle third of the esophagus with poor pulmonary function.
2. Previous thoracic surgeries and severe adhesions in the right hemithorax.
3. Tumors with tracheobronchial invasion and those showing axis deviation on barium studies and aortic involvement.

Investigations

The preoperative investigations done are: Barium-swallow studies, endoscopy, and biopsy. Positron emission tomography (PET), MRI, EUS and bronchoscopy may be done in addition. CT (computerized tomography) and EUS (endoscopic ultrasonography) can determine the anatomic location and enlargement of the mediastinal, perigastric, or coeliac lymph nodes. A CT scan is necessary to rule out tracheobronchial invasion. A 2D echocardiography is done whenever necessary.

Routine blood chemistry and medical evaluation for pulmonary and cardiac status is done.

Pulmonary function tests should be performed.

Preoperative Preparation

The patient is admitted 2 days prior to the surgery.

Pulmonary exercises in the form of incentive spirometry, steam inhalation, and nebulisation are started.

A central venous access is taken. The patient is hydrated. With CVP monitoring as the guideline a CVP of 6–7 mm is to be maintained. Intravenous antibiotics are started a day prior to the surgery. A pint of blood is reserved.

Anesthesia

General anesthesia in combination with thoracic epidural anesthesia is used.

Single lung ventilation is mandatory for the thoracic part and is achieved by using a left-sided double lumen endotracheal tube. The right lung is collapsed by blocking of the right-side arm of the tube. The double lumen tube is replaced by the regular endotracheal tube once the thoracic part of dissection is over, and the patient is placed in supine position.

Surgical Technique

Thoracoscopic and laparoscopic esophagectomy is performed in three stages.

1. In the first stage the patient is positioned in the left lateral decubitus position for *thoracoscopic esophageal mobilization.*
2. In the second stage, the patient is placed in a supine position for *laparoscopic stomach mobilization.* The specimen is retrieved by a small epigastric incision, and the stomach tube is created extracorporeally through the same incision.
3. The third stage is performed simultaneously by the second team. The *cervical esophagus is mobilized* and the stomach tube is placed intra-thoracically. The *esophagogastric anastomosis* is performed in the neck.

Instrumentation

1. Two 10 mm and two 5 mm ports
2. Bipolar forceps-two
3. Needle holder
4. Scissors
5. Suction canula
6. Two atraumatic fenestrated graspers
7. Clip applicator (10 mm vascular locking clips – plastic)
8. ACE harmonic
9. A 0 or 30° scope

Stage 1: Thoracoscopic Mobilization of the Esophagus

Patient, Port, and Surgeon Positions

(a) Patient Position

The patient is placed with the right side up at an angle of 60° with the horizontal plane. The right shoulder and elbow joints are flexed. A bolster is used to support the patient's back. The left leg is slightly flexed at the hip and knee joints and the patient is strapped to the table at the level of iliac crest and at the tip of the shoulder. The position of the primary port is marked at the angle of scapula (6th or 7th intercostal space) in the posterior axially line. Patient, surgeon, and monitor positions are shown in Fig 4.1.

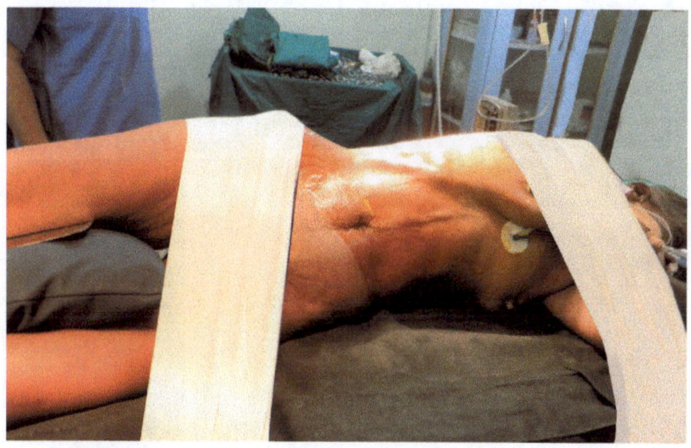

Fig. 4.1 Patient, surgeon and monitor positions

The surgeon stands on the right side, facing the patient's back. Single-lung ventilation through a double lumen endotracheal tube is initiated by occluding ventilation to the right lung. The camera assistant stands to the left of the operating surgeon. The assistant surgeon stands on the left side of the patient.

(b) Port Position

1. The primary port is inserted in the 6th or 7th intercostal space in the posterior axillary line remaining close to the upper border of the lower rib. The anesthetist uses the

suction to deflate the right lung at this moment to prevent injury to the right lung. A 10 mm 0°-scope is passed to confirm intrapleural placement of the port and CO_2 is insufflated. The pressure is maintained at 7 mm of Hg so as not to interfere with the venous return (Photo 4.2a, b).

2. The secondary ports are inserted under vision as shown in Photo 4.2. A 10-mm port is placed in the 8th–9th intercostal space in the mid-axillary line and a 5 mm port is placed in the 2nd intercostal space in the mid or anterior axillary line to achieve triangulation with the camera port. These two ports are the right (10 mm) and left (5 mm) hand working ports of the operating surgeon (Photo 4.2c, d).
3. A fourth port is inserted in a diamond configuration in the 5th intercostal space in the mid-clavicular line; this is used by the assistant to retract the right lung.

A diagnostic thoracoscopy is first performed to inspect the pleural cavity and the surface of the lung for any suspicious lesion. The right lung is retracted anteriorly to expose the thoracic esophagus.

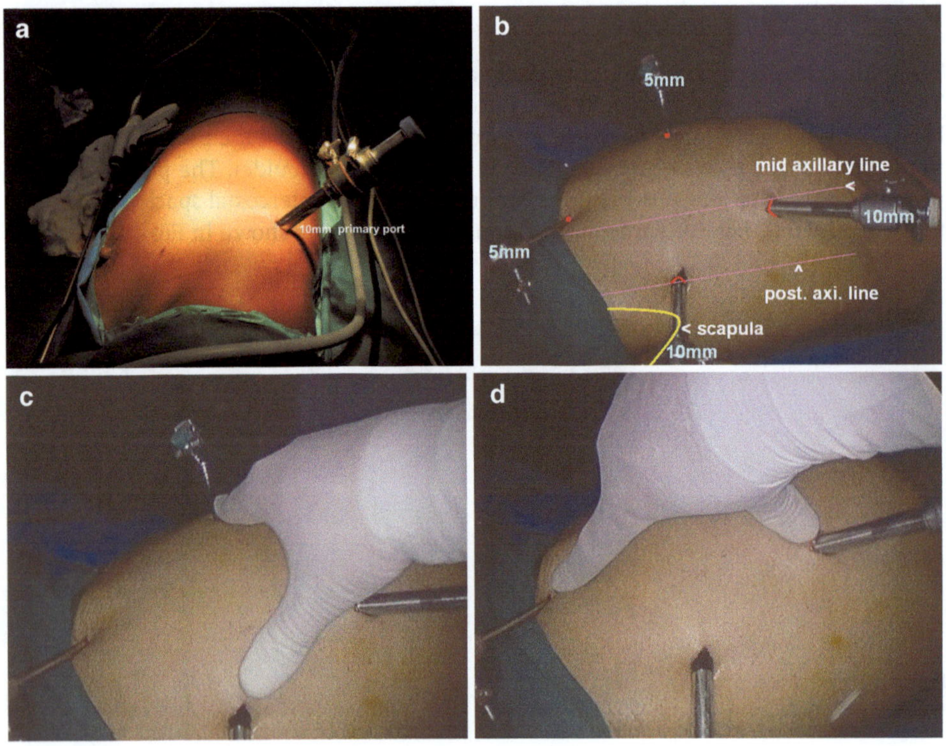

Photo 4.2 (a-d)

Procedure

(a) Infra Azygous Dissection

Dissection Anterior to the Esophagus

The visceral pleura that covers the esophagus is grasped and the esophagus is pulled laterally. This exposes the anterior space between the esophagus and the pericardium. A pleural cut is taken with the bipolar forceps or the Ace Harmonic (Ethicon Endo-surgery Inc. Cincinnati, OH) and the cut is extended cranially and caudally remaining parallel to the esophagus.

The anterior vagus is seen clearly as it traverses along the esophagus. The principle of dissecting "outside" the vagus and not between the esophagus and vagus is applied, and the esophagus is pushed laterally. The use of a gauze strip at this point helps to dissect the nodes off the underlying pericardium. These can be removed en-bloc with the esophagus, or may be removed separately at this stage through the 10 mm port using the stone holding forceps.

Dissection of the Right Hilar, Subcarinal, and Left Hilar Nodes

The vagus is pulled laterally and the cardiac fibers of the vagus passing anteriorly and to the left are cut. The right main bronchus is identified passing upward. Further lateral retraction of the vagus and esophagus exposes the right hilar and subcarinal nodes. These nodes are dissected with the bipolar forceps. The nodes are supplied by small veins and these are coagulated carefully.

The dissection between the esophagus and the pericardium is continued caudally. The paraesophageal nodes are dissected and removed along with the esophagus. The pericardium is completed stripped of fibro-fatty tissue and the pericardial nodes. The dissection is achieved by blunt dissection with the suction canula and is facilitated by the CO_2 insufflation. The left pleura is again seen in this region as a shining membrane and is prone to injury. By retracting the esophagus laterally, a clear plane between the pleura and esophagus can be seen. There are a few nodes at this level and these are included in the dissection. The esophagus is continuously pulled further laterally with the left hand while the right hand performs the dissection. The assistant pulls the lung medially to give counter traction. The caudal end point of dissection is the hiatus.

Dissection Posterior to the Esophagus

The procedure starts by taking a cut on the visceral pleura between the esophagus and the aorta in the infra-azygous part. The CO_2 insufflation helps in opening the plane between the esophagus and the aorta. The medial end of the pleura is held up by the left-hand grasper. This lifts the esophagus and the posterior vagus nerve is seen. The pleural cut is extended caudally up to the level of the diaphragm. The plane of dissection always lies outside the vagus and not between the vagus and the esophagus. This is the oncologically correct plane and results in complete paraesophageal tissue clearance. This plane is relatively avascular and so bleeding is minimized. The vagus can be used for upward traction, so that tethering of the esophageal muscle fibers is avoided. The vagus is held up with the left hand and the fibro-fatty tissue and the lymph tissue is swept toward the esophagus. Thus all the paraesophageal nodes are removed. Preferably a bipolar instrument is used here, since it is better at coagulating the small blood vessels going to the lymph nodes. Further upward traction on the esophagus exposes the direct branches of the aorta. These are usually two or three in number. They are clipped with vascular clips (Hemlock plastic locking clips) and cut.

The esophagus is separated upward (anteriorly) and cranially and the left inferior pulmonary vein is identified. It is more clearly seen medially, when the anterior and posterior dissections are completed. The traction is always maintained by pulling on the pleura overlying the esophagus, or on the vagus to avoid tethering of the esophagus. This posterior dissection is continued further, cranially lifting up all the fibro fatty tissue till the aorta is bared. The direction of the aorta is followed cranially and the esophagus is lifted from the arch of the aorta. The arch lies at a level just below the azygous vein. The left main bronchus crosses anterior to the descending aorta. Utmost care is taken not to injure the posterior wall of the left bronchus while lifting esophagus from the arch of the aorta. The left hilar nodes are exposed at this level and can be dissected from the bronchus at this stage or at a later stage when the subcarinal nodes are removed.

Caudally, the dissection is continued toward the hiatus. At this stage, the opposite pleura is identified by careful blunt dissection using the suction canula. The paraesophageal nodes and those at the hiatus are removed completely. The thoracic duct is identified as a white glistening structure over the descending aorta at the hiatus. This can be clipped or can be separated completely from the esophagus.

This completes the posterior dissection. The sign of completed posterior dissection is absence of fibro fatty tissue on the aorta, complete removal of paraesophageal nodes, clear visualization of the arch of aorta, the left main bronchus, and the inferior pulmonary vein.

Medial and Circumferential Dissection

The esophagus at the level of the pericardium is retracted laterally with the left hand, and a strip of gauze is pushed from the medial side of the esophagus, to aid identification of the plane of dissection. The dissection is continued using the suction canula or the bipolar forceps. The strip of gauze is then retrieved by lifting the esophagus from the aorta posteriorly, thus achieving separation of the esophagus along its entire circumference.

Once such a window is created at one point, and the left-hand grasper is passed through the window to pull the esophagus laterally. The tip of the grasper should rest on the vertebrae so that no vital structure is damaged. This helps in dissecting the esophagus on the medial side and freeing it further.

The esophagus is manipulated by the left-hand grasper and the organ is separated along its length and all around. The assistant surgeon continues to give counter traction so that the tissues are put under stretch.

Cranially, the anterior dissection ends at the level of the azygous vein. The vagus is seen parallel to the esophagus. On completion of the anterior dissection, the carina is clearly seen with the left and right main bronchi.

The infra azygous dissection achieves complete removal of paraesophageal, subcarinal, hilar, and the hiatal nodes. The esophagus is also separated all around from the pericardium and the left pleura medially, arch of the aorta, and the descending aorta posteriorly, and the azygous vein laterally. At the end of dissection, all these structures should be identified. They should be free of any fibro-fatty and lymphoid tissue.

A few nodes lie along the inferior pulmonary vein and are dissected and removed. A strip of gauze is kept, for some time, in the gutter between the esophagus and the aorta. Complete hemostasis is achieved before proceeding for the supra-azygous dissection. The thoracic duct area is inspected for any damage.

(b) Supra-Azygous Dissection

The next step is the supra-azygous dissection. The apex of the lung is pulled down by the assistant to expose this area. Once the lung is retracted, one can see the entire supra-azygous anatomy. The pleura that covers the esophagus is lifted with the left-hand grasper and a cut is taken. This cut is extended upward to the root of the neck.

The vagus nerve is identified. The vagal fibers going to the bronchus are preserved, and the rest of the vagus is cut at the level of the azygous vein.

The dissection begins posterior to the esophagus; the right-hand grasper pulls the esophagus upward and a plane is created between it and the vertebrae. This dissection is done either with the suction canula or with the bipolar forceps. The use of the bipolar is recommended, as small vessels can be easily coagulated. A few small vessels arising from the intercostal vessels and supplying the esophagus are coagulated and cut. The entire fibro-fatty tissue along with the nodes is pushed with the esophagus.

At this stage the infra-azygous esophagus is lifted, and dissection is performed in the posterior plane with a suction canula. The left hand is used to pull the esophagus caudally and anteriorly; the supra- and infra-azygous planes are joined. Thus the entire esophagus is freed posteriorly.

The pleura on the lateral wall of the azygous vein is held and cut. The lymphovascular tissues along the azygous vein are cleared at this stage. The azygous vein is freed along its entire length. The bronchial artery is posterior to the azygous vein and can be seen by retracting the vein downward. We usually preserve the azygous vein and the azygous is dissected completely by creating a plane between the esophagus and the vein. This allows for a complete separation of the vein. The vein is then retracted slightly and then the nodes along with the fibro-fatty tissue are removed. These nodes can be removed en-block, or can be removed separately.

Once the azygous vein is freed or cut, the supra-azygous esophagus is pulled laterally, this exposes the plane between the posterior wall of the trachea and the esophagus. The dissection should be done with extreme caution; especially so, if the tumor involves the esophagus at this level. We recommend the use of a blunt dissector like a suction canula, since the membranous trachea is to be protected against injury. The dissection should always be done parallel to the esophagus as well as to the trachea. A clear plane is identifiable, and this plane is further exposed by pulling the esophagus laterally. A strip of gauze can be used to complete the dissection. Once the infra azygous esophagus has been freed completely, the dissection between the esophagus and the trachea is easier. A medial window, similar to that made earlier is made and the left-hand grasper pulls the esophagus further laterally. The entire esophagus is thus separated. There are a few nodes in the paratracheal region which are dissected and removed. The esophagus is dissected around the circumference in the surpa-azygous region and these planes are joined with those in the infra-azygous region, thus completely freeing the esophagus. This can be confirmed by pulling the esophagus cranio-caudally ("the shoe-shine sign").

Once the esophagus is completely freed, it is pulled laterally to expose the left recurrent laryngeal nerve lying in the trachea–esophageal groove. Nodes along this nerve are removed. The use of bipolar or any other energy sources is not recommended near the nerve. The right recurrent laryngeal nerve is also identified at the thoracic inlet near the innominate artery.

The esophageal dissection is continued cranially to the root of the neck. The sign of complete dissection is the appearance of fat, as seen thoracoscopically, or subcutaneous emphysema felt by the assistant in the left supra-clavicular area. It is essential to dissect the esophagus completely from the posterior wall of the trachea and to the root of the neck, thus obviating the need of blind finger dissection in the neck. The esophagus is then moved cranio-caudally and medio-laterally to confirm complete esophageal mobilization. The nodal areas are examined for the complete removal of the nodes. A thorough wash is given and the damage to the left pleura is checked under water; if damaged an intercostal drain needs to be placed on the left side too. Complete haemostasis is achieved by additional use of clips or bipolar energy.

On the right side, an intercostal drain is inserted through the working 10mm port and is placed near the apex, with the help of the left-hand grasper. The 5 mm ports are removed under vision, as the intercostal vessels may have been damaged during the insertion of the ports and this is to be checked. The lung is inflated and the camera port is removed under vision. The intercostal drainage tube should be open and not clamped, to push out all the air during lung inflation.

At the end of the thoracoscopic procedure, the drain is fixed and the incisions are closed. The patient is turned and positioned for the laparoscopic and neck dissection.

Stomach Mobilization and Nodal Dissection

The gastrocolic omentum is opened, taking care to remain outside the gastroepiploic arcade. The greater curve is mobilized from the pylorus to the spleen. The right gastroepiploic artery must be preserved. When proceeding toward the spleen, the short gastric vessels are clamped close to the stomach wall, taking care not to injure the splenic hilum. These are taken with the Harmonic Ace. The left crus is again seen when the short gastric vessels are divided and the fundus is mobilized medially.

The greater omentum is divided, but complete resection is not necessary. Congenital adhesions between the pancreas and stomach are released and the stomach is now completely lifted off the pancreas. Duodenal mobilization is performed only if the stomach is not of sufficient length. It is sometimes/usually not necessary. The author does not routinely perform a drainage procedure. If deemed necessary, a pyloromyotomy can be performed laparoscopically or extracorporeally during specimen removal.

The nodal dissection at the coeliac axis is performed using the bipolar forceps or the Harmonic Ace. Nodes around the base of the left gastric vessels are dissected to delineate the left gastric artery and vein separately. The left gastric vein is clipped and cut. The common hepatic artery and the splenic artery are identified. The areolar tissue and nodes along the common hepatic artery are dissected and taken medially, along with the gastric nodes. There is sometimes some bleeding from the small vessels supplying the nodes. The bleeding usually stops once the node has been completely removed. This bleeding can be temporarily controlled by packing with a piece of gauze for some time; alternatively, the bleeders can be coagulated or clipped. The nodes along the splenic artery are then taken. For this, the assistant on the left side has to gently depress the cranial part of the head of pancreas. This helps the camera to reach the celiac axis and show the splenic vessels well during the lymph node clearance. The Para-aortic nodes in this region are cleared, again proceeding toward the hiatus. Completed nodal dissection bares the celiac axis entirely; this is seen as the "Mercedes Benz" sign. The magnification offered by the laparoscopic approach greatly aids the lymph node dissection and improves precision.

The left gastric artery is ligated or clipped and cut. The vessels along the lesser curve are clipped, for an adequate distance distally. This can also be done extracorporeally during specimen removal.

The stomach tube can be fashioned intra-corporeally (using staplers) or extracorporeally. The author prefers the latter method, since the aim of the procedure is not to do everything laparoscopically, but to complete the operation with minimum morbidity.

Mobilization of the Esophagus in the Neck

The neck dissection is commenced by a second team, to mobilize the esophagus in the neck and upper mediastinum.

A left horizontal supra-clavicular incision is taken, extending just beyond the lateral border of the left sternocleidomastoid muscle. The platysma and the omohyoid muscles are cut to expose the internal jugular vein. Dissection remains medial to the carotid sheath. The middle thyroid vein is divided and the thyroid gland is retracted medially. The esophagus is identified and dissection is continued posteriorly up to the prevertebral fascia. The posterior wall of the esophagus is separated from the prevertebral fascia. Anteriorly the esophagus is gently separated from the trachea, remaining close to the esophageal wall, taking care not to injure the left recurrent laryngeal nerve. A cotton tape is passed around the esophagus. This sling helps to maintain traction on the esophagus for further mobilization in the mediastinum. A finger-dissection, remaining close to the esophageal wall is used to mobilize the upper thoracic esophagus. Special care is taken anteriorly not to tear the membranous trachea. Deeper into the mediastinum, the pleura is separated from the esophagus as far as possible. The entire intrathoracic esophagus is thus freed, and is accompanied by a give-away sensation perceived by the left hand pulling on the esophagus.

The naso-gastric (Levine) tube is removed and the esophagus is transected in the neck. On the proximal end, the mucosal and submucosal level of transection is kept 2–3 mm distal to the transection of the muscle layers. Two lateral stay sutures are placed on the proximal esophagus. The distal cut end of the esophagus is tied and a nasogastric tube is transfixed to it.

Specimen Delivery and Creation of the Stomach Tube

The pneumoperitonum is reestablished and the esophagus is pulled into the abdominal cavity.

A small midline incision (usually 5 cm in thin patients) is used to deliver the specimen and the stomach outside the abdomen. The author prefers to fashion the stomach tube extracorporeally, using linear staplers. The lesser curve is excised in such a way that the stomach tube is of 5-6cm width. The Levine tube attached to the esophagus and brought down through the thorax is now disconnected from the esophagus, and the specimen is removed. The staple-line is reinforced by continuous 3:0 running sutures (silk or PDS). A very wide stomach tube leads to gastric stasis, and is therefore avoided. The Levine tube is transfixed to the upper end of the stomach tube. The conduit is thus pulled into the neck by rail-roading it to the Levine tube.

We routinely perform a feeding jejunostomy in all patients. The abdomen is closed in layers.

Hand-Sewn Anastomosis in the Neck

The esophagus is anastomosed to the posterior wall near the apex of the gastric conduit to create an inverted ink-bottle effect. This effect prevents anastomotic leakages. The posterior seromuscular layer is taken using interrupted 3:0 silk sutures. An opening is made on the stomach wall with a diathermy. Continuous full-thickness sutures of 4:0 PDS/Vicryl are taken. This is the second layer and includes the full thickness of the posterior wall of the stomach and full-thickness of the posterior wall of the esophagus. A nasogastric tube is passed across the anastomosis and the second layer is continued anteriorly as the third layer. A fourth layer of interrupted 3:0 silk/PDS seromuscular sutures completes the anastomosis.

A soft corrugated drain is placed adjacent to the anastomosis and the neck incision is closed.

Postoperative Management

The patient is shifted to recovery with endotracheal tube in situ. Postoperative X-ray of the chest is done serially to confirm lung expansion. Jejunostomy feeding is started 48 h later. Patient is extubated on the next day. IV antibiotics are continued for 3 days postoperatively. Epidural analgesia is continued for 2 days, and later pain relief is achieved with NSAIDs. The intercostal drainage tube is removed, usually on the 2nd or 3rd post-operative day, after ensuring complete lung expansion, if intercostal drain output is <100ml on 2 consecutive days. Water soluble Gastrograffin swallow is performed between 7th and 9th day. If no leak, the nasogastric tube is removed and oral feeds started.

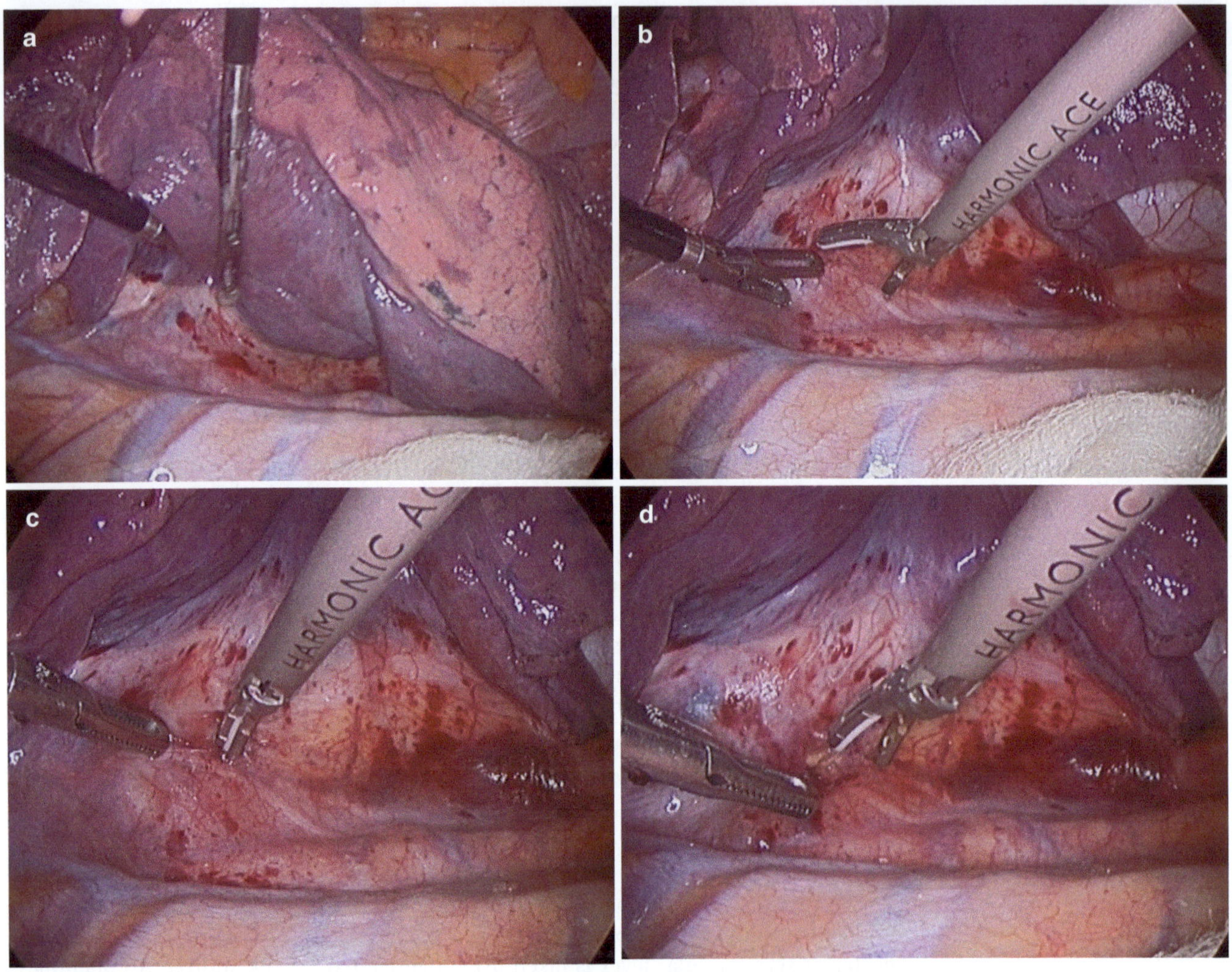

Photo 4.3 (a-d)

Atlas of the Operative Procedure

Thoracoscopic Part

1. The procedure starts in the infra-azygous portion of esophagus by taking a cut on the visceral pleura between the esophagus and the pericardium (Photo 4.3a–d).

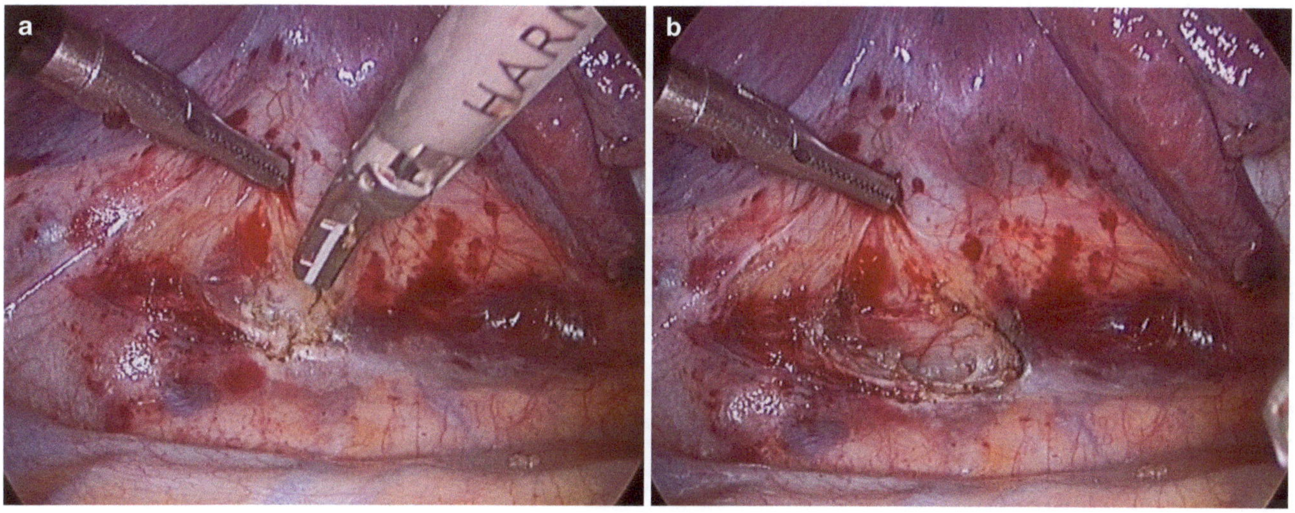

Photo 4.4 (a, b)

2. The CO_2 insufflation opens the plane between the esophagus and the pericardium (Photo 4.4a, b).

3. The pleural cut is extended cranially and caudally with the harmonic scalpel remaining parallel to the esophagus (Photo 4.5a–d).

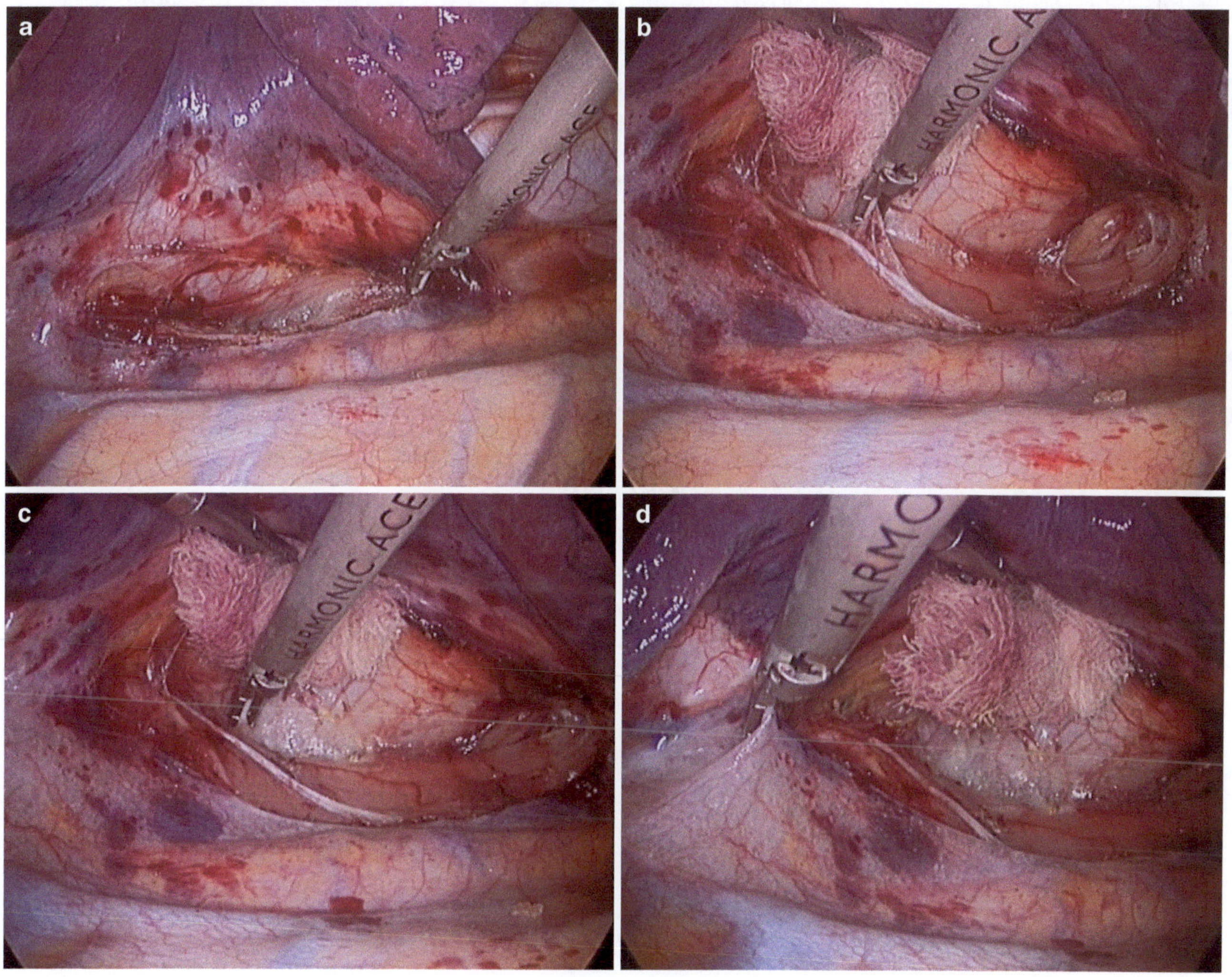

Photo 4.5 (a-d)

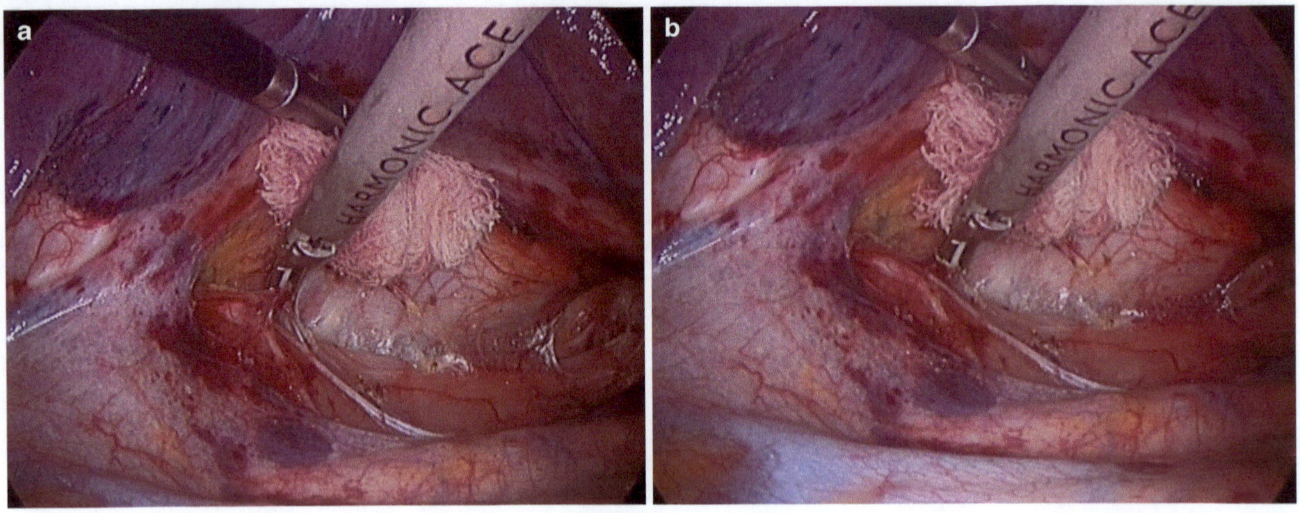

Photo 4.6 (a, b)

4. The anterior vagus is seen clearly as it traverses the esophagus (Photo 4.6a, b).
5. The plane of dissection should remain outside the vagus nerve that is between the vagus nerve and pericardium, and not between the vagus and esophagus (Photo 4.7a–e).

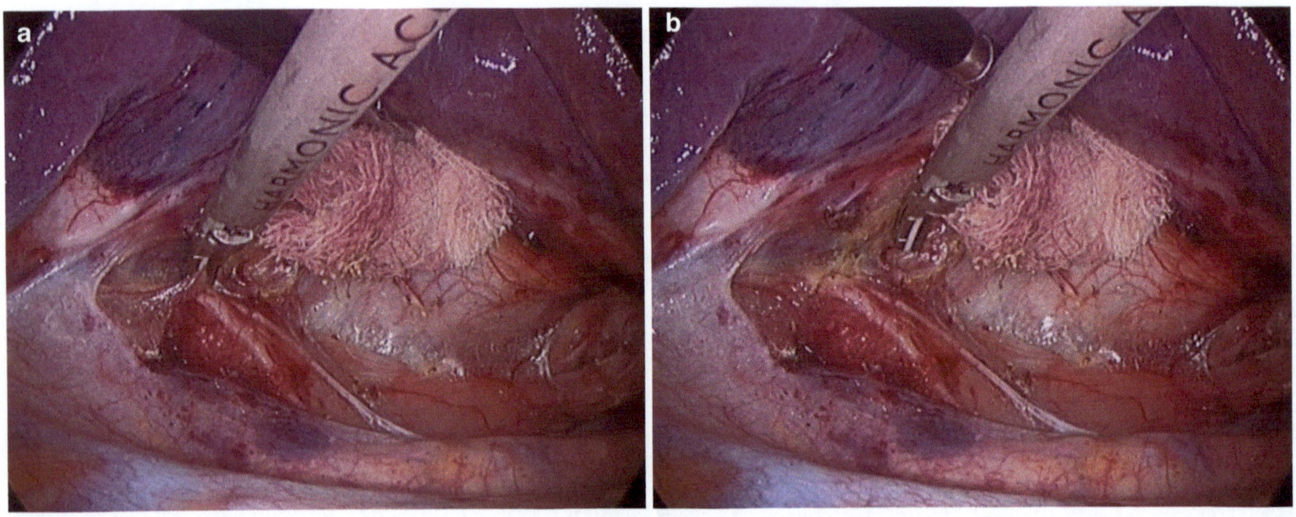

Photo 4.7 (a-e)

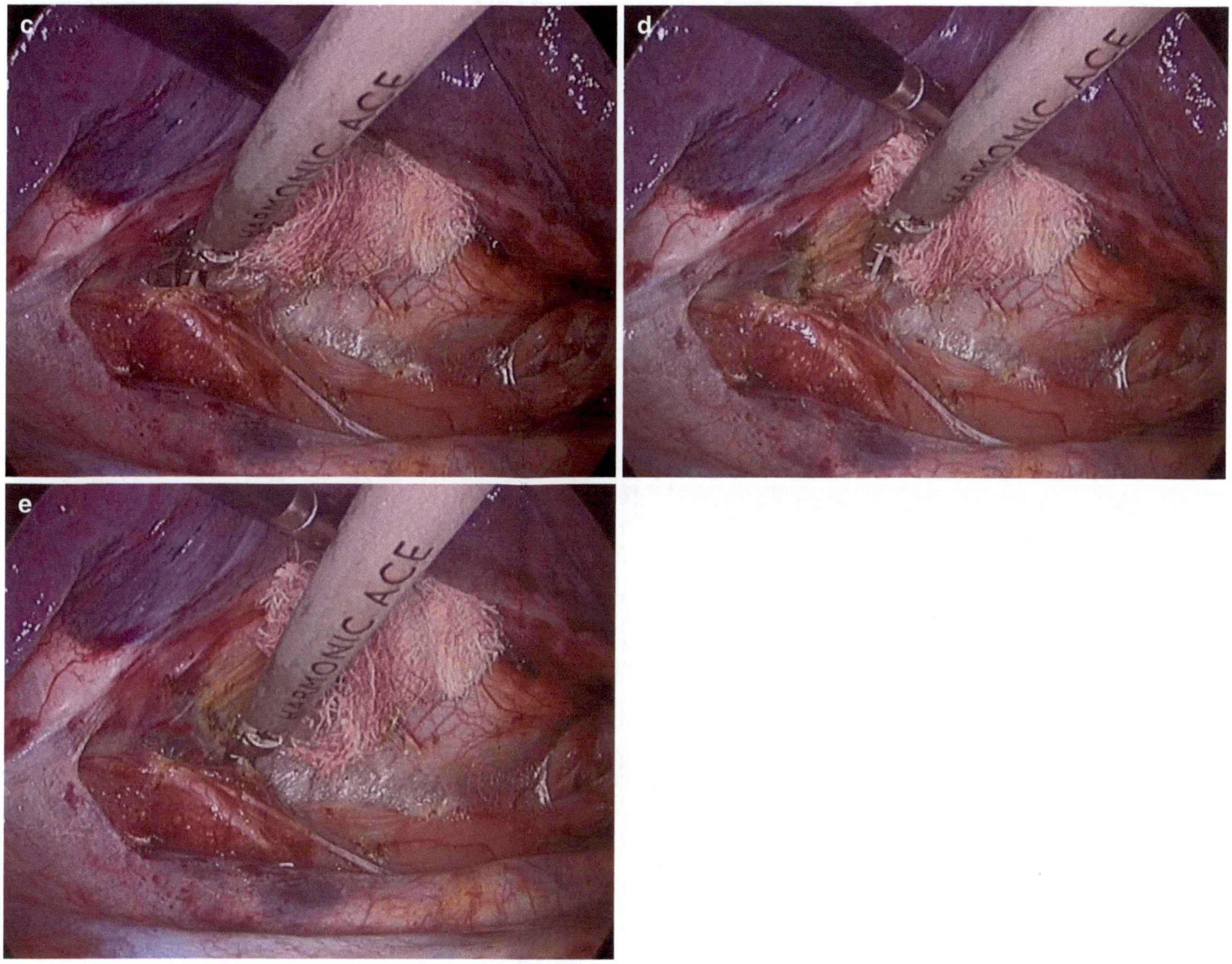

Photo 4.7 (Continued)

6. At this stage, the right main bronchus is seen along with the subcarinal nodes (Photo 4.8a, b).

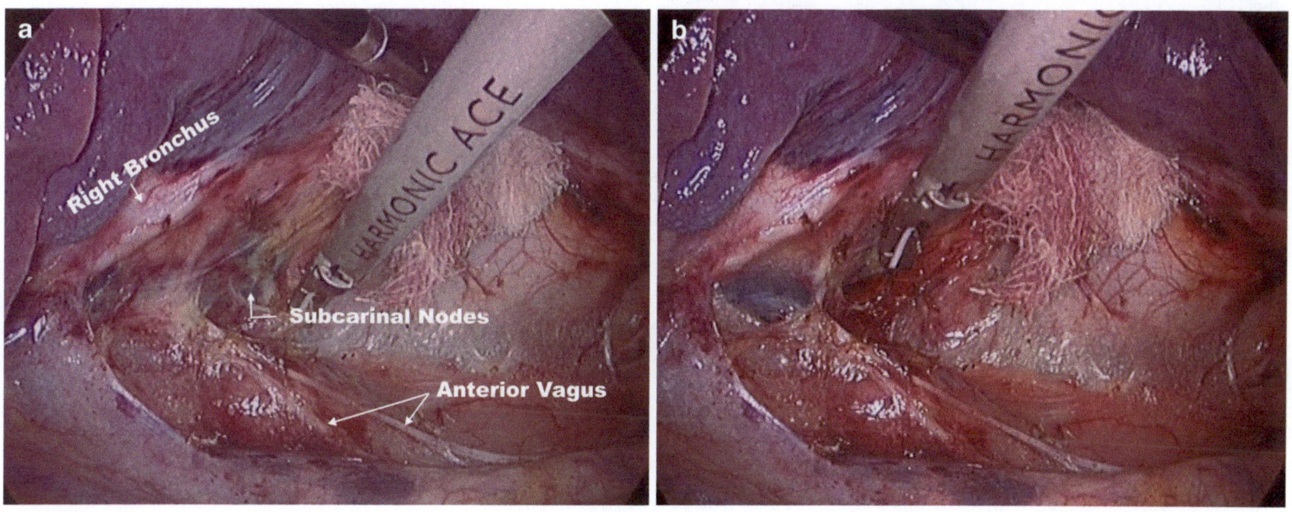

Photo 4.8 (a, b)

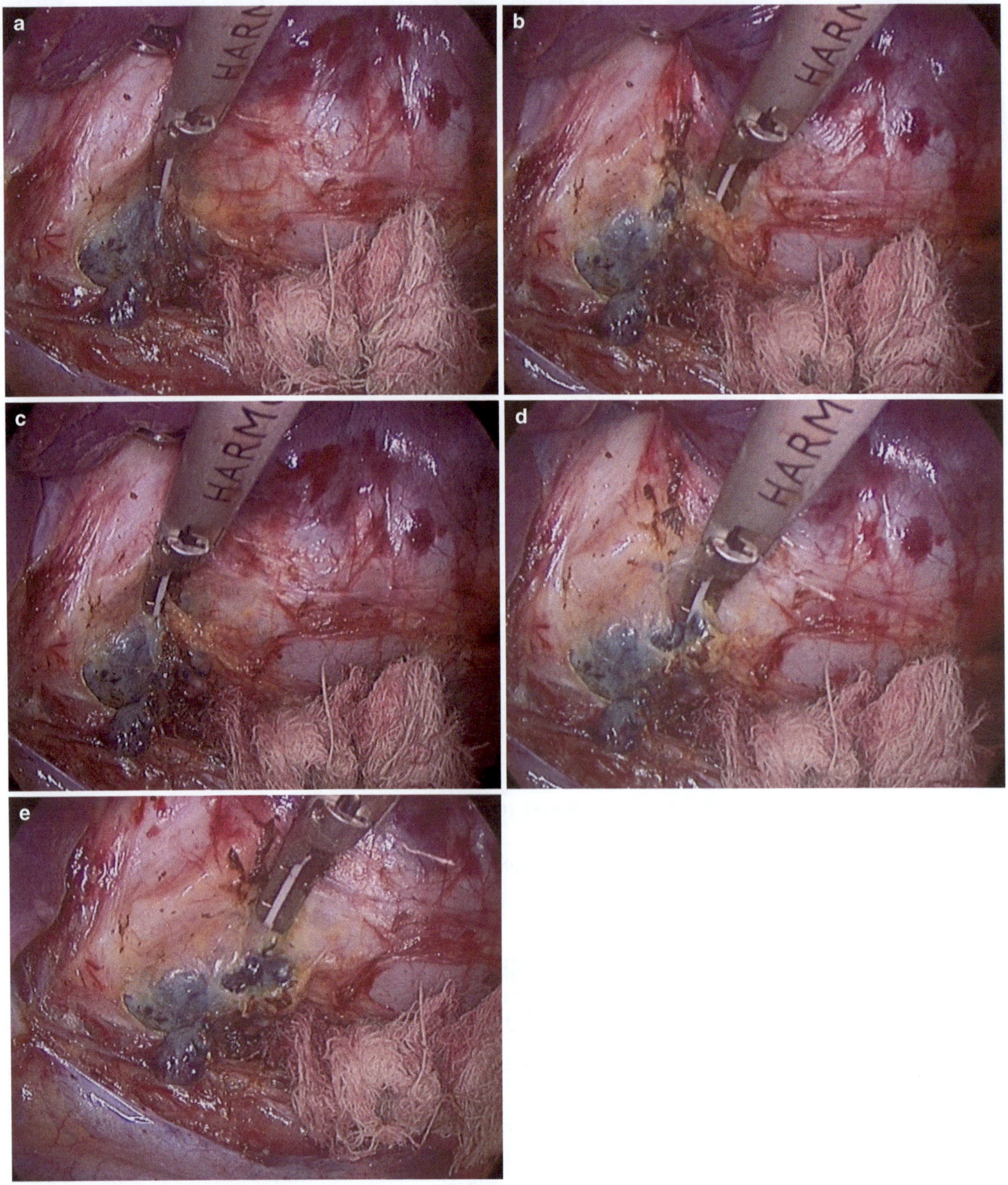

Photo 4.9 (a-e)

7. Subcarinal nodes are now dissected with harmonic scalpel and taken with the esophagus so as to remove en bloc (Photo 4.9a–e).

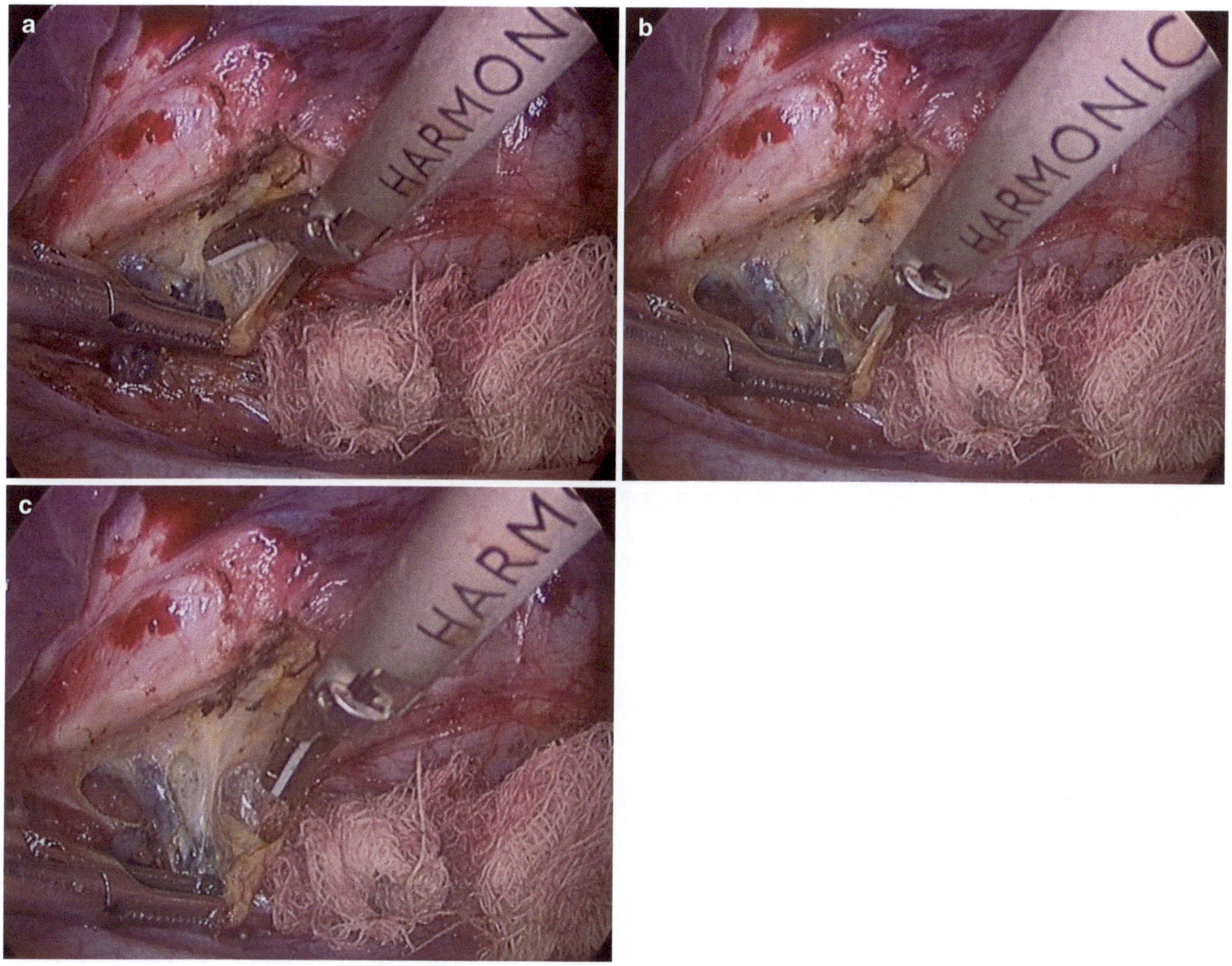

Photo 4.10 (a-c)

8. The subcarinal nodes are supplied by small veins, and these should be coagulated carefully (Photo 4.10a–c).

9. A use of gauze strip helps to push the subcarinal nodes toward the esophagus (Photo 4.11).

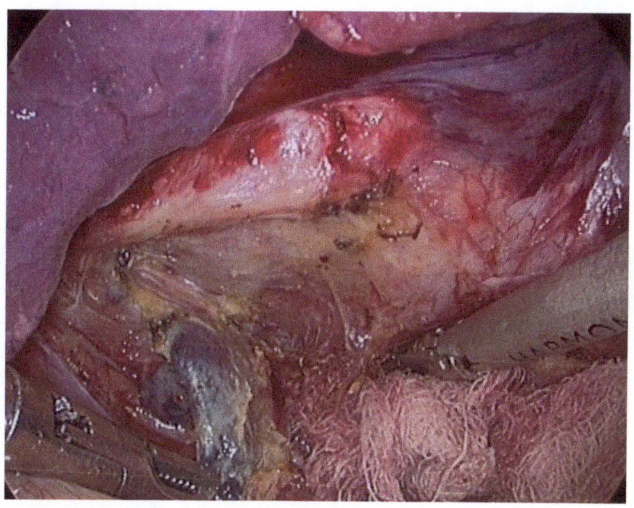

Photo 4.11

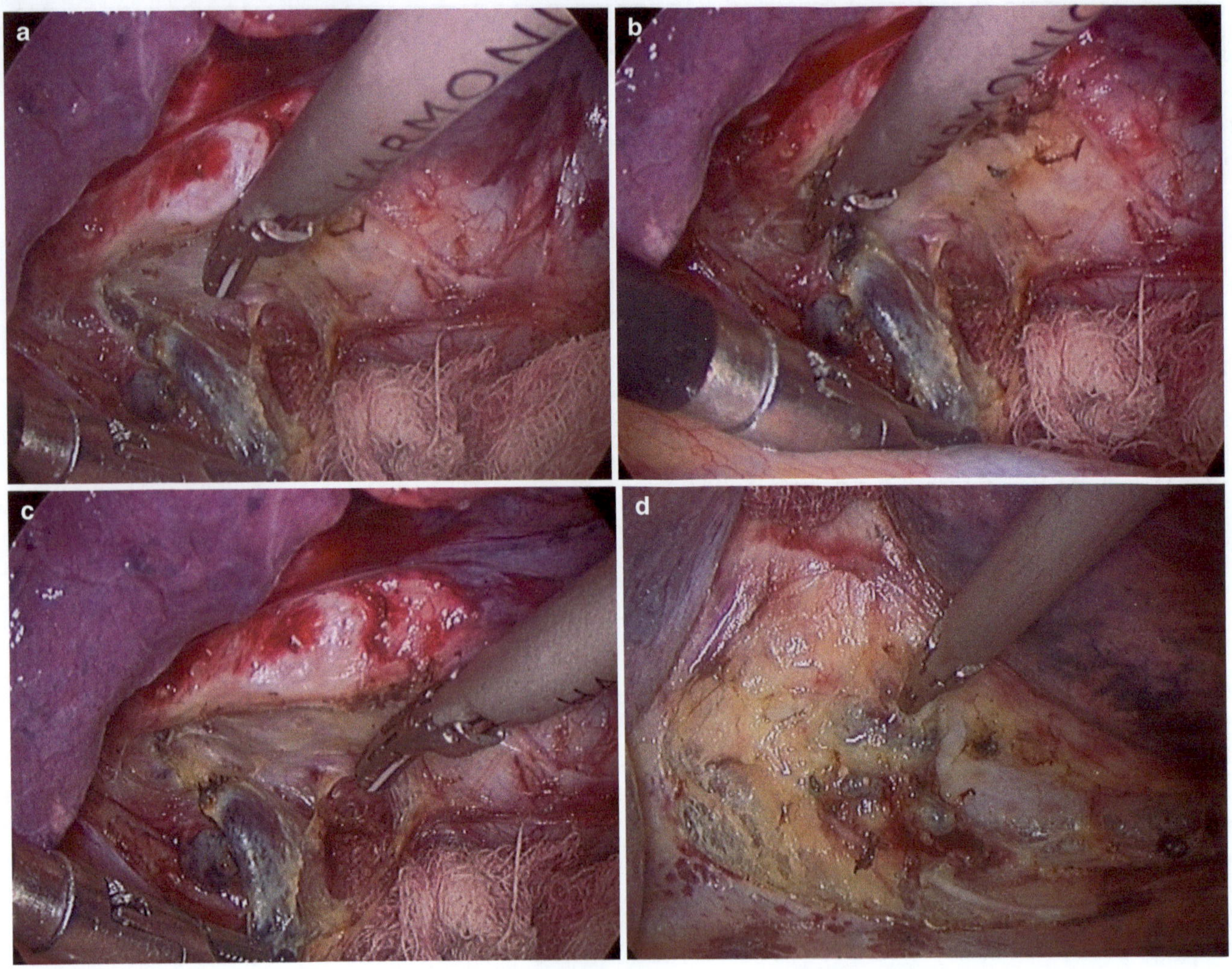

Photo 4.12 (a-d)

10. The dissection is further carried to the subcarinal region and all the nodal tissue is removed from that area (Photo 4.12a–d).

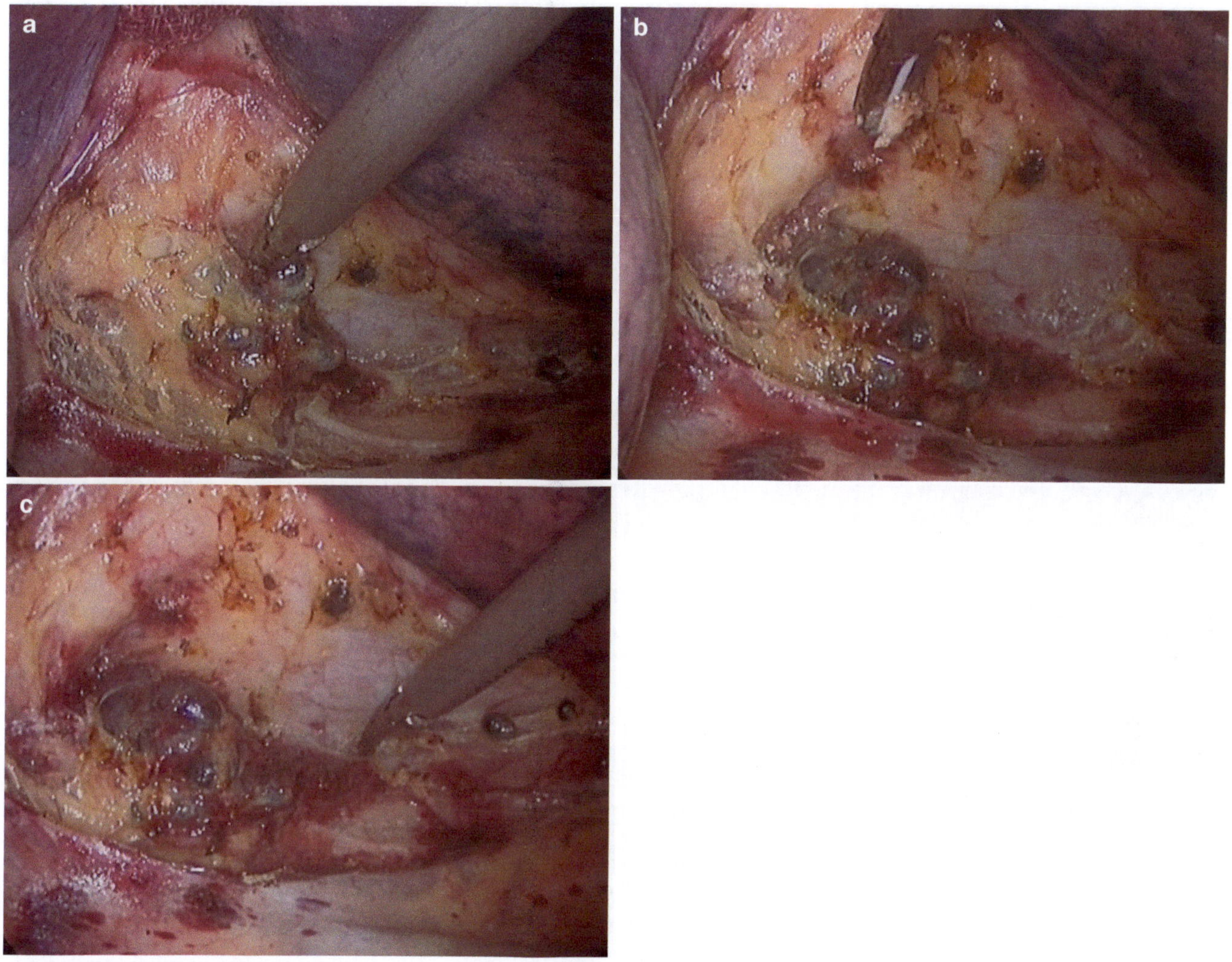

Photo 4.13 (a-c)

11. The dissection between the esophagus and the pericardium is done using sharp and blunt dissection (Photo 4.13a–c).

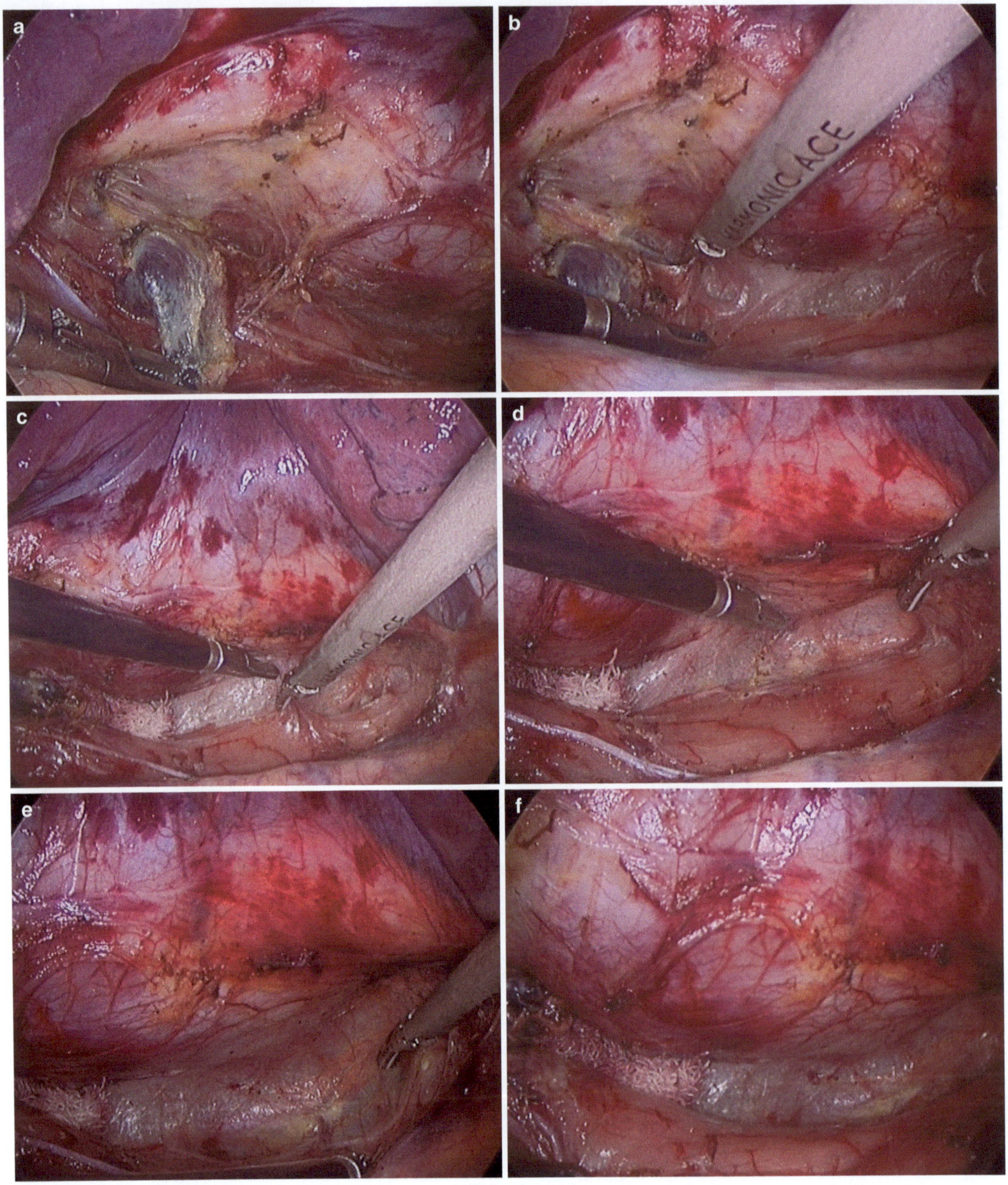

Photo 4.14 (a-f)

12. The pericardium is stripped off the fibro-fatty tissues and the esophagus is mobilized up to the hiatus (Photo 4.14a–f).

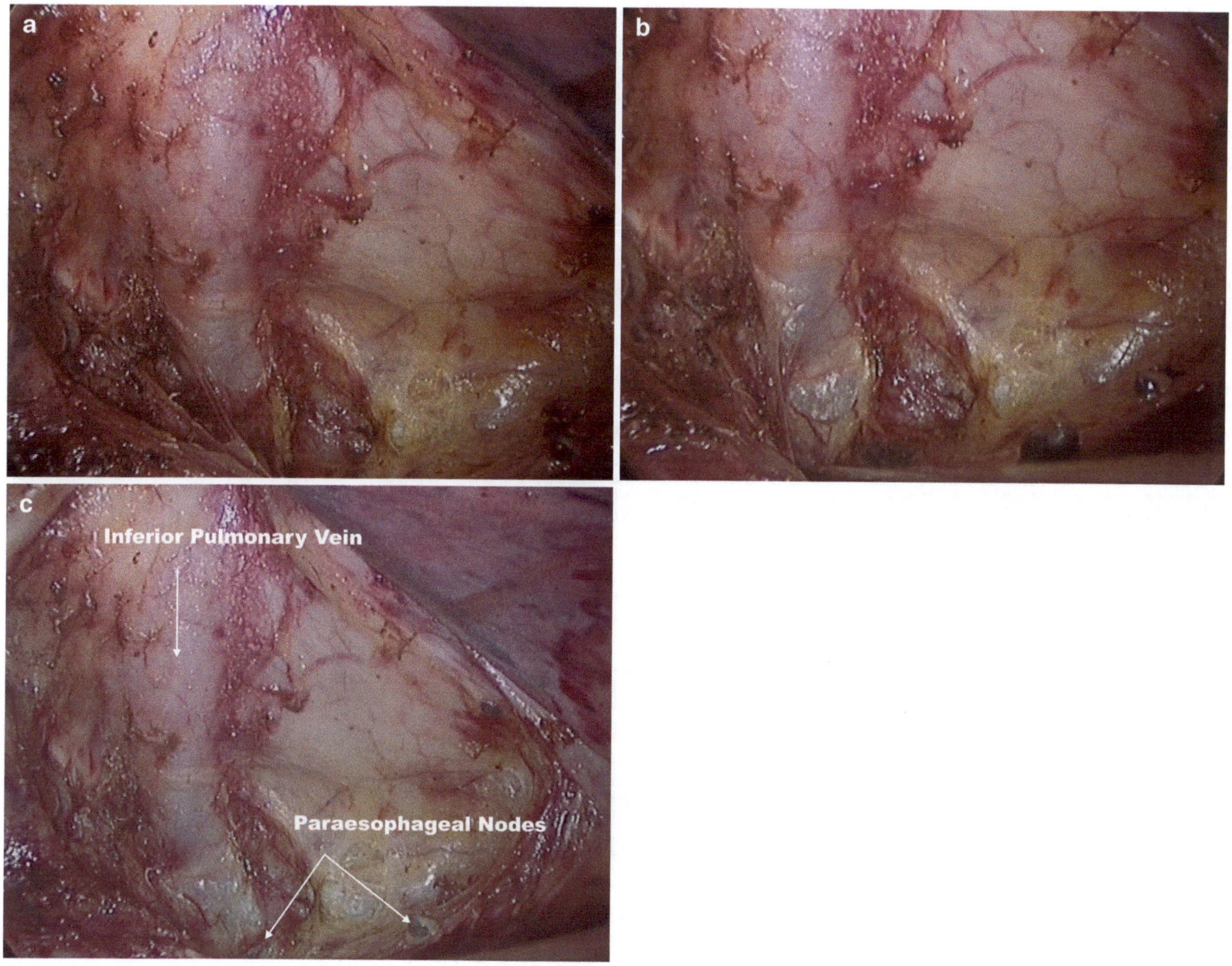

Photo 4.15 (a-c)

13. The lateral traction on the esophagus exposes the left inferior pulmonary vein and the paraesophageal nodes. The paraesophageal nodes are removed en bloc (Photo 4.15a–c).

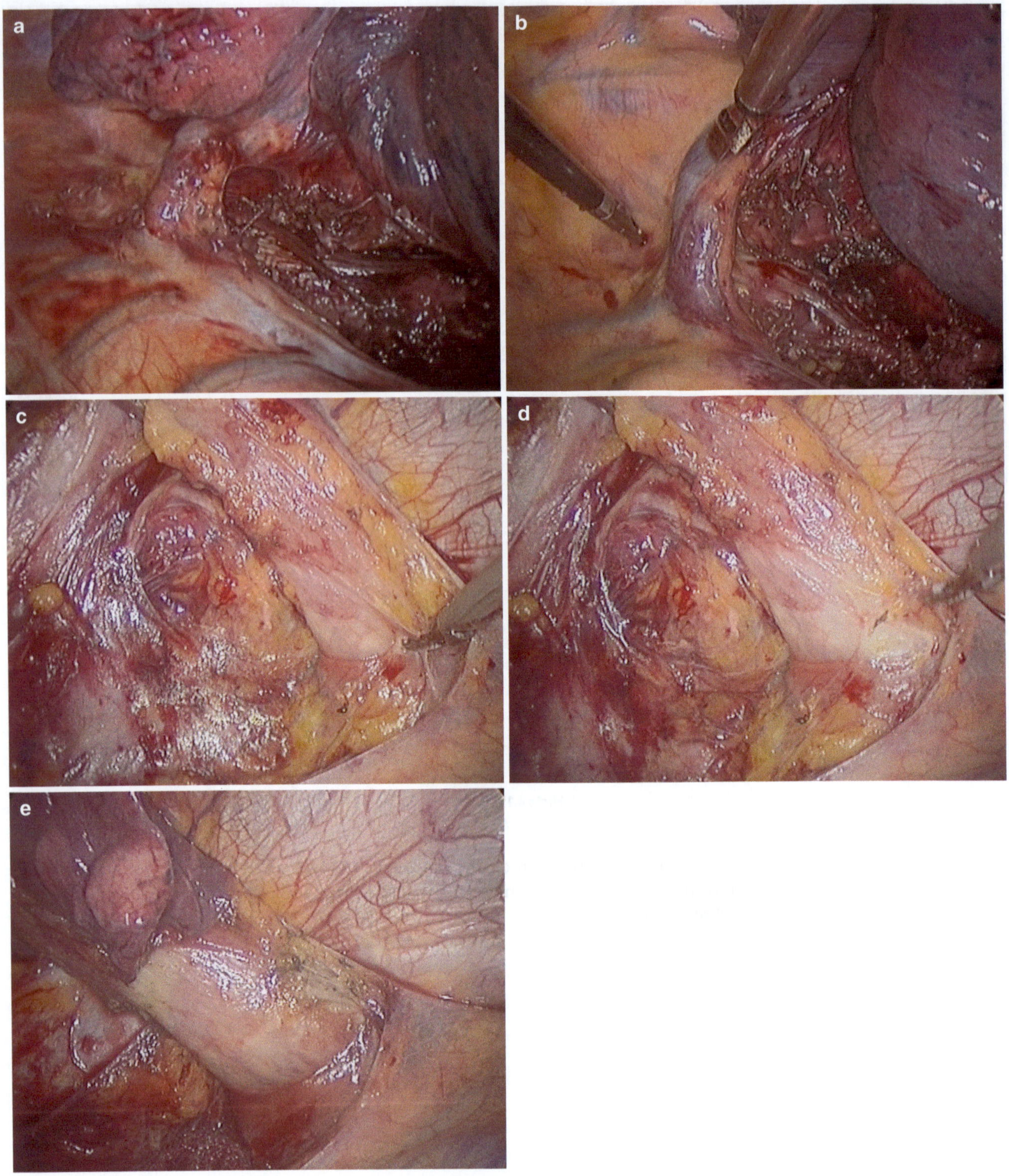

Photo 4.16 (a-e)

14. The upper limit of the infra-azygous dissection is the azygous vein while the lower limit is the crural fibers of the hiatus (Photo 4.16a–e).

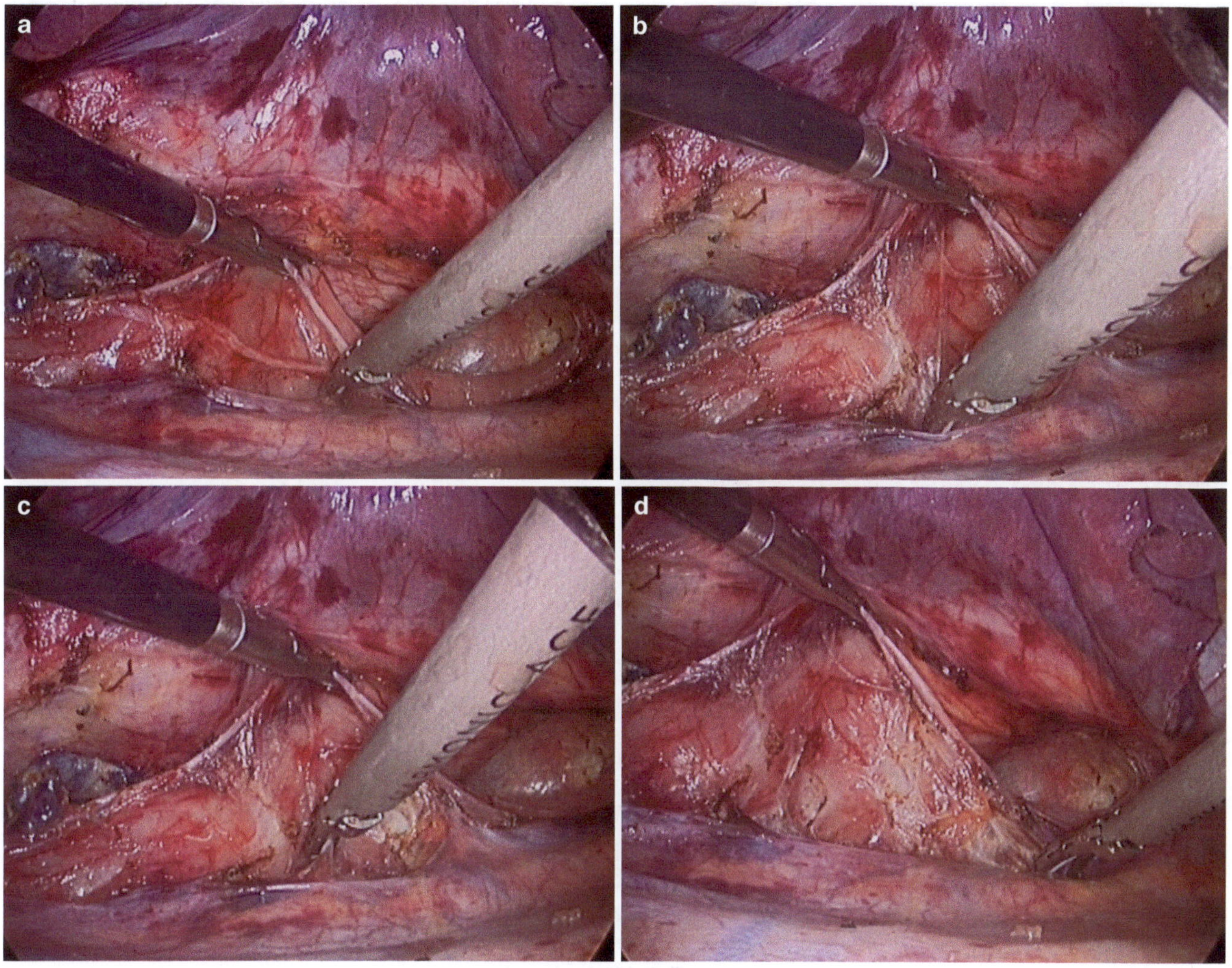

Photo 4.17 (a-d)

15. The next step is to cut the pleura between the esophagus and descending aorta. This cut is then extended upward up to the azygous vein and downward up to the hiatus (Photo 4.17a–d).

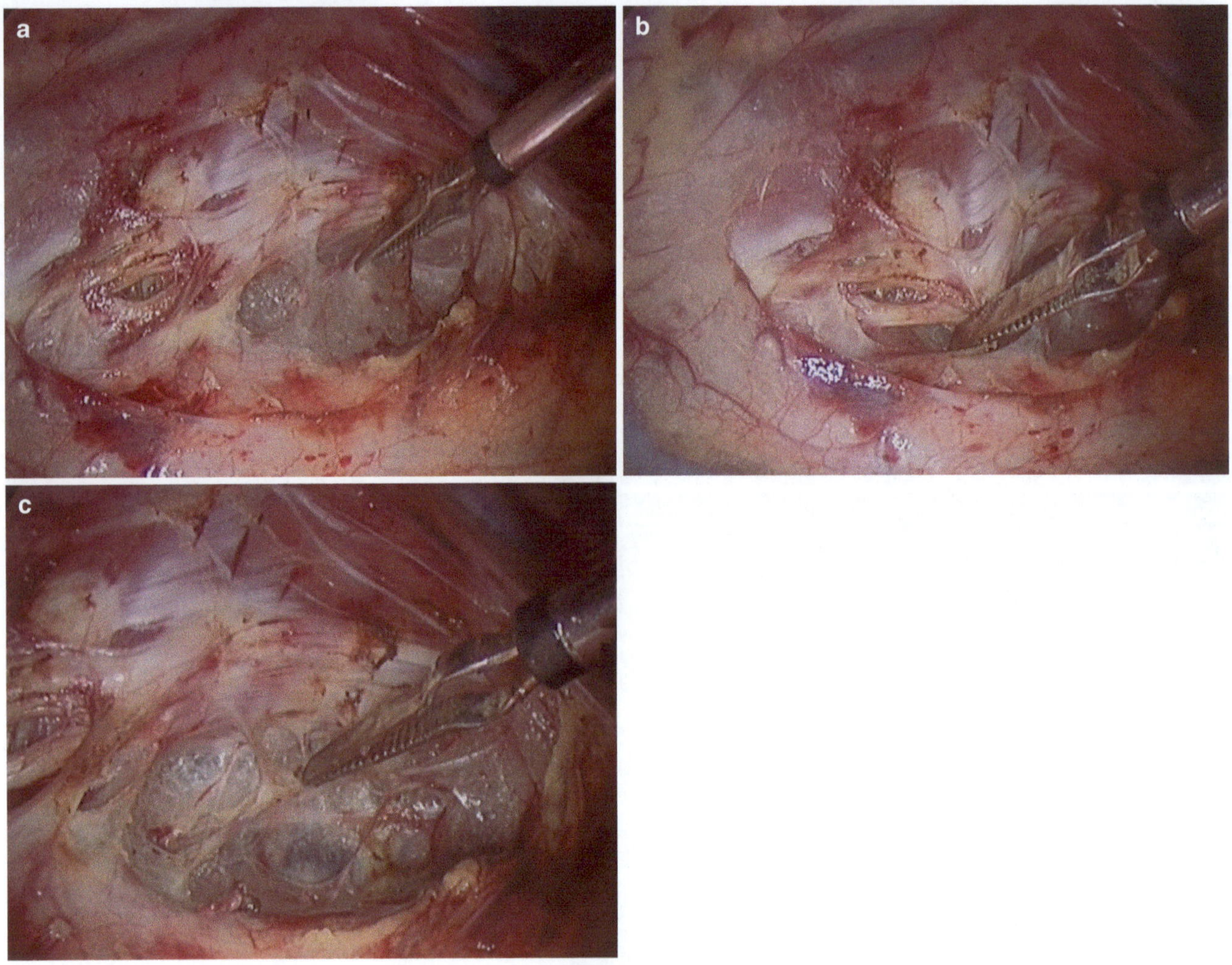

Photo 4.18 (a-c)

16. The esophagus is lifted with the left hand and the posterior vagus is visualized (Photo 4.18a–c).

17. The plane of dissection always lies outside the vagus, and not between the vagus and the esophagus. This ensues less blood loss. The vagus can be used for traction, thus assisting the removal of all the paraesophageal nodes (Photo 4.19a-f).

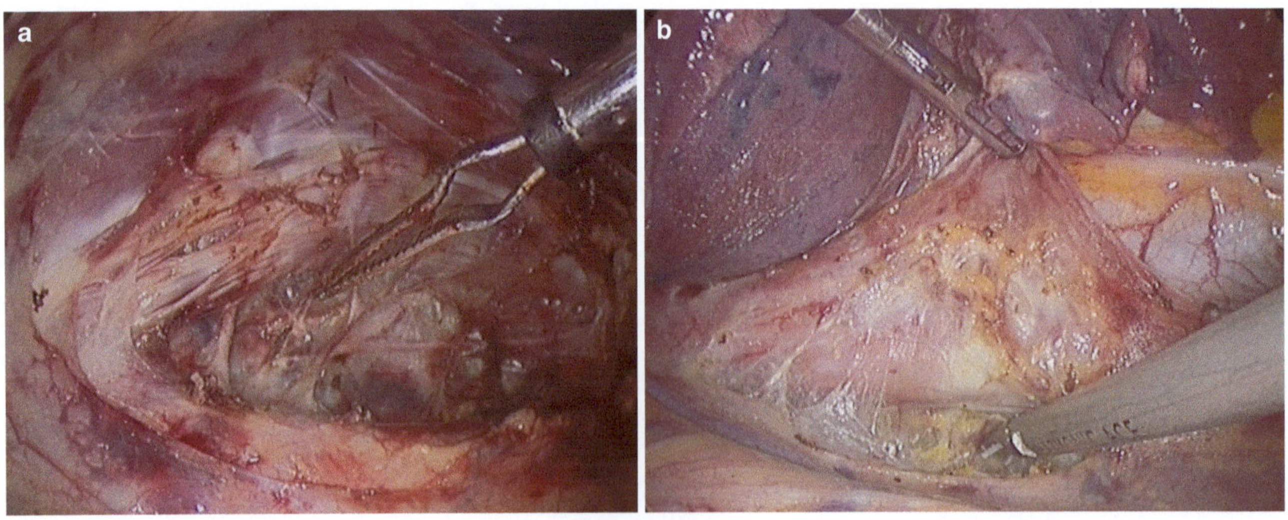

Photo 4.19 (a-f)

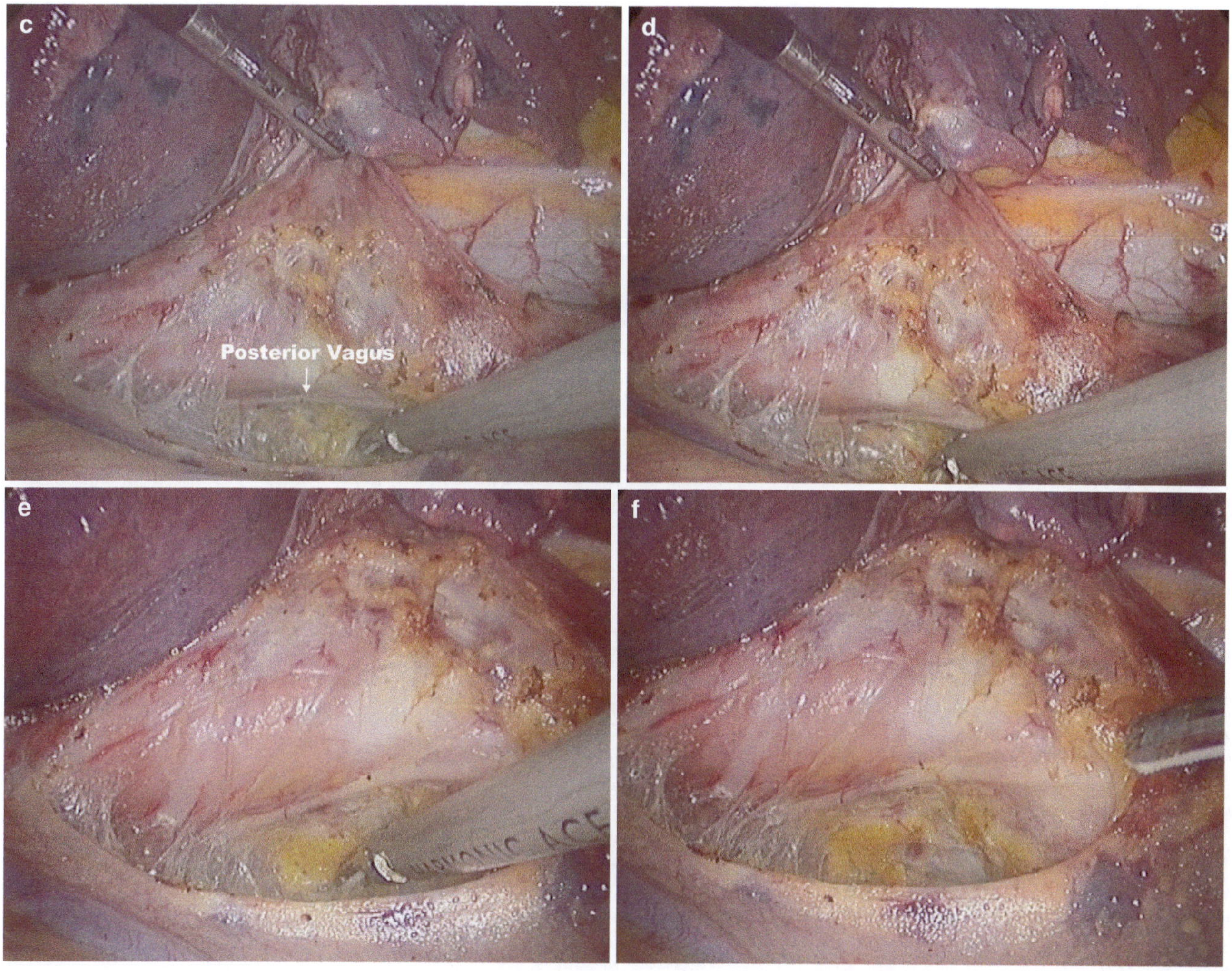

Photo 4.19 (Continued)

18. The left hand gives upward traction to the esophagus. The fibro-fatty and the lymph tissue are swept toward the esophagus. Small blood vessels going to the lymph nodes are visualized and coagulated (Photo 4.20a–g).

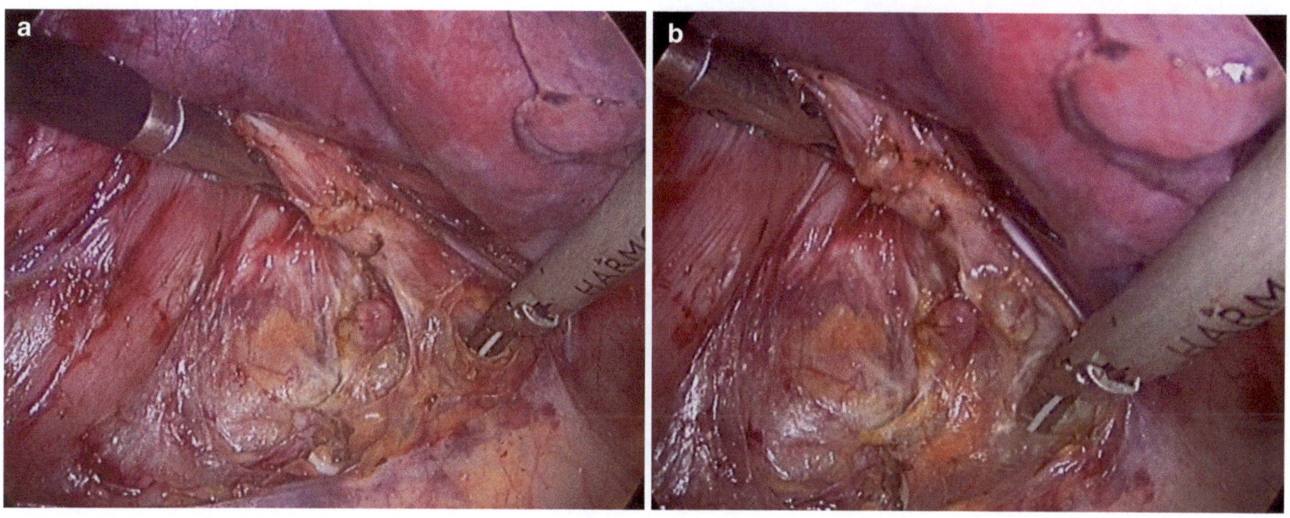

Photo 4.20 (a-g)

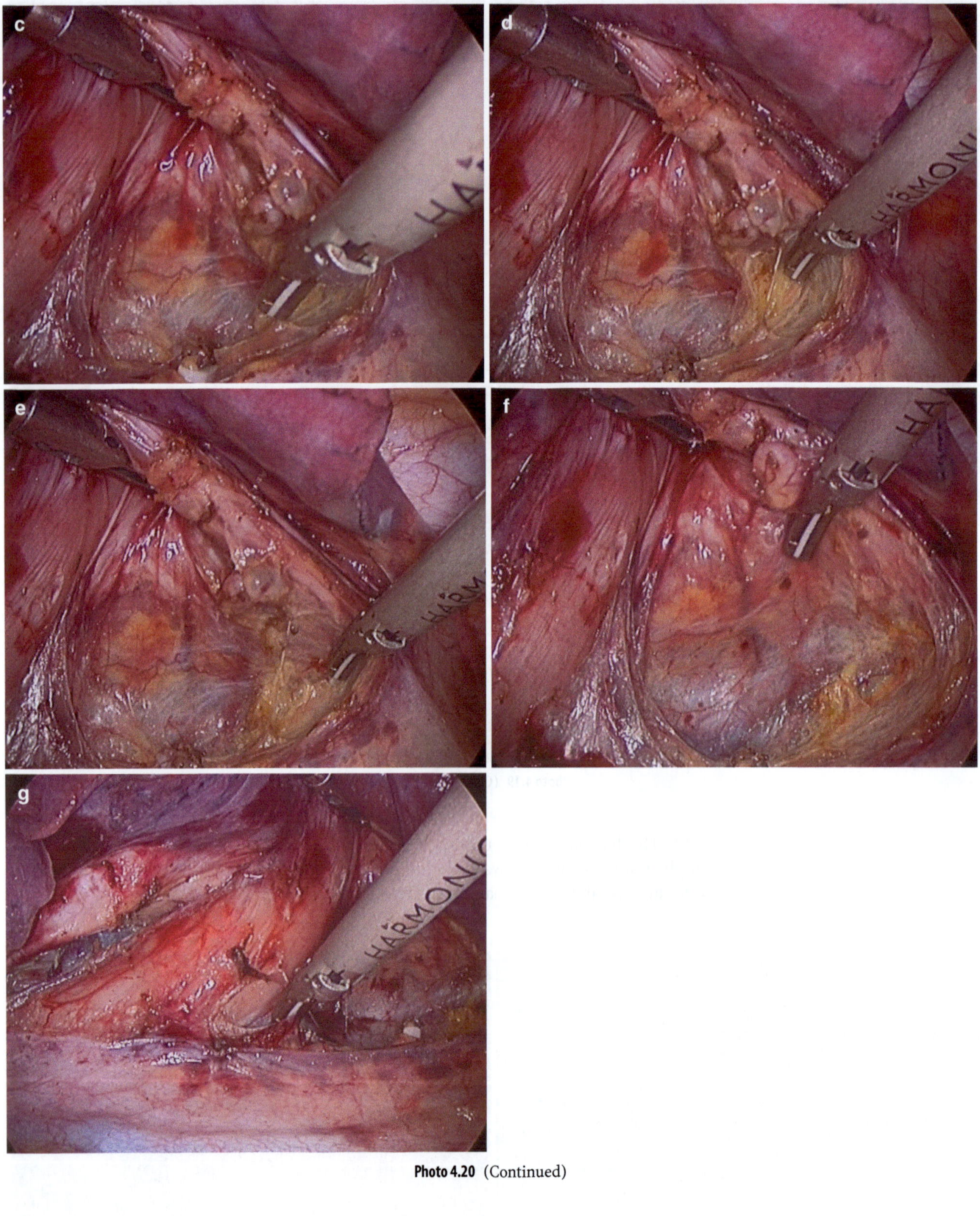

Photo 4.20 (Continued)

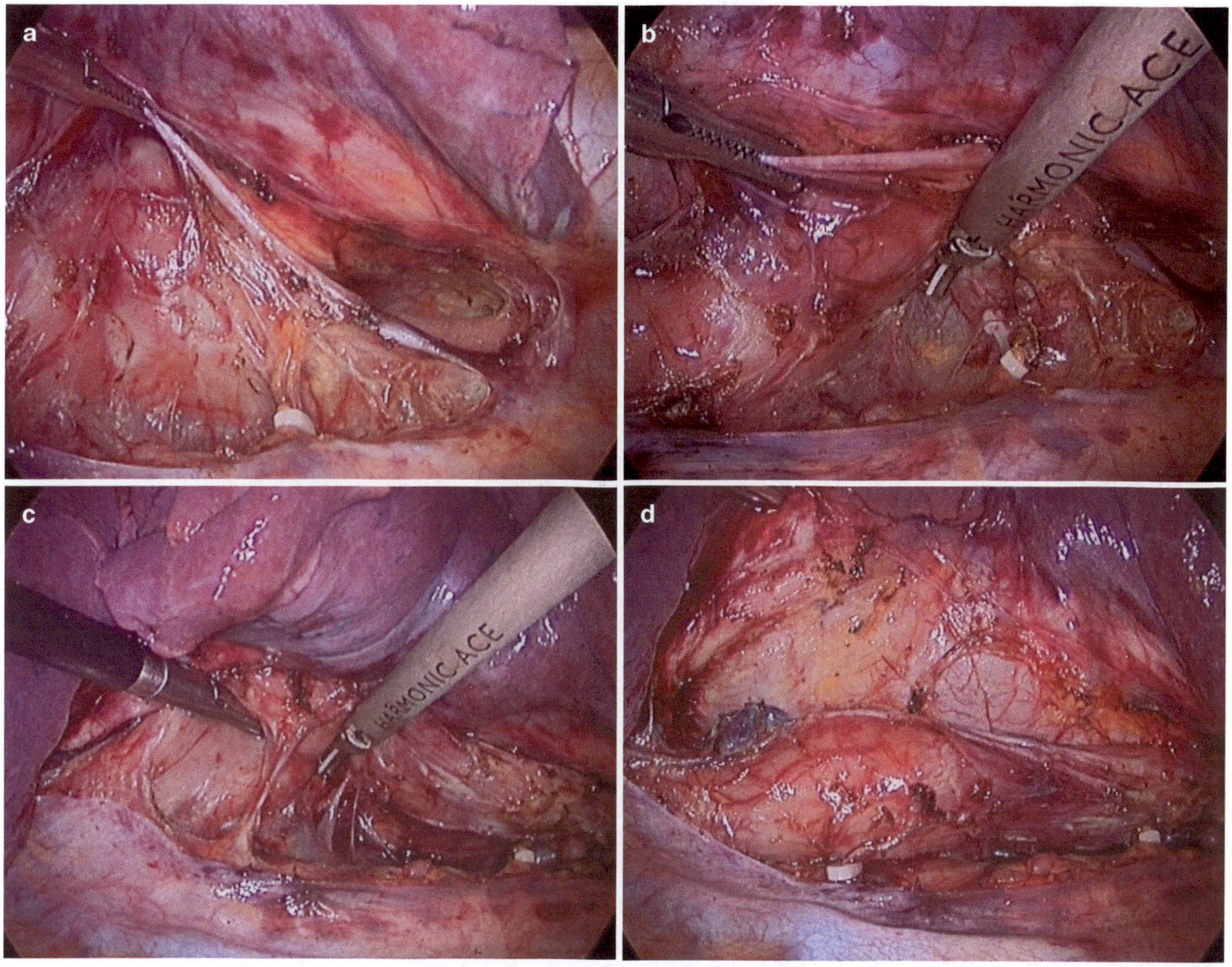

Photo 4.21 (a-d)

19. A further upward traction on the esophagus exposes the direct branches of the aorta which are usually two or three in number. They are clipped with vascular clips and cut (Photo 4.21a–d).

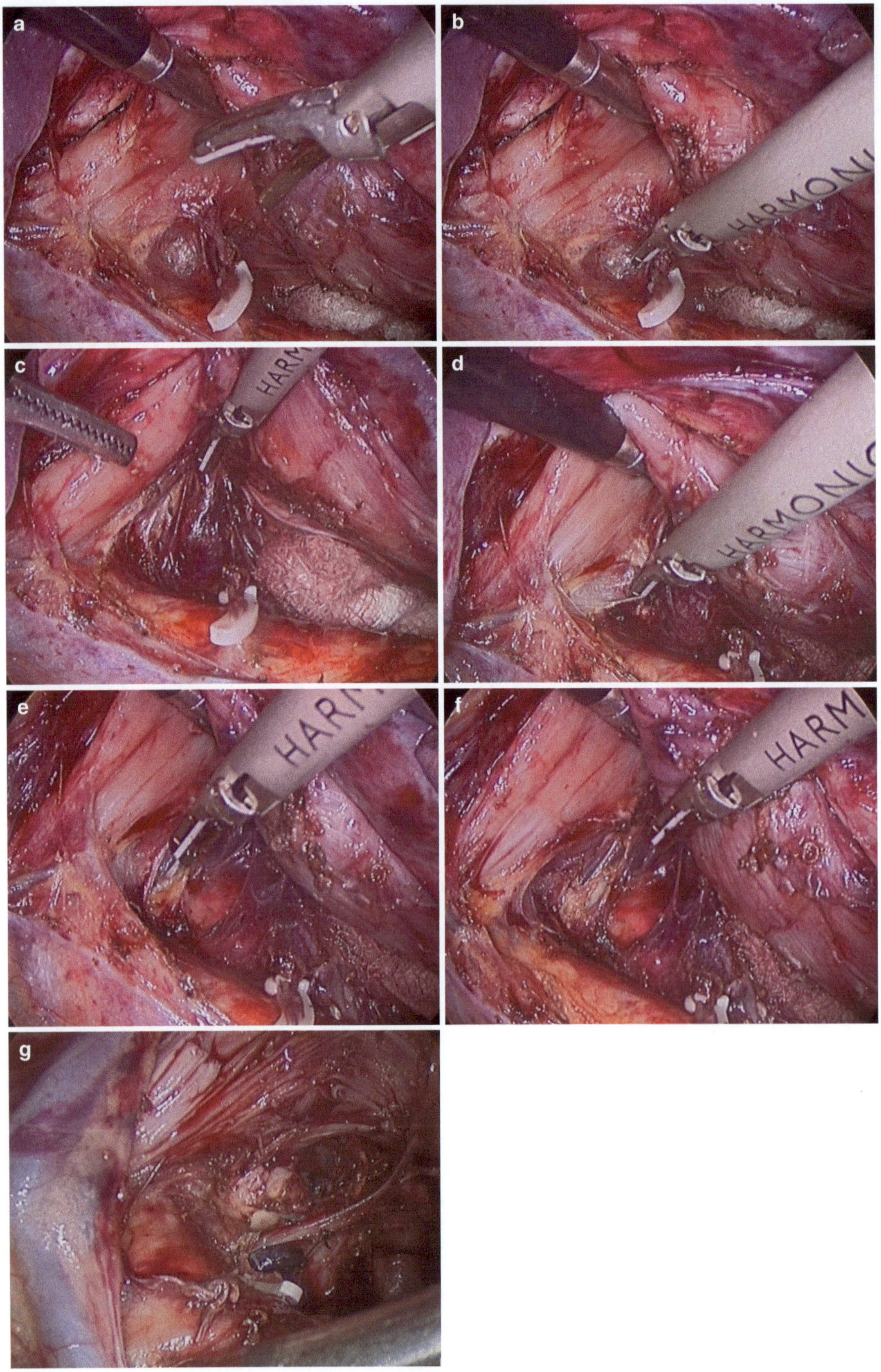

Photo 4.22 (a-g)

20. This posterior dissection is carried cranially, lifting up all the fibrofatty tissue till the aorta is bare. The esophagus is lifted from the arch of the aorta which is seen at the level just below the azygous vein (Photo 4.22a–g).

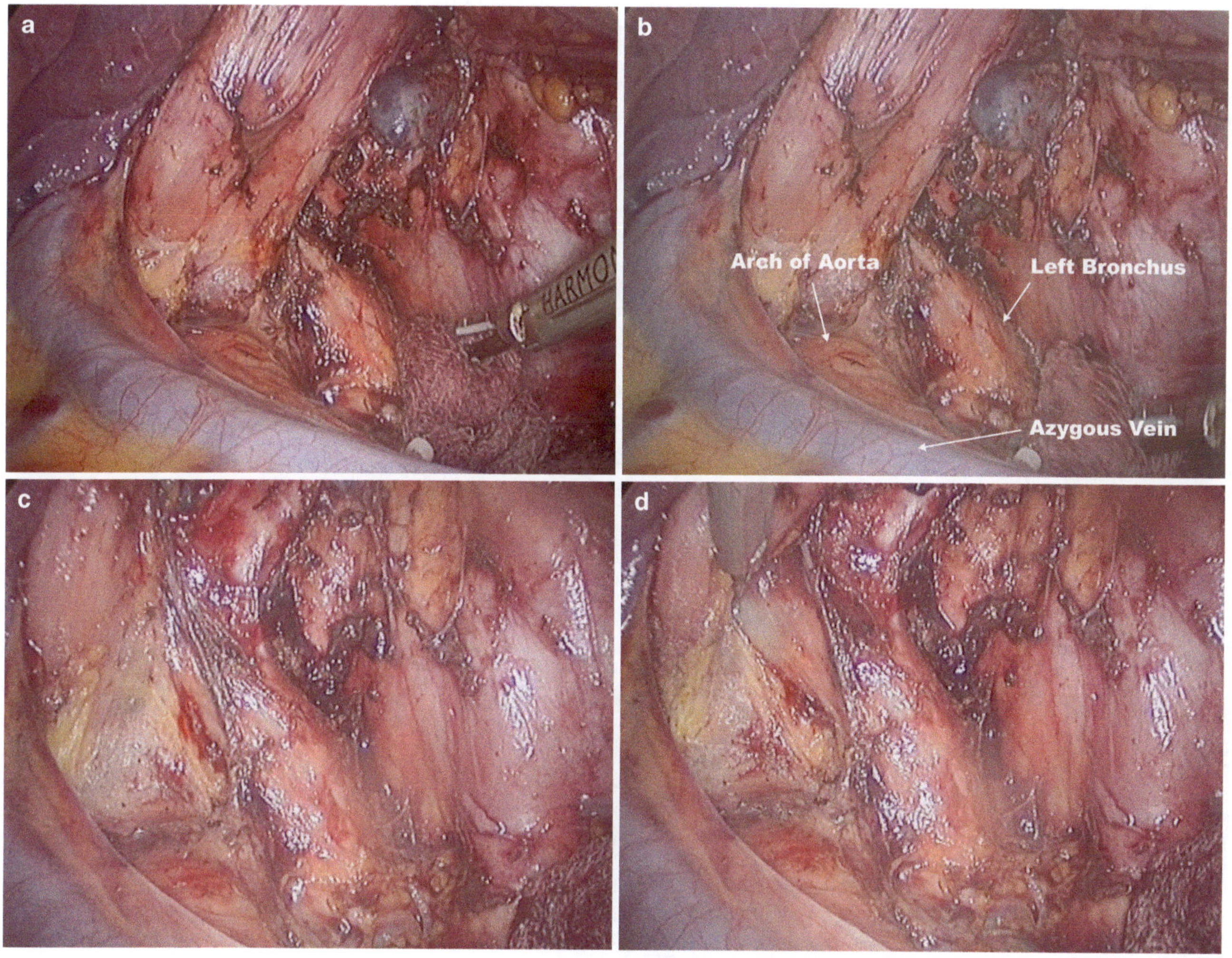

Photo 4.23 (a-d)

21. The left main bronchus crosses anterior to the descending aorta. Thus, while lifting esophagus from the arch of the aorta, one has to be careful of the posterior wall of the left main bronchus (Photo 4.23a–d).

22. The mobilized esophagus is then pushed laterally by the left-hand grasper, thus exposing the left hilar nodes and the remaining subcarinal nodes. The descending aorta can be seen postero-medially, while the inferior pulmonary vein can be seen medially (Photo 4.24a–g).

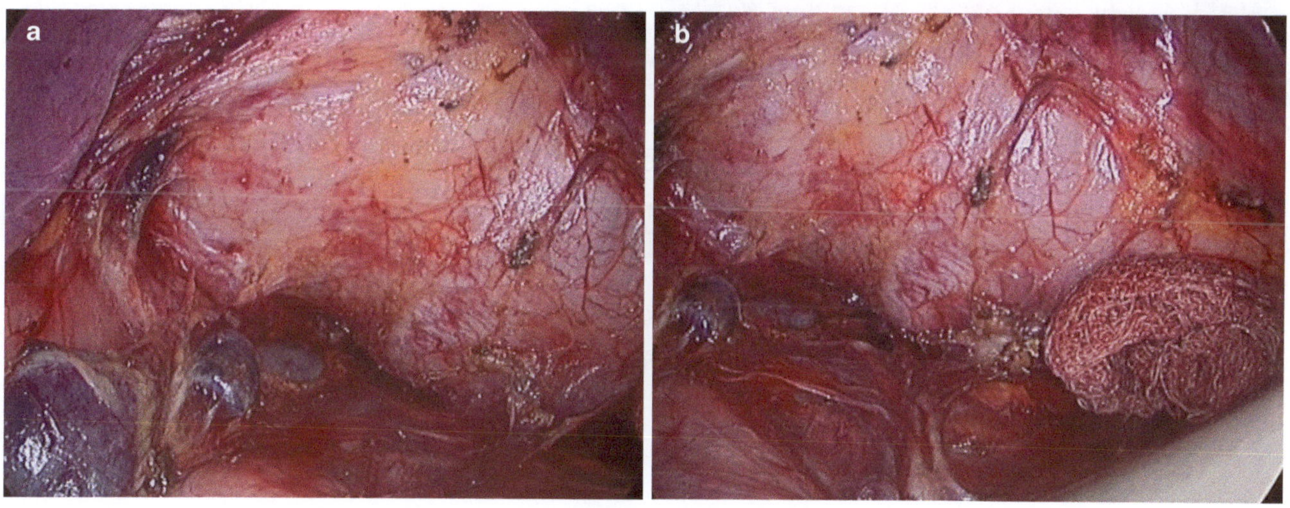

Photo 4.24 (a-g)

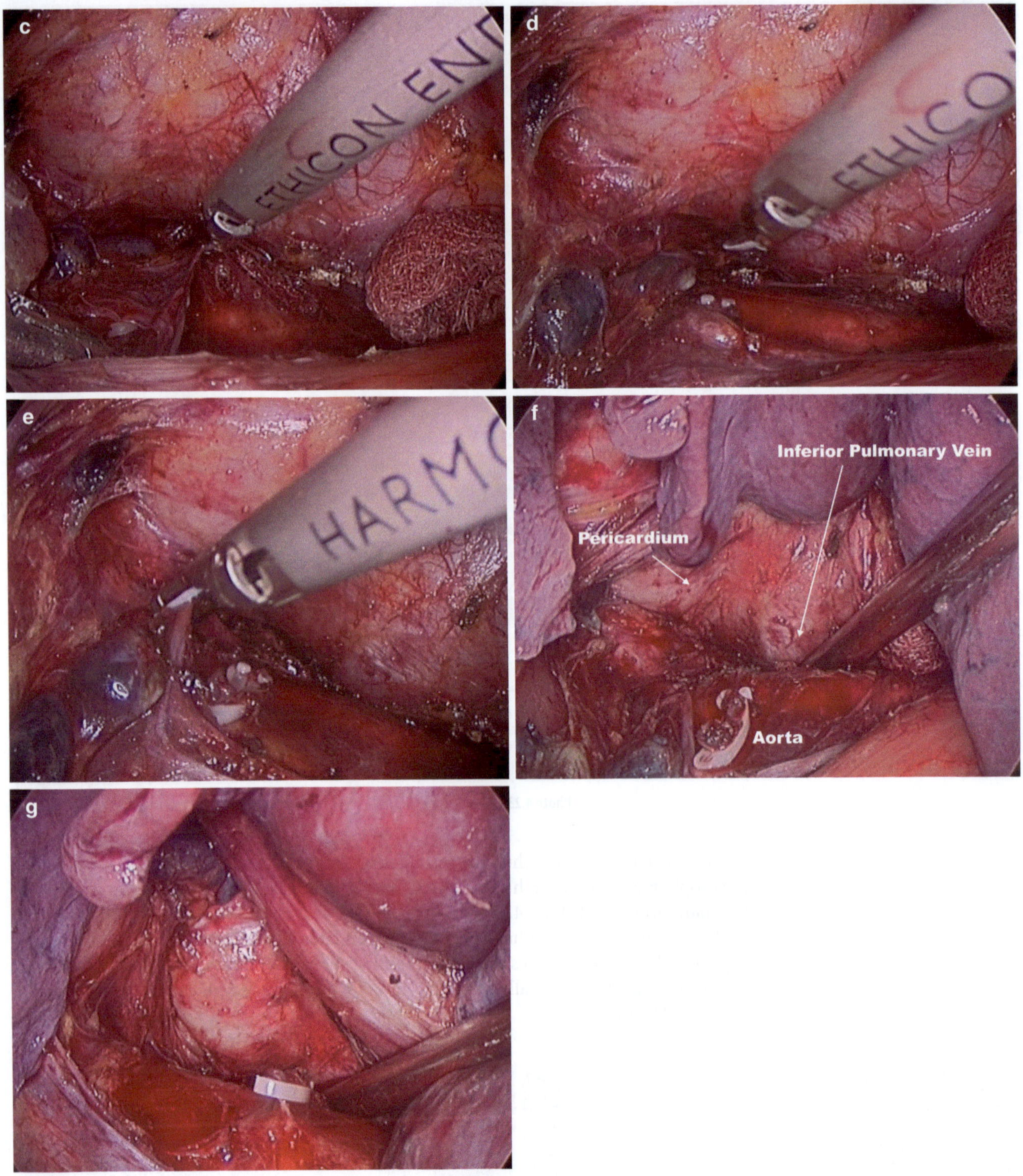

Photo 4.24 (Continued)

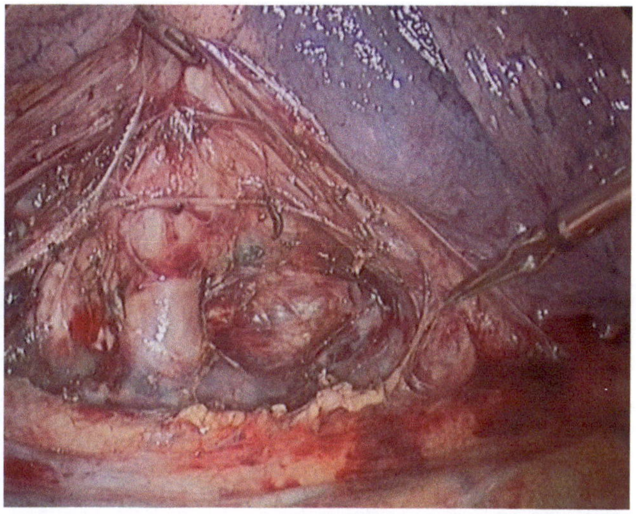

Photo 4.25

23. The inferior pulmonary vein can also be seen by lifting the esophagus upward (Photo 4.25).

24. At this stage the opposite pleura can be seen clearly. One has to be careful to avoid damage as inserting a left intercostal drain is difficult. The paraesophageal nodes and those at the hiatus are removed completely (Photo 4.26a–b).

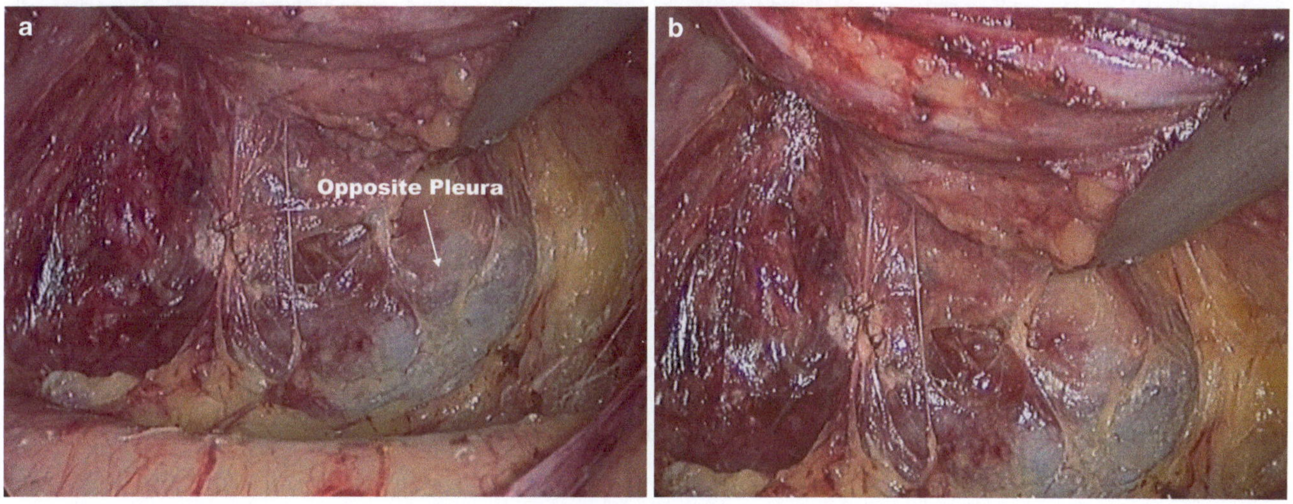

Photo 4.26 (a, b)

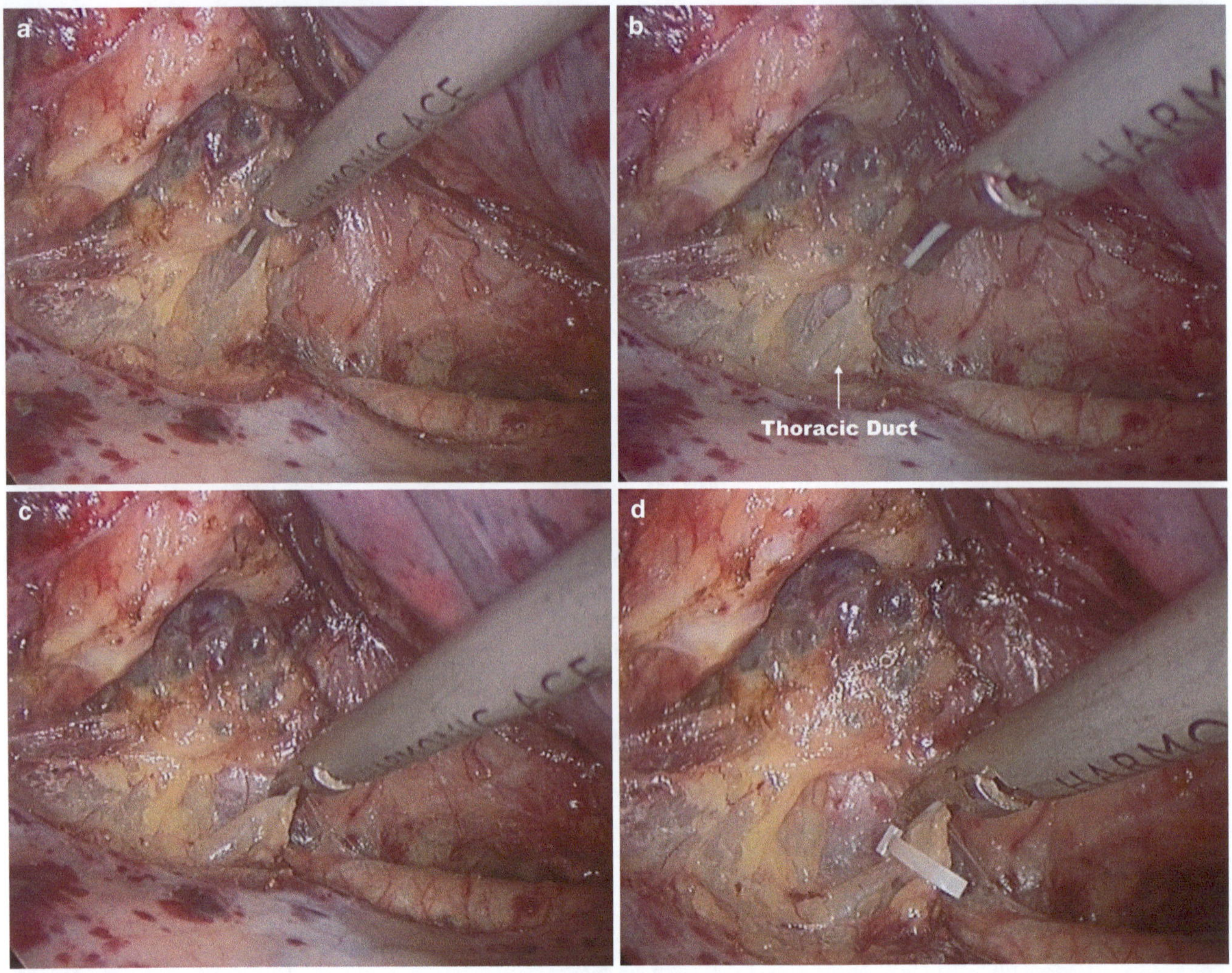

Photo 4.27 (a-d)

25. The thoracic duct can be identified as a white glistening structure over the descending aorta over the hiatus. This can be clipped, or can be separated completely from the esophagus (Photo 4.27a–d).

26. This completes the posterior dissection. The sign of completed posterior dissection is absence of fibro-fatty tissue on the aorta, complete removal of paraesophageal nodes, and clear visualization of the arch of aorta, the left main bronchus, and the inferior pulmonary vein (Photo 4.28a–e).

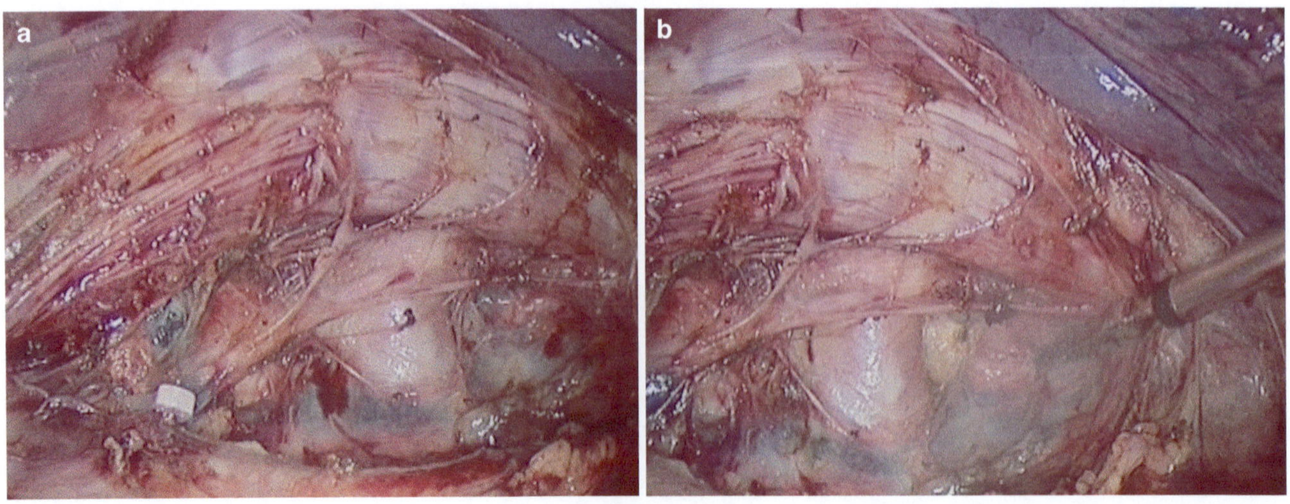

Photo 4.28 (a-e)

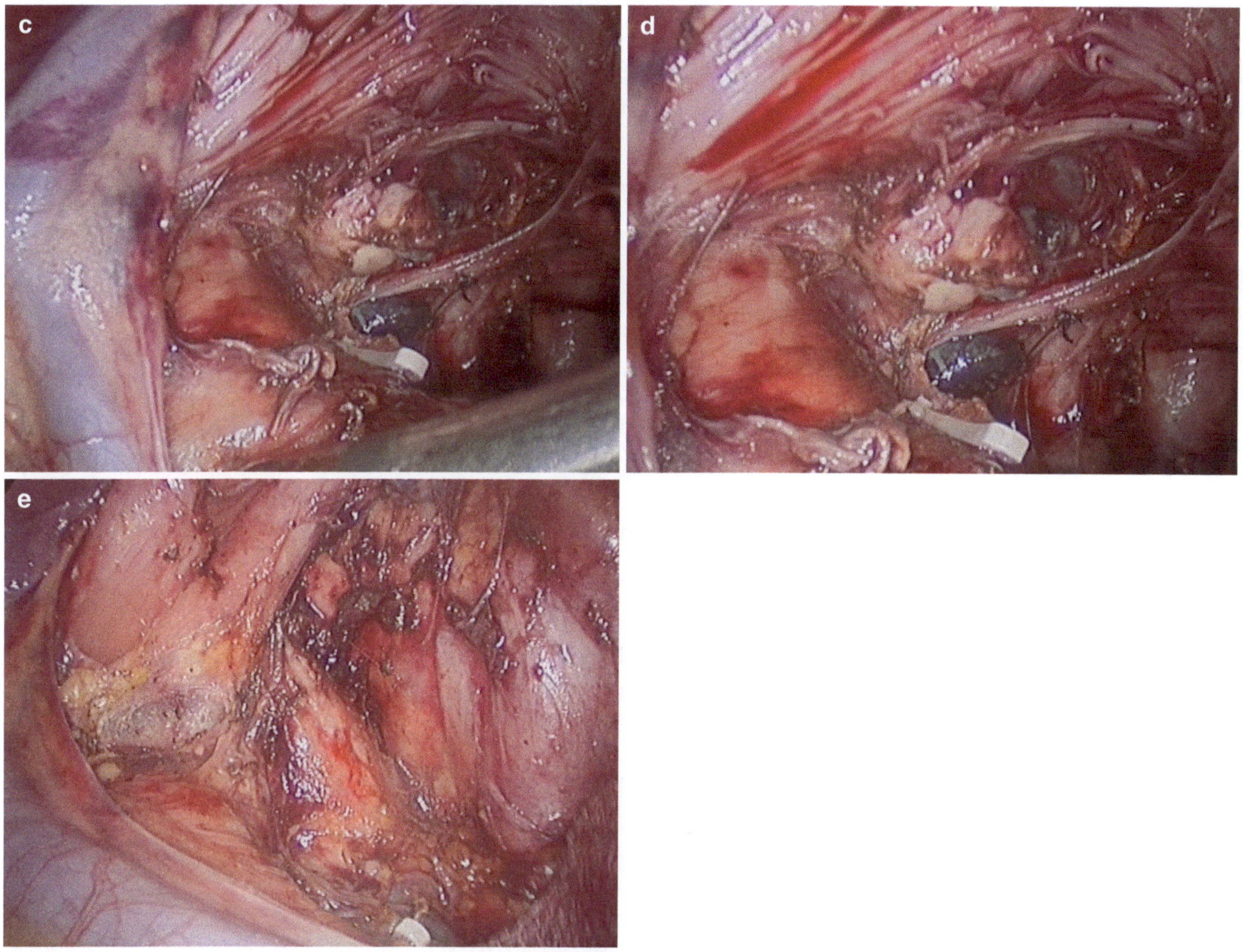

Photo 4.28 (Continued)

27. The esophagus can be manipulated by the left-hand grasper, thus confirming that it is separated all-around (Photo 4.29).

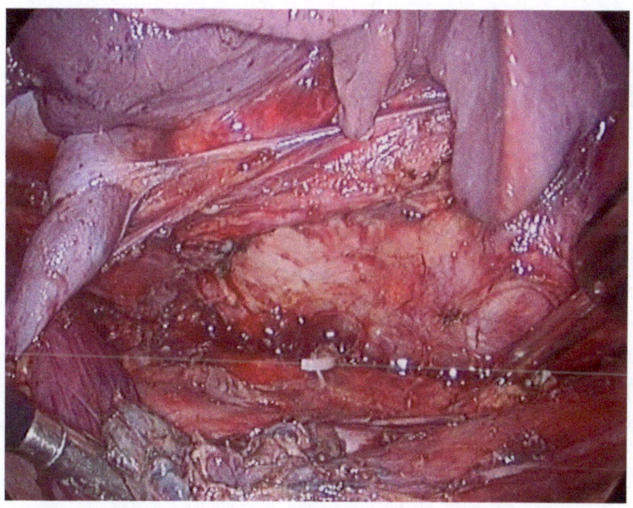

Photo 4.29

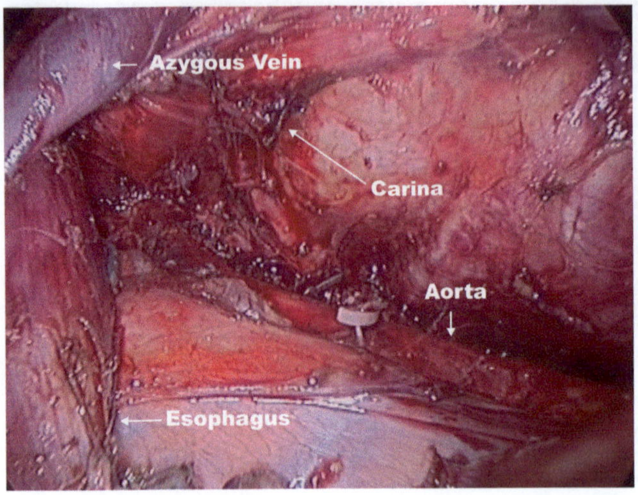

Photo 4.30

28. At this stage, the carina can be clearly seen with left and right main bronchus devoid of any nodal tissues (Photo 4.30).

29. The infra azygous dissection achieves complete removal of paraesophageal, subcarinal, hilar, and the hiatal nodes. The esophagus is separated all around from the pericardium and the left pleura medially, arch of the aorta, and the descending aorta posteriorly and the azygous vein laterally. At the end of dissection, all these structures should be identified. They should be free of any fibro-fatty and lymphoid tissue (Photo 4.31a–c).

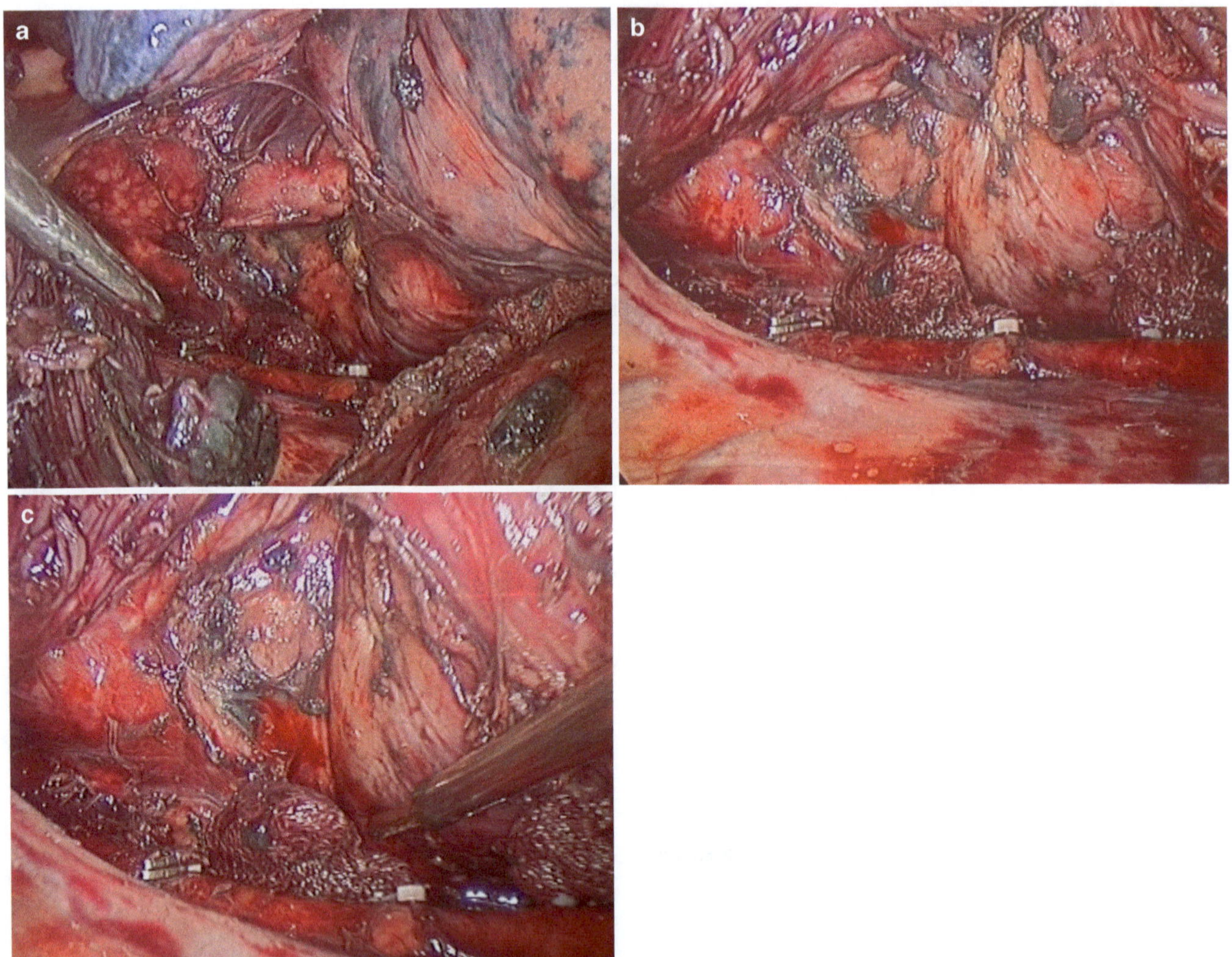

Photo 4.31 (a-c)

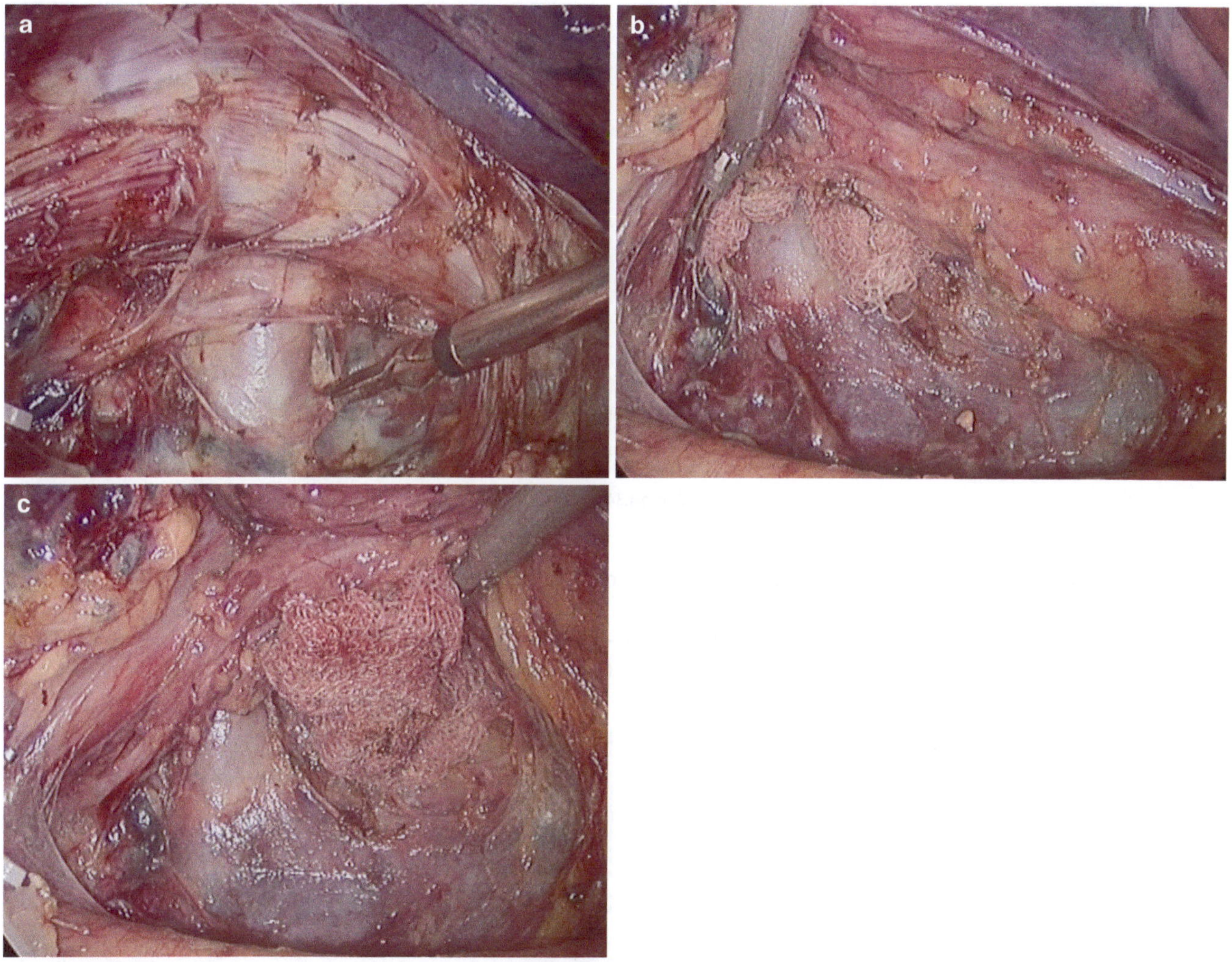

Photo 4.32 (a-c)

30. A few nodes along the inferior pulmonary vein can be dissected and removed. A strip of gauze should be kept in the gutter between the esophagus and the aorta (Photo 4.32a–c).

31. The next step is to do the supra-azygous dissection. The apex of the lung is pulled down by the assistant to expose this area (Photo 4.33).

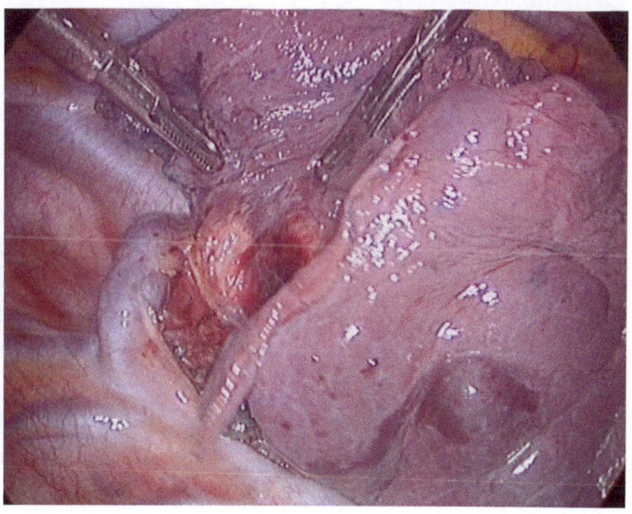

Photo 4.33

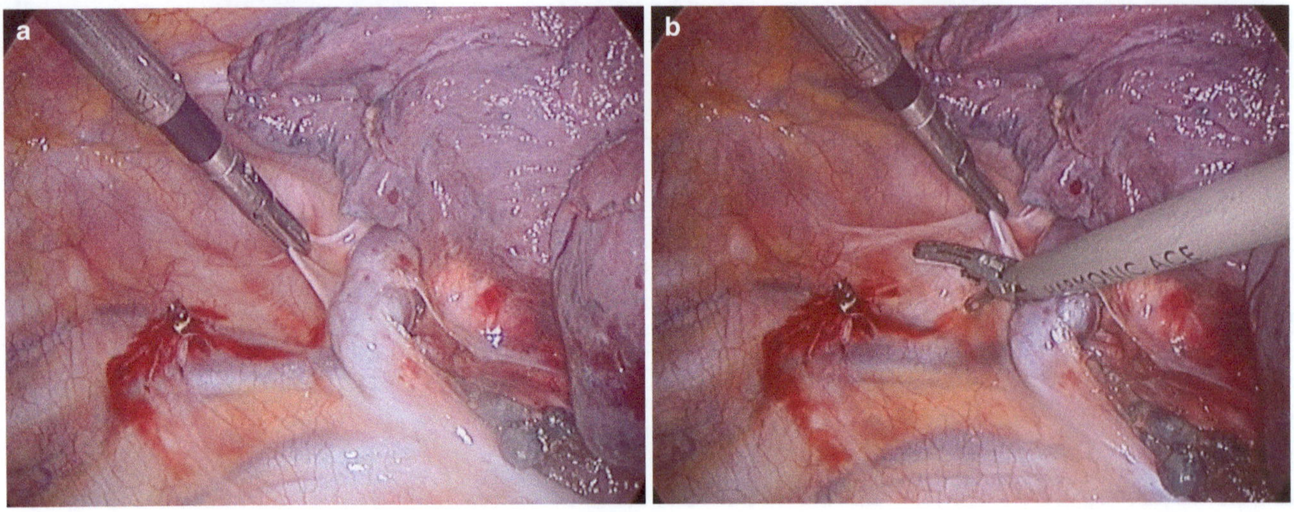

Photo 4.34 (a, b)

32. Once the lung is retracted, supra-azygous pleura is stretched and can be grasped (Photo 4.34a, b).

33. The pleura over the esophagus is lifted with the left-hand grasper and a cut is taken. This cut is extended upward upto the root of the neck (Photo 4.35a–d).

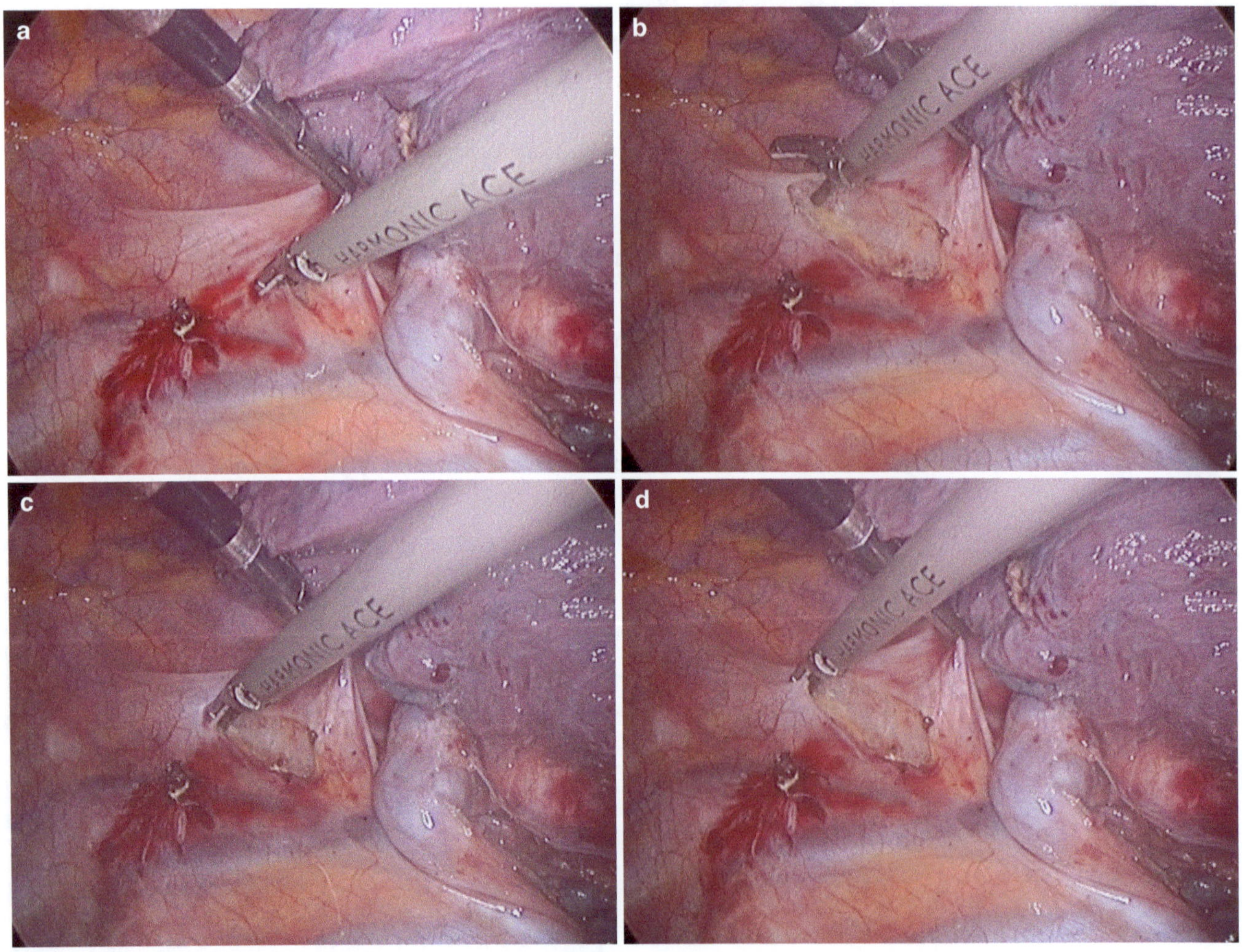

Photo 4.35 (a-d)

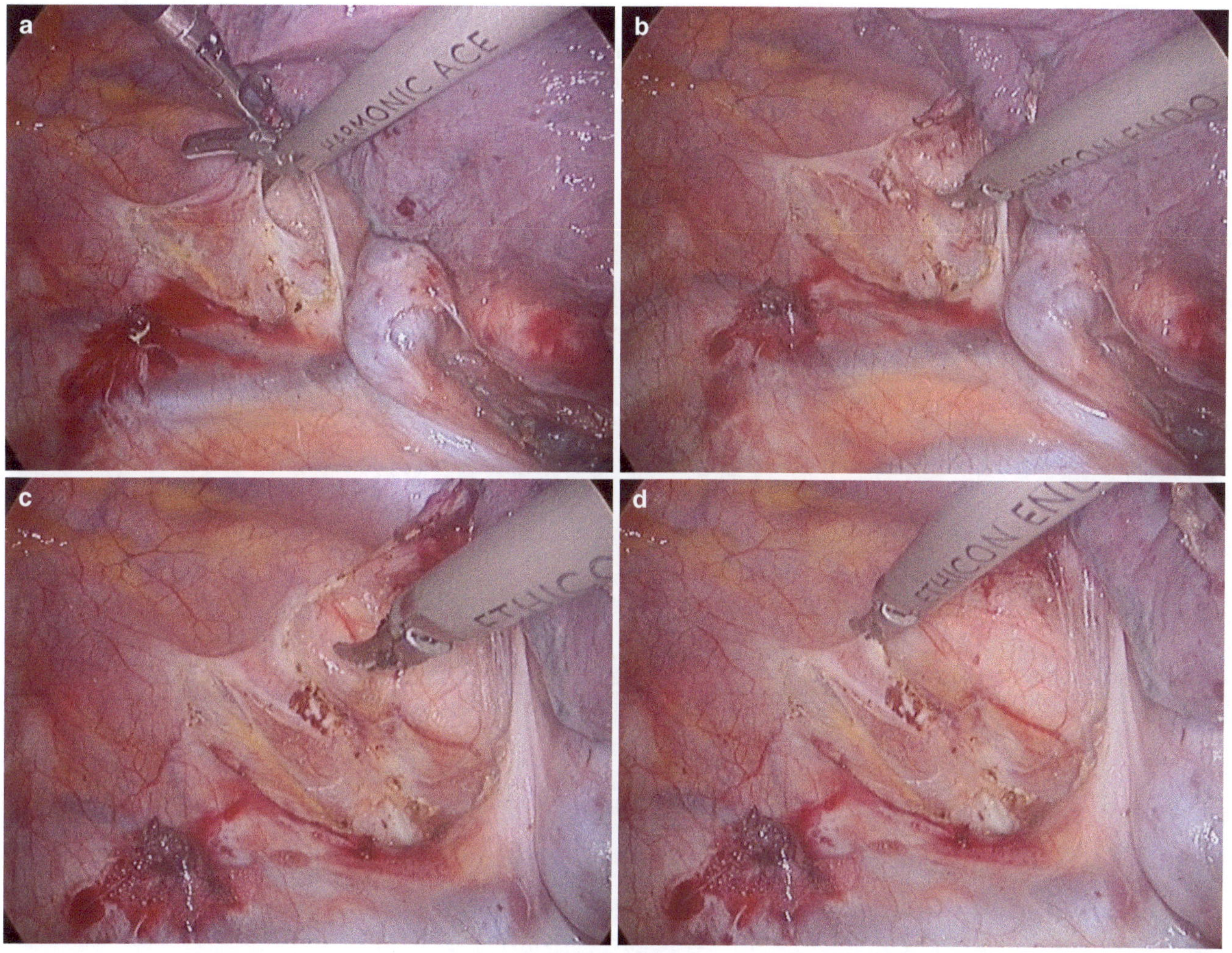

Photo 4.36 (a-d)

34. The anterior pleural cut is taken. This exposes the medial wall of esophagus and posterior wall of trachea. This cut is extended up to the root of the neck (Photo 4.36a–d).

35. The dissection starts posteriorly, the left-hand grasper pulls the esophagus and a plane is created between it and the vertebrae. This dissection is done either with a suction cannula or with bipolar forceps (Photo 4.37a, b).

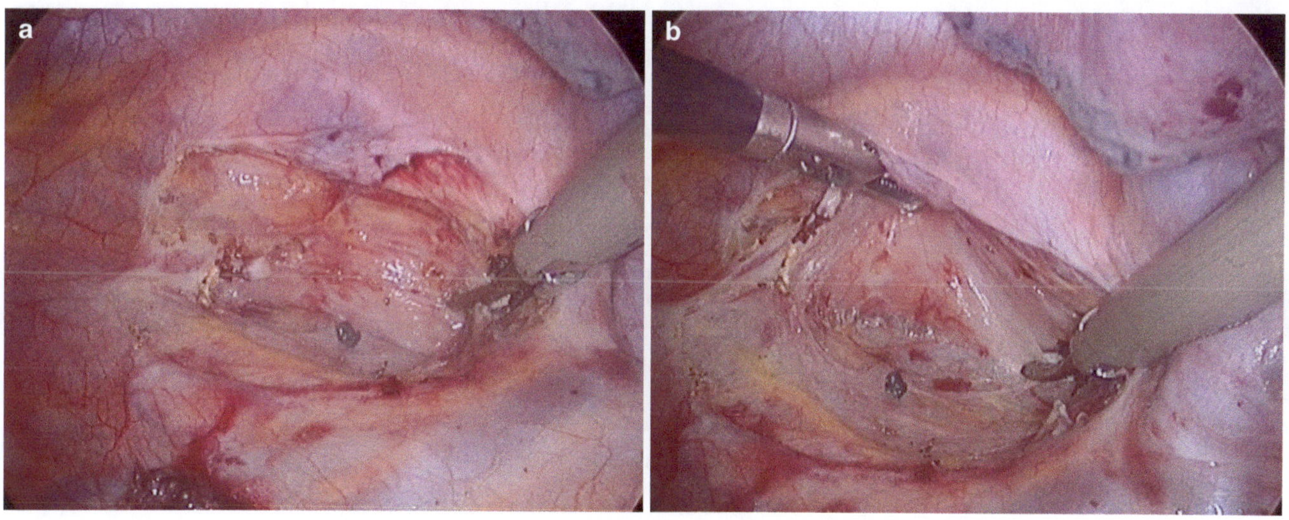

Photo 4.37 (a, b)

36. The esophagus is grasped and pulled laterally. The plane medial to the esophagus is exposed and the dissection is carried out between the esophagus and the posterior wall of trachea. Any perpendicular dissection may lead to the damage of the posterior wall of the trachea. We recommend the use of blunt dissector like a suction cannula in the learning face (Photo 4.38a–l).

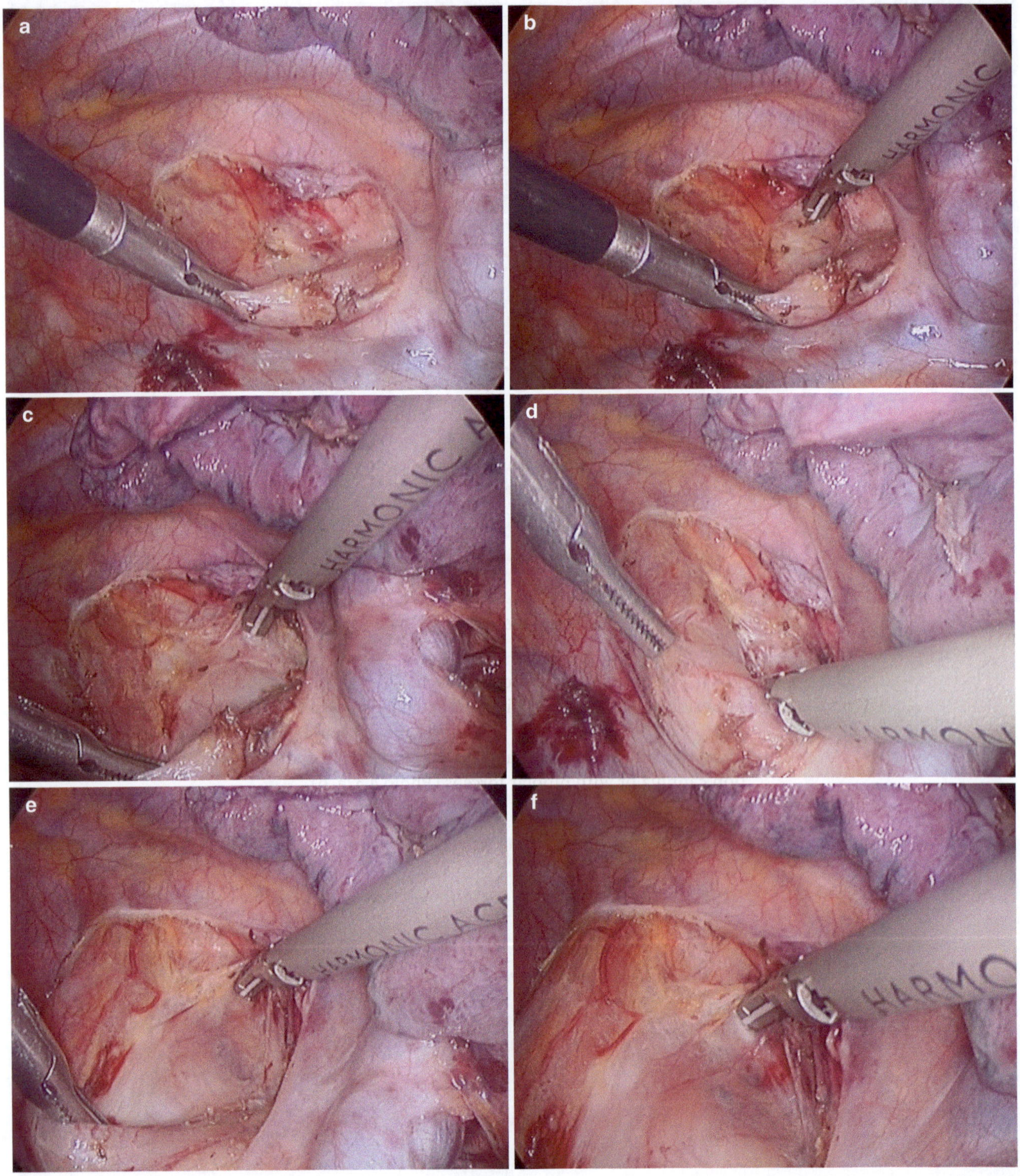

Photo 4.38 (a-l)

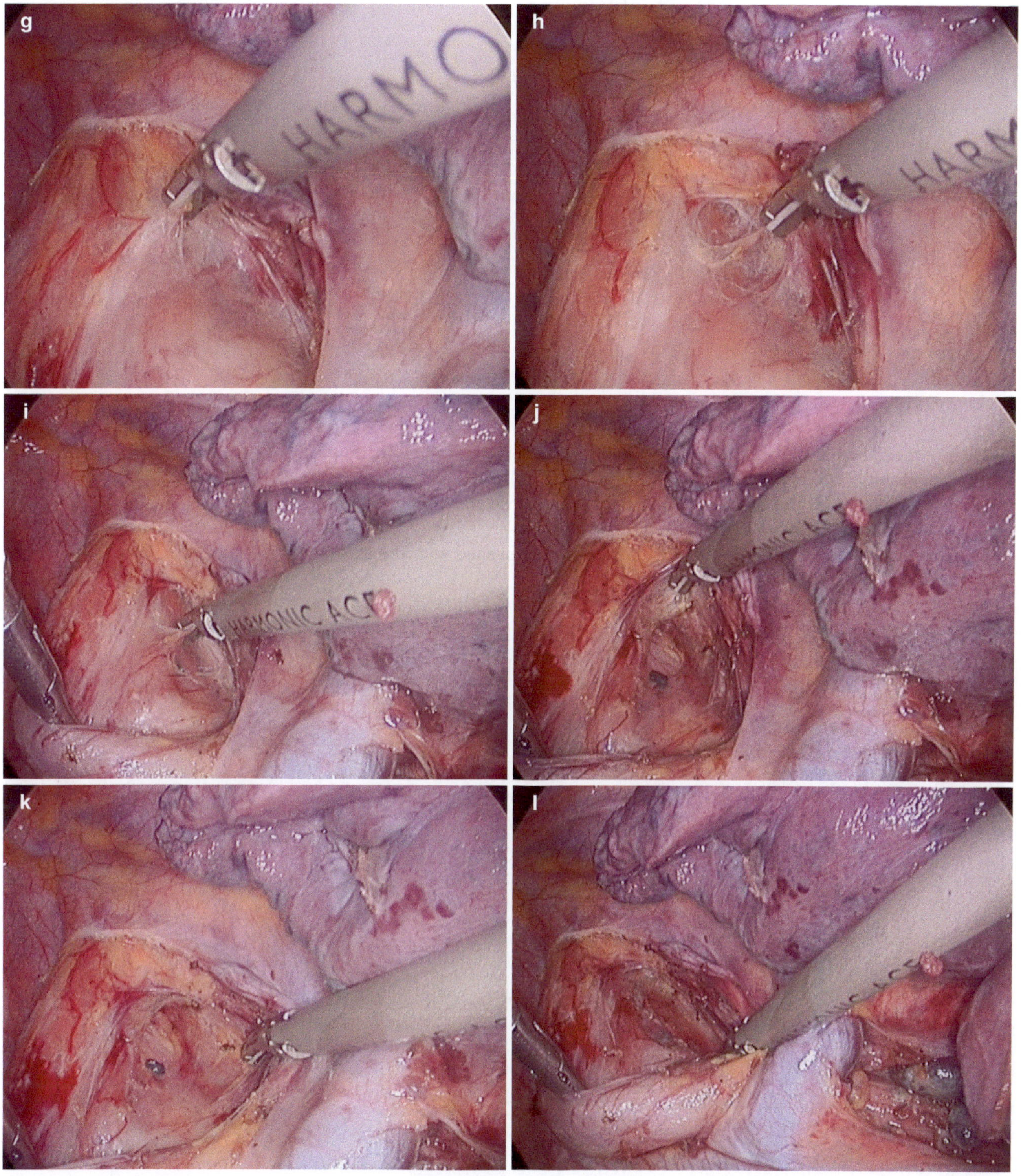

Photo 4.38 (Continued)

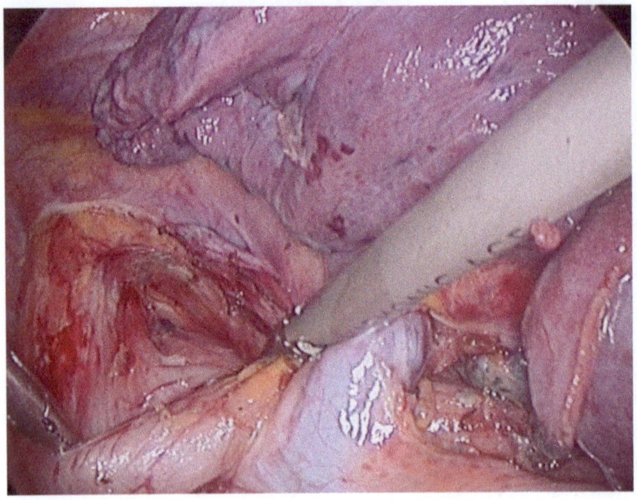

Photo 4.39

37. The medial separation of the esophagus allows further lateral traction, thus separating it all around (Photo 4.39).

38. The esophagus is pulled upward and further posterior dissection is done. The pleura of the opposite lung can be visualized (Photo 4.40a–d).

39. The entire fibro-fatty tissue along with the nodes is pushed with the esophagus.

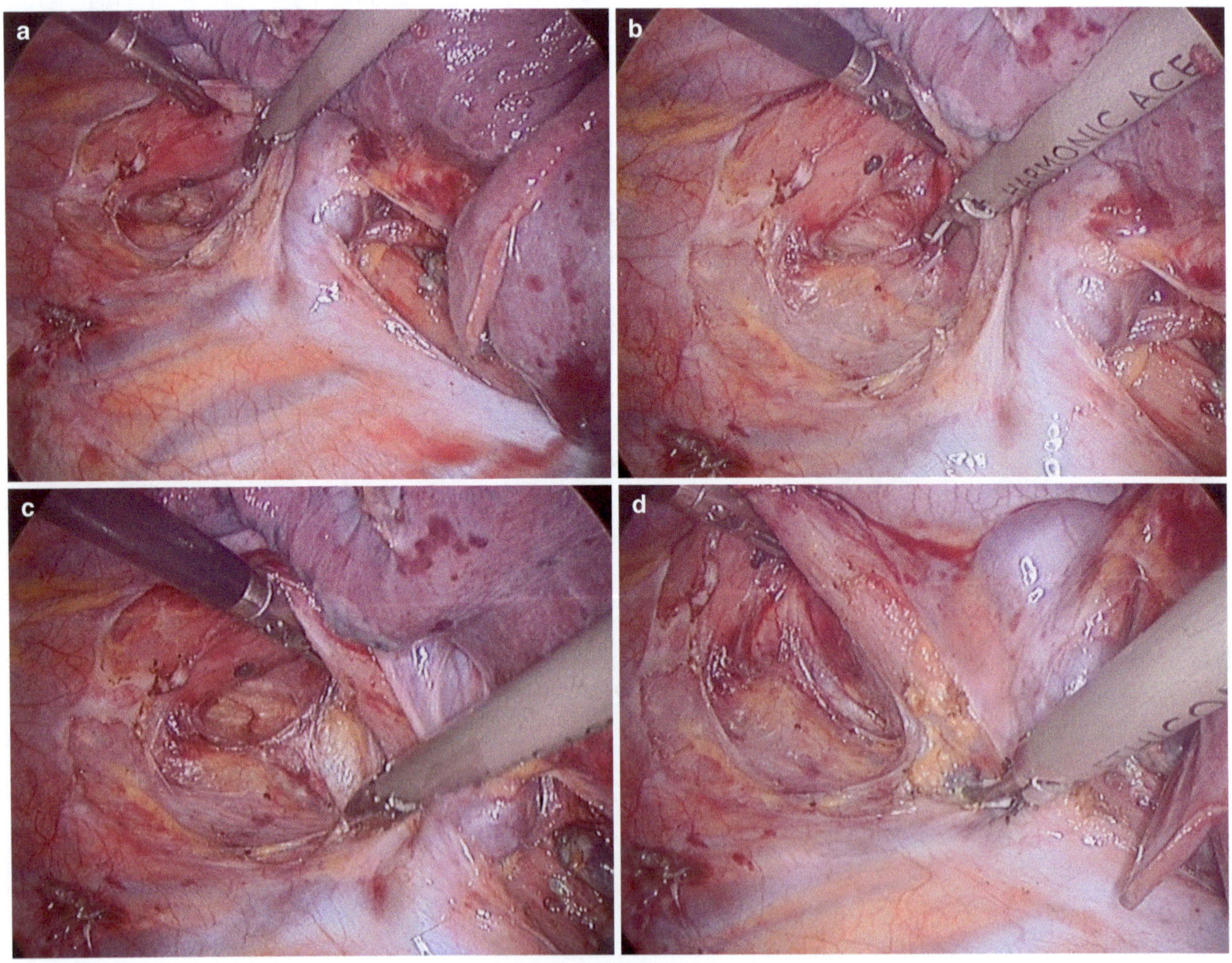

Photo 4.40 (a-d)

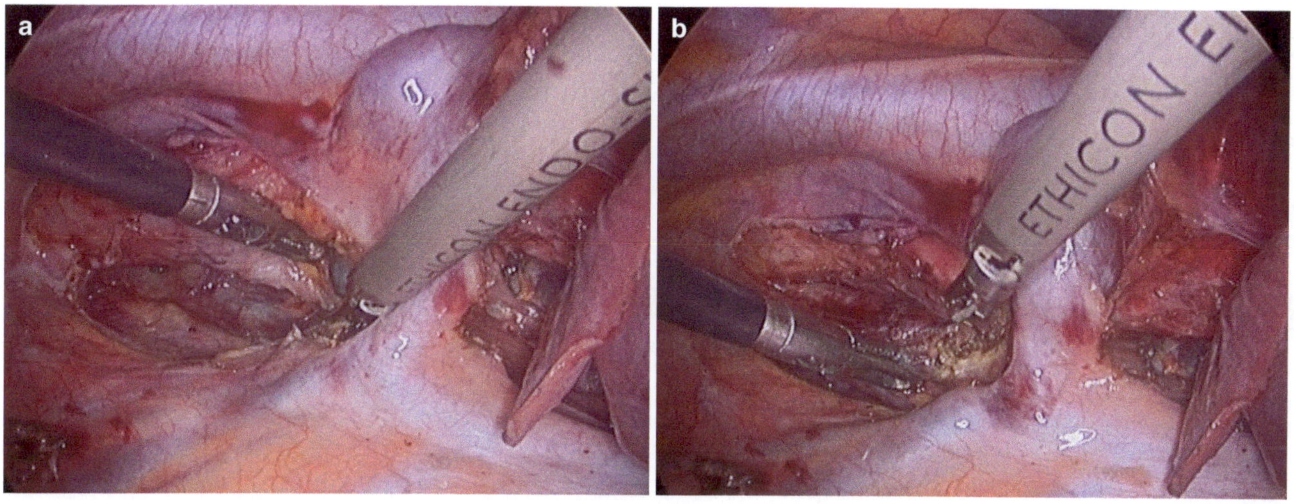

Photo 4.41 (a, b)

The esophagus is separated posteriorly (Photo 4.41a, b).

40. The pleura over the azygous vein is held, and the azygous vein is freed along its entire length of all fibrofatty tissue. The bronchial artery is posterior to the azygous vein and can be seen by retracting the vein downward (Photo 4.42a–i).

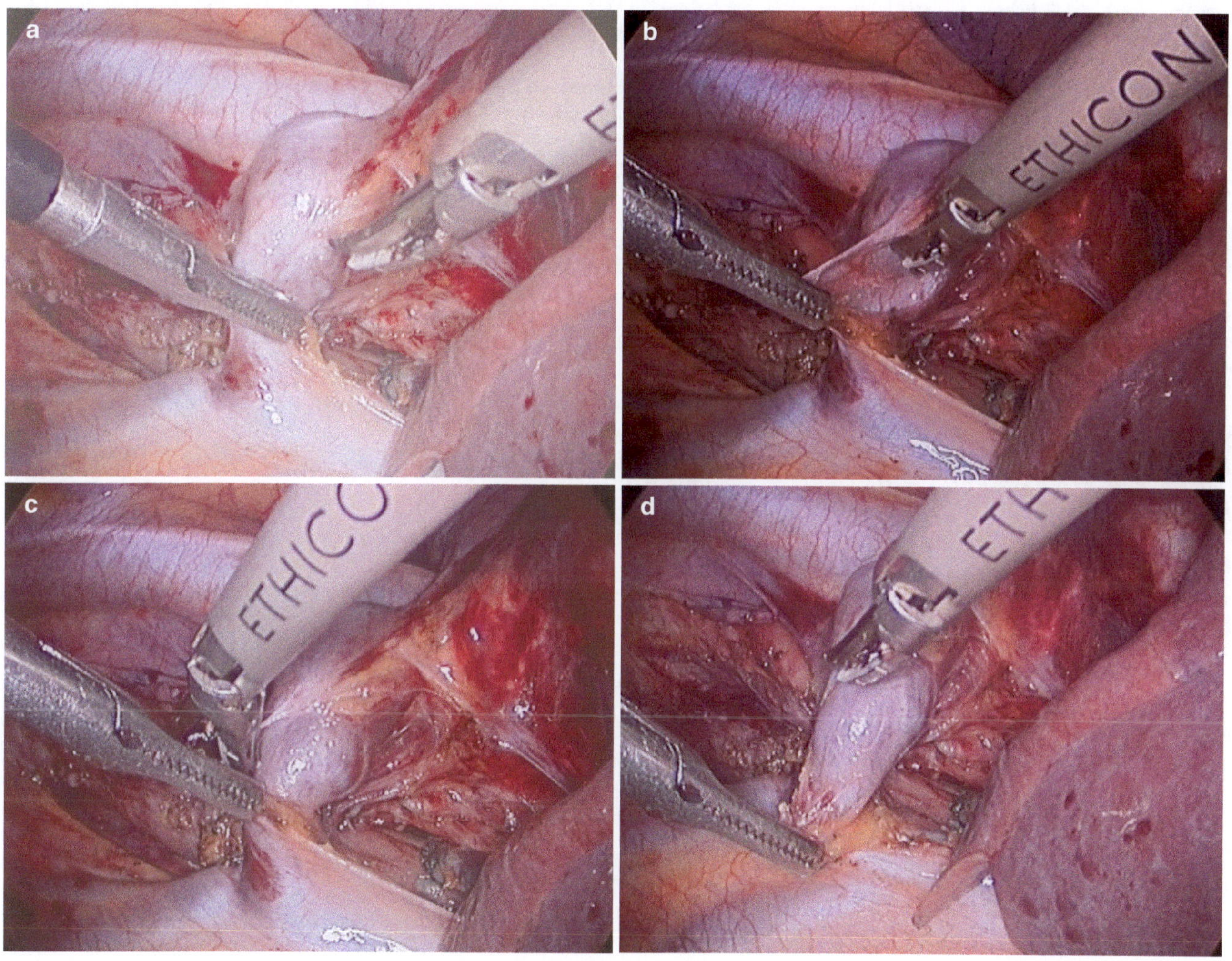

Photo 4.42 (a-i)

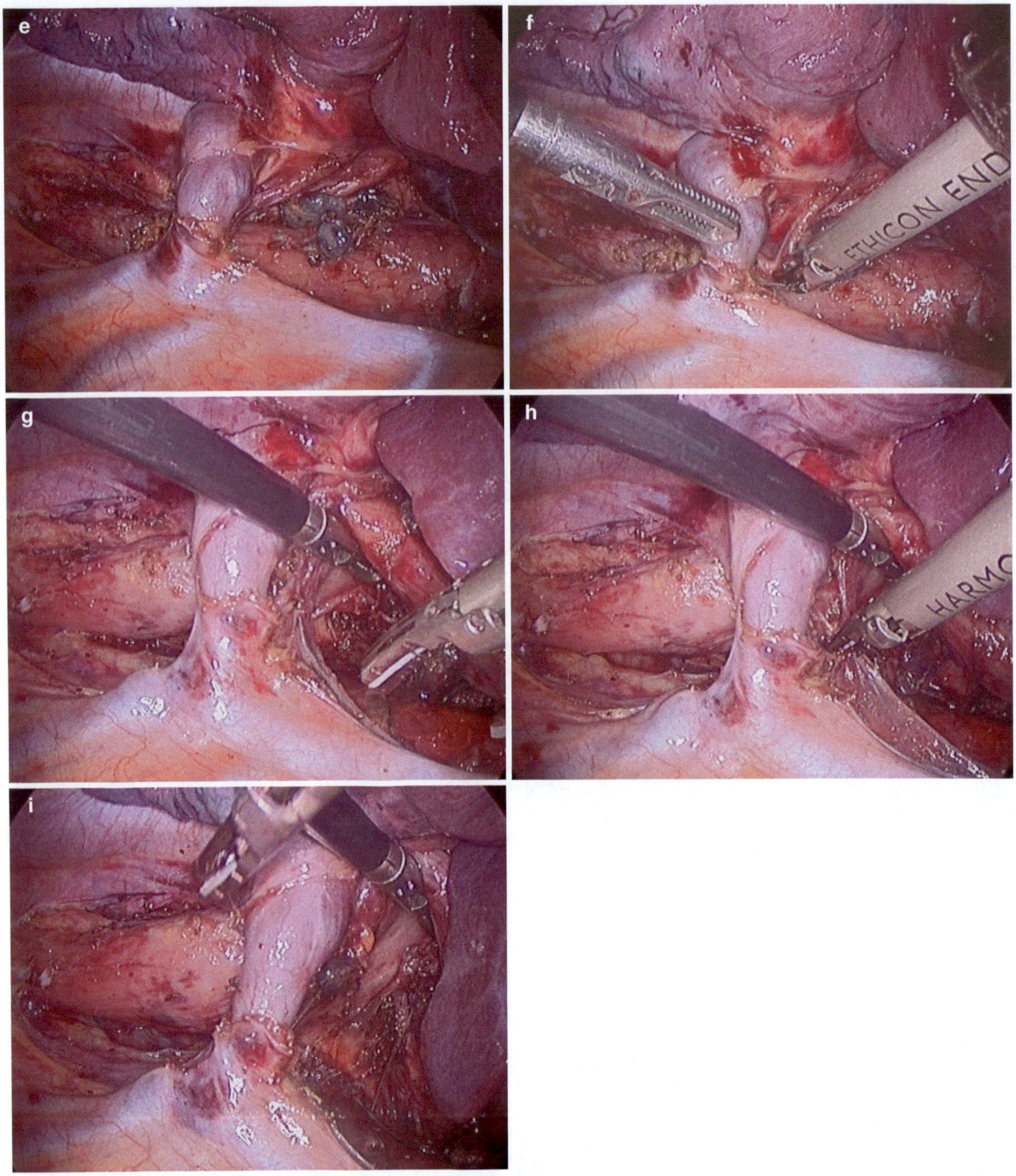

Photo 4.42 (Continued)

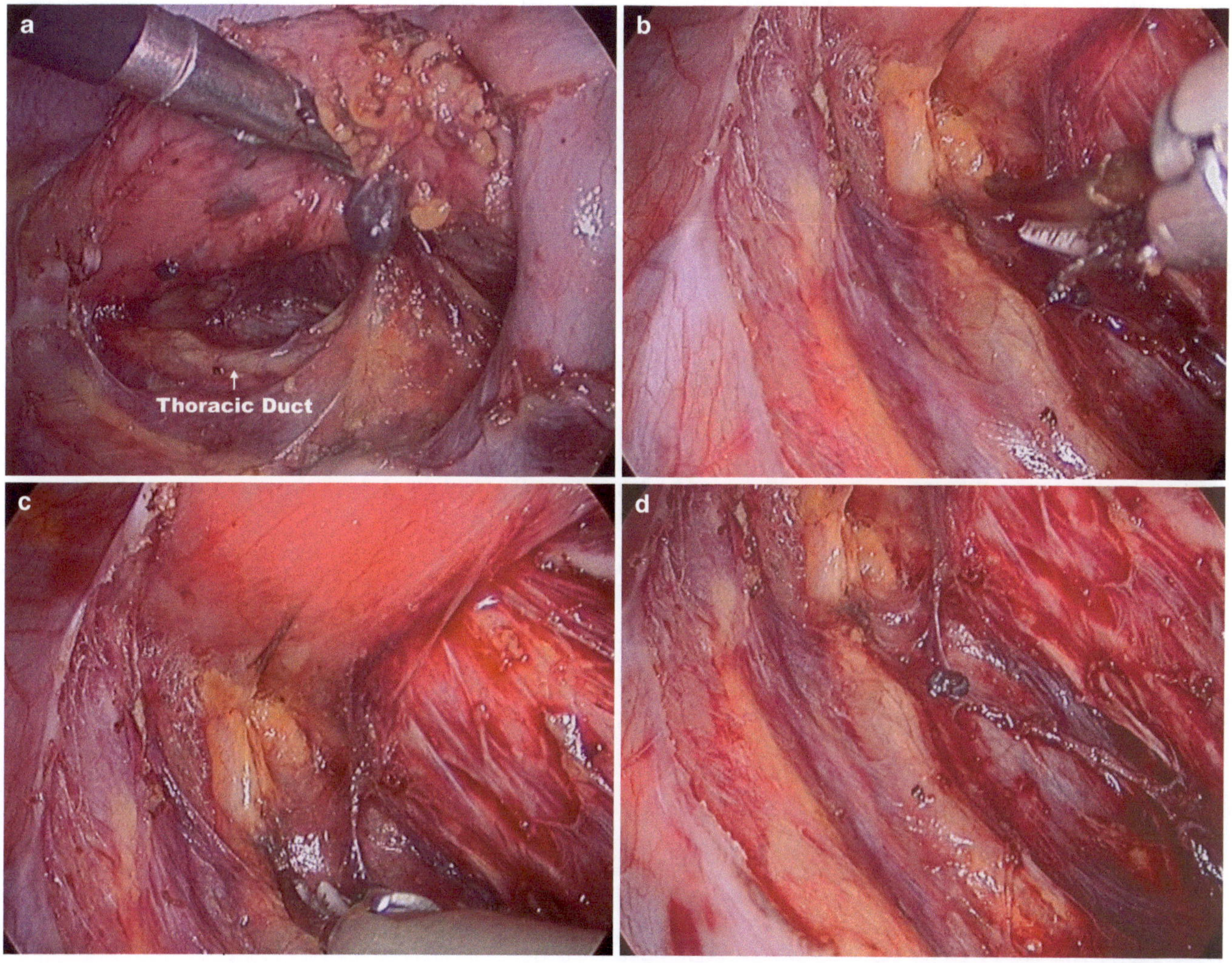

Photo 4.43 (a-d)

41. The esophagus is lifted to visualize the upper course of thoracic duct which can be seen resting on the opposite pleura as a shiny structure (Photo 4.43a–d).

42. The azygous vein is seen completely bare of pleura. The supra- and infra-azygous esophagus can be seen separated from its bed (Photo 4.44).

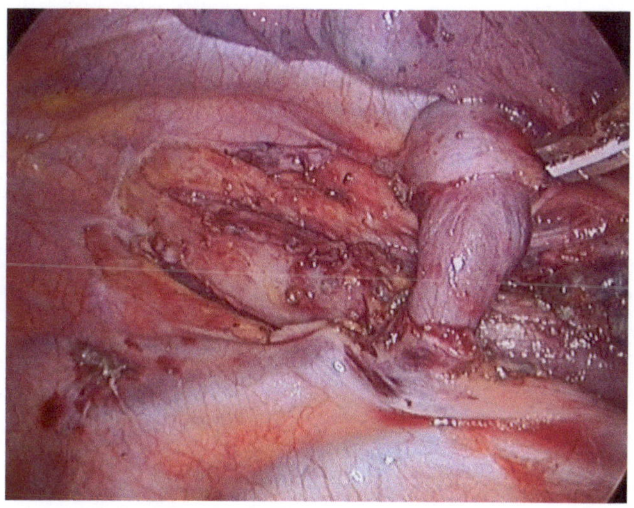

Photo 4.44

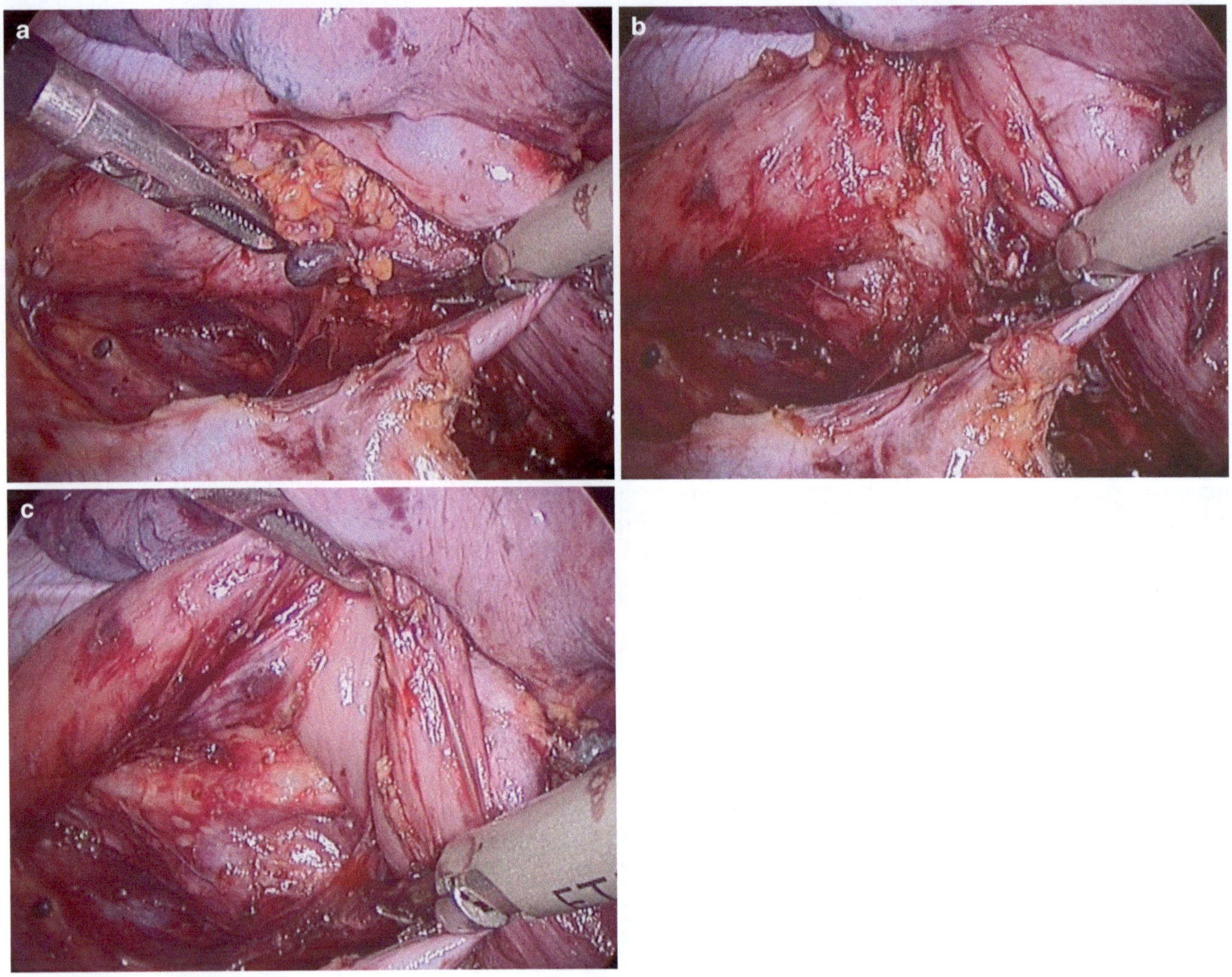

Photo 4.45 (a-c)

43. The esophagus is lifted upward by the left-hand grasper and further dissection is done to separate it all around (Photo 4.45a–c).

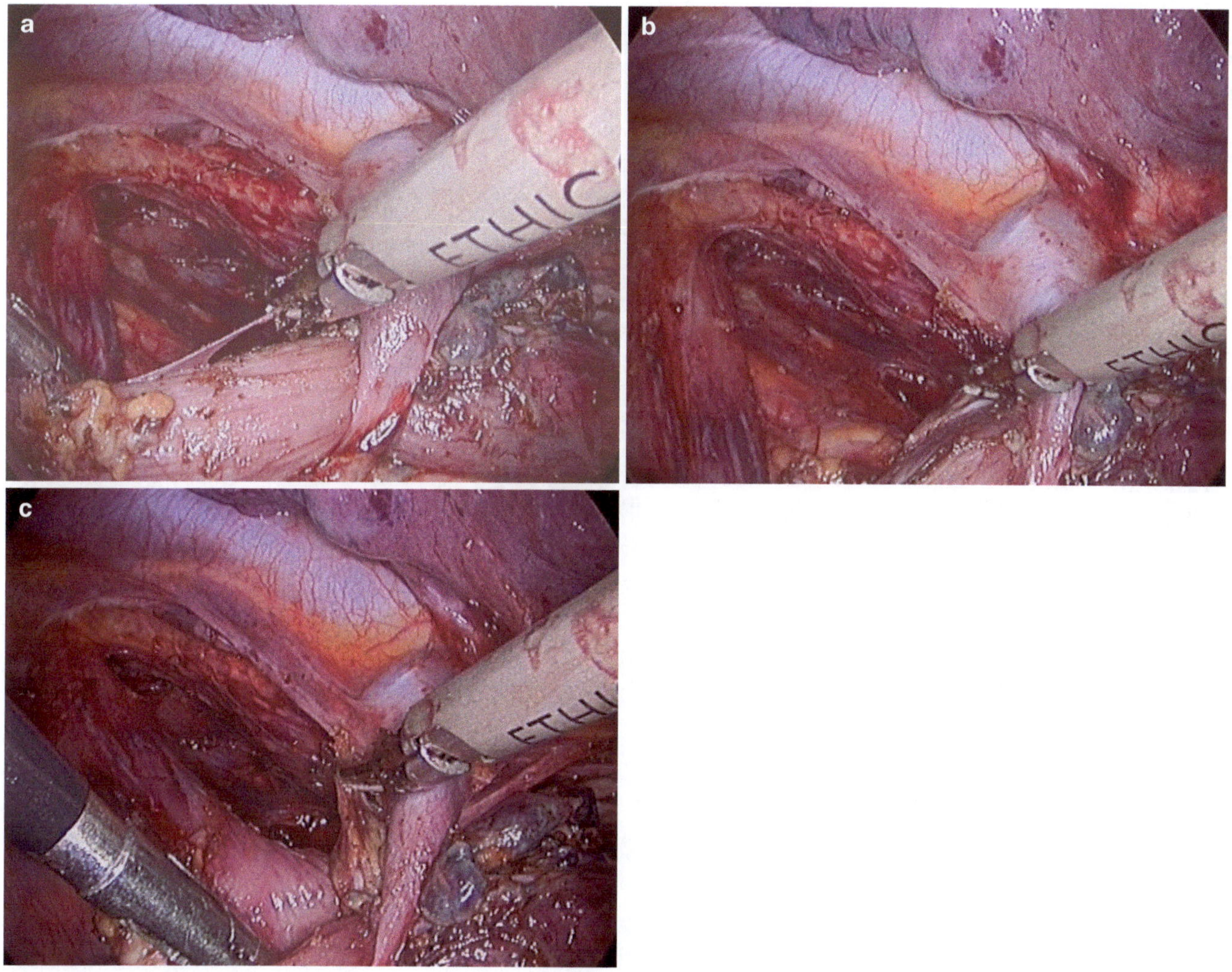

Photo 4.46 (a-c)

44. The separated esophagus is retracted laterally and all the nodes along the azygous vein are removed (Photo 4.46a–c).

45. The mobilized esophagus is pushed upward along with the paraesophageal and carinal nodes. The posterior wall of the trachea and its bifurcation can be seen. The cuff of the left bronchial endobronchial tube can be visualized (Photo 4.47a–f).

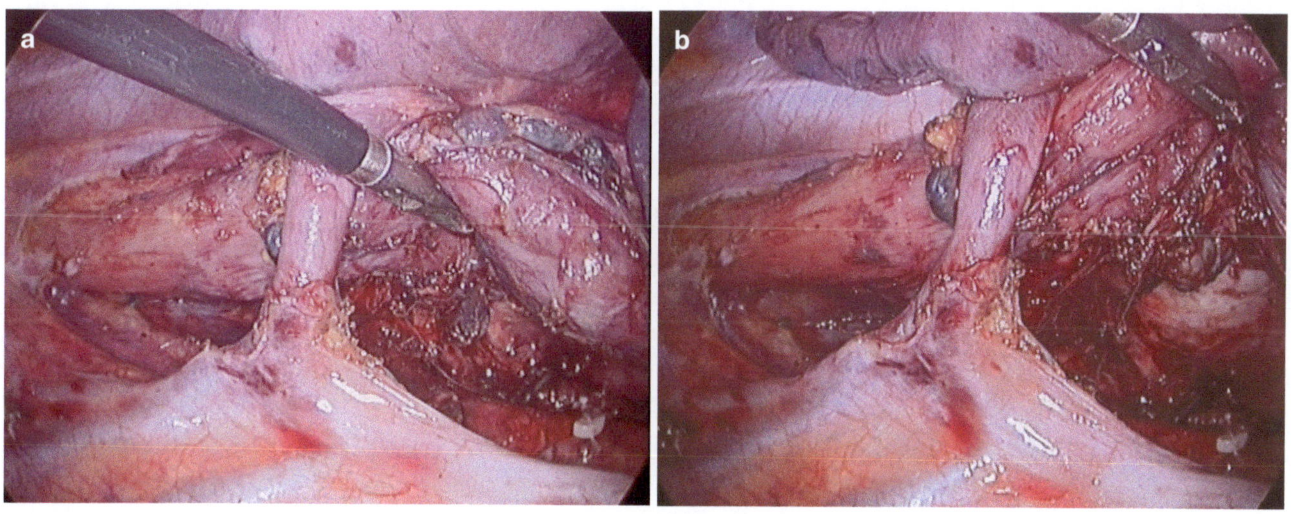

Photo 4.47 (a-f)

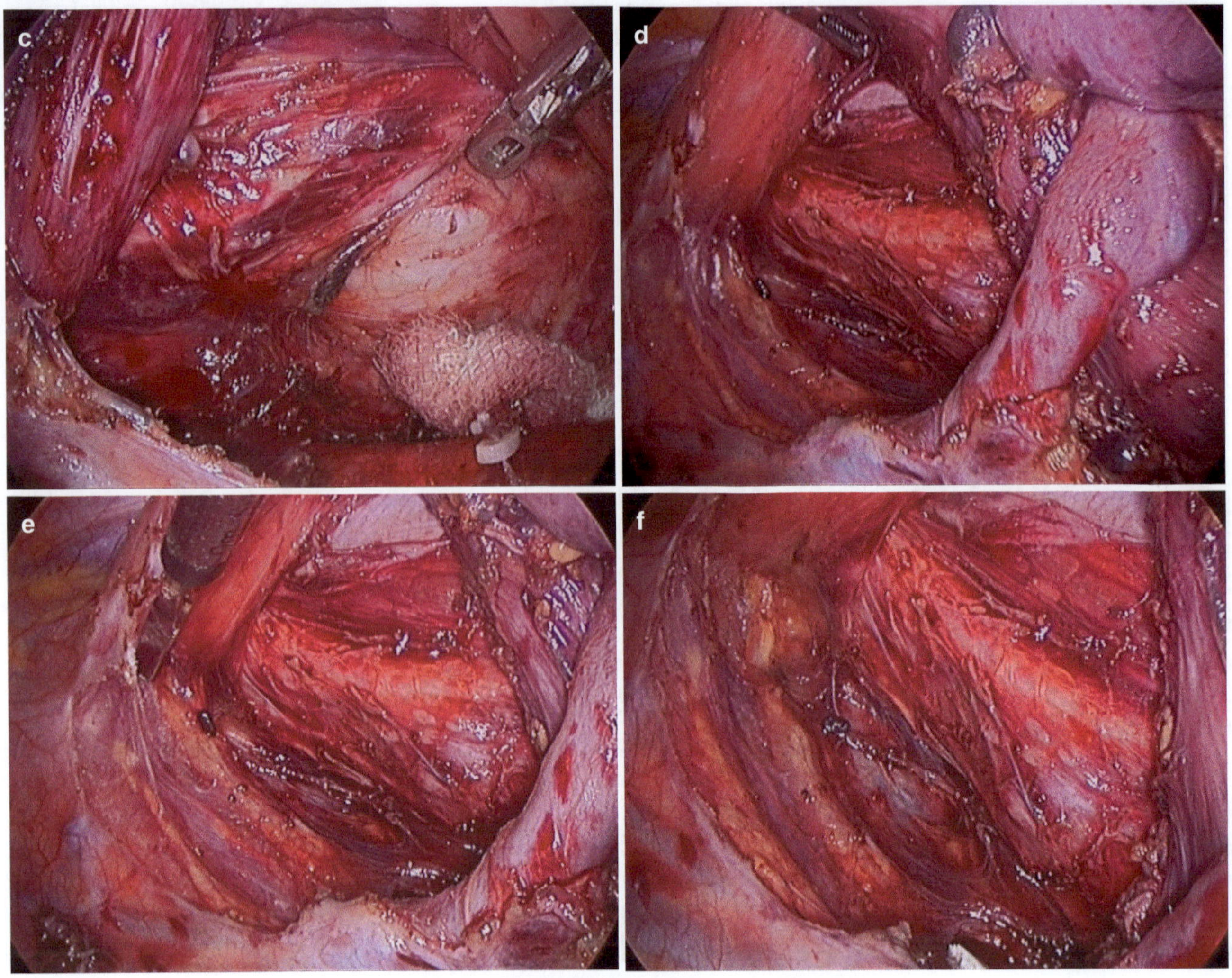

Photo 4.47 (Continued)

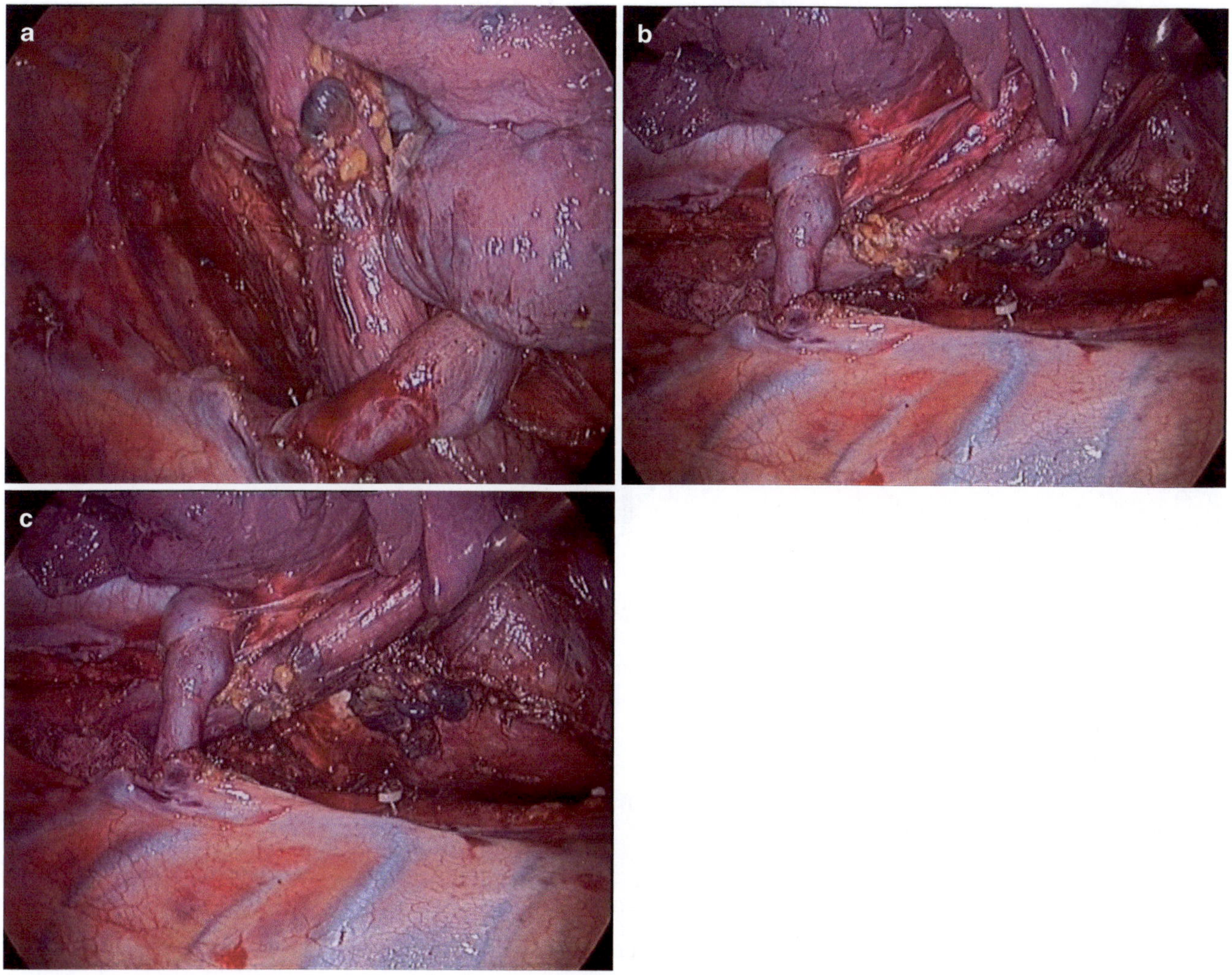

Photo 4.48 (a-c)

46. The esophagus is dissected around the circumference in the surpa-azygous region, and these planes are joined with those in the infra-azygous region, thus completely freeing the esophagus. This can be confirmed by pulling the esophagus cranio-caudally (like the "shoe-shine sign") (Photo 4.48a–c).

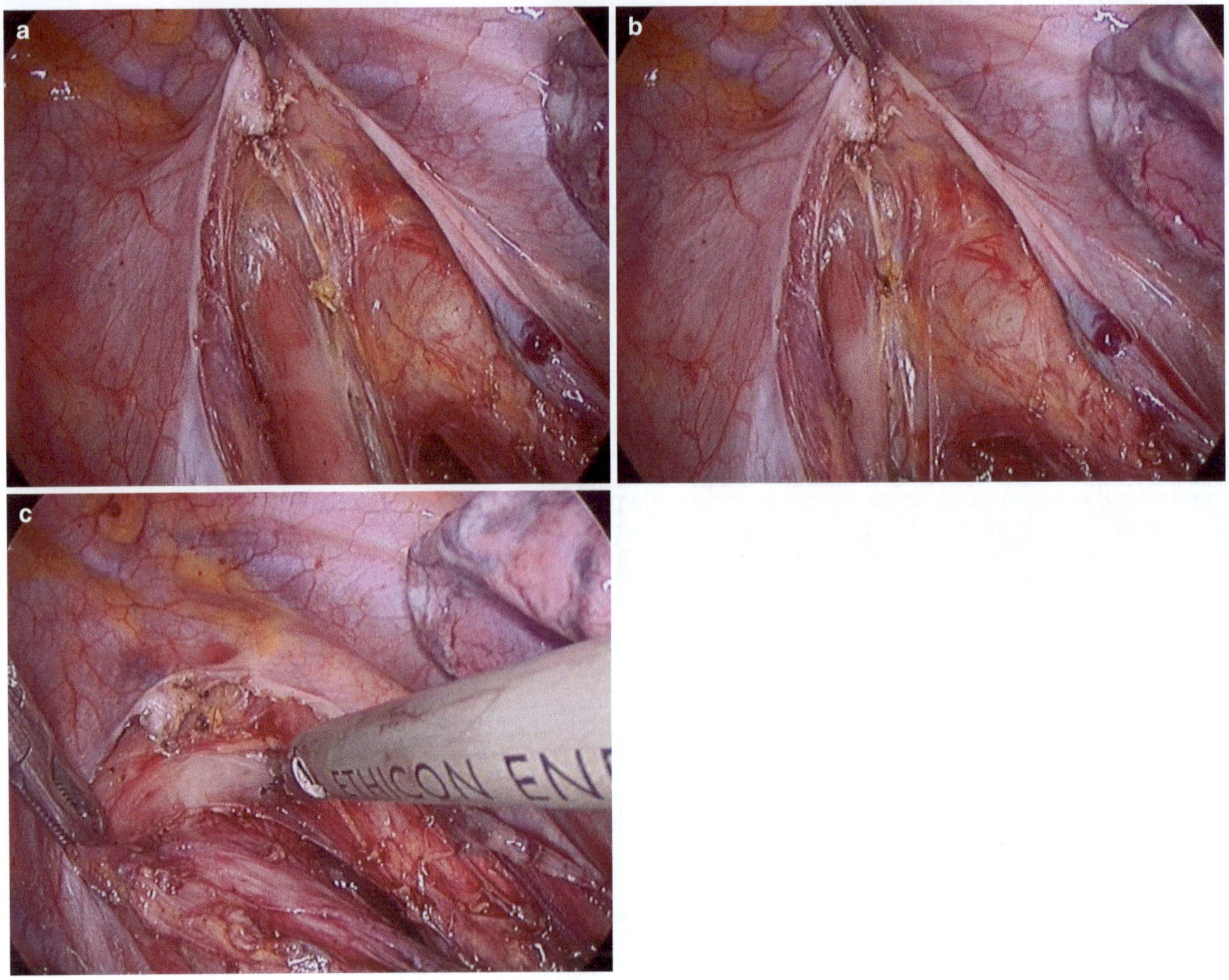

Photo 4.49 (a-c)

47. The esophageal dissection is carried cranially till the root of the neck. The sign of complete dissection is the appearance of neck pad of fat and/or subcutaneous emphysema felt by the assistant in the supra-clavicular area. It is essential to dissect the esophagus completely from the posterior wall of the trachea and reaching upto the root of the neck, thus obviating the need of a blind finger dissection in the neck (Photo 4.49a–c).

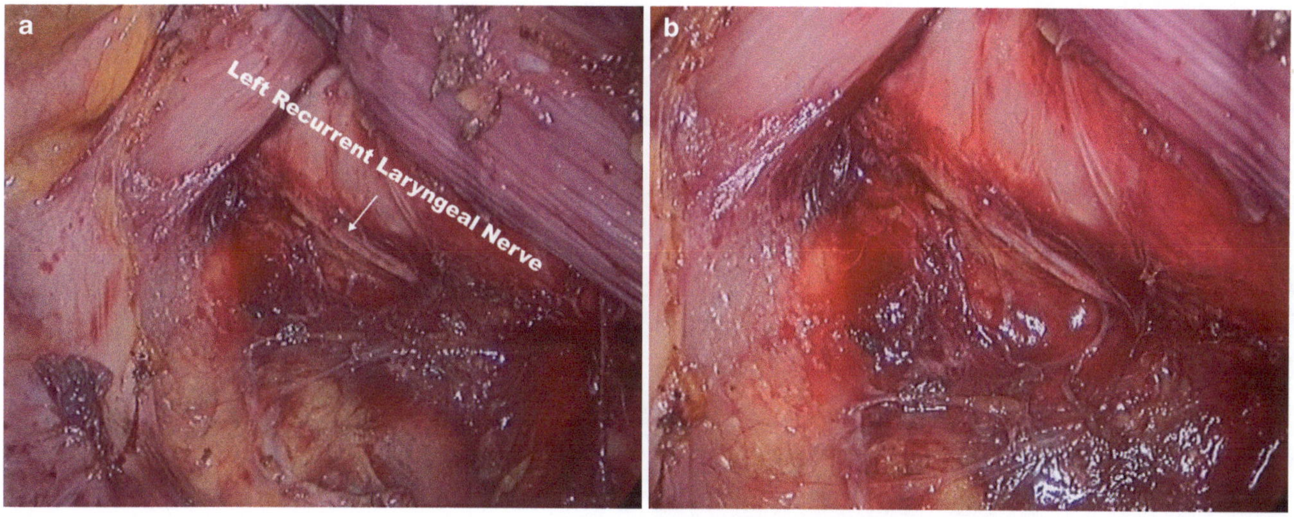

Photo 4.50 (a, b)

48. Once the esophagus is completely freed, it is pulled laterally to expose the left recurrent laryngeal nerve lying in the trachea-esophageal groove. A few nodes along this nerve can be removed. The use of bipolar or any other energy sources are not recommended (Photo 4.50a, b).

49. The right recurrent laryngeal nerve can be identified at the thoracic inlet near the inominate artery (Photo 4.51a, b).

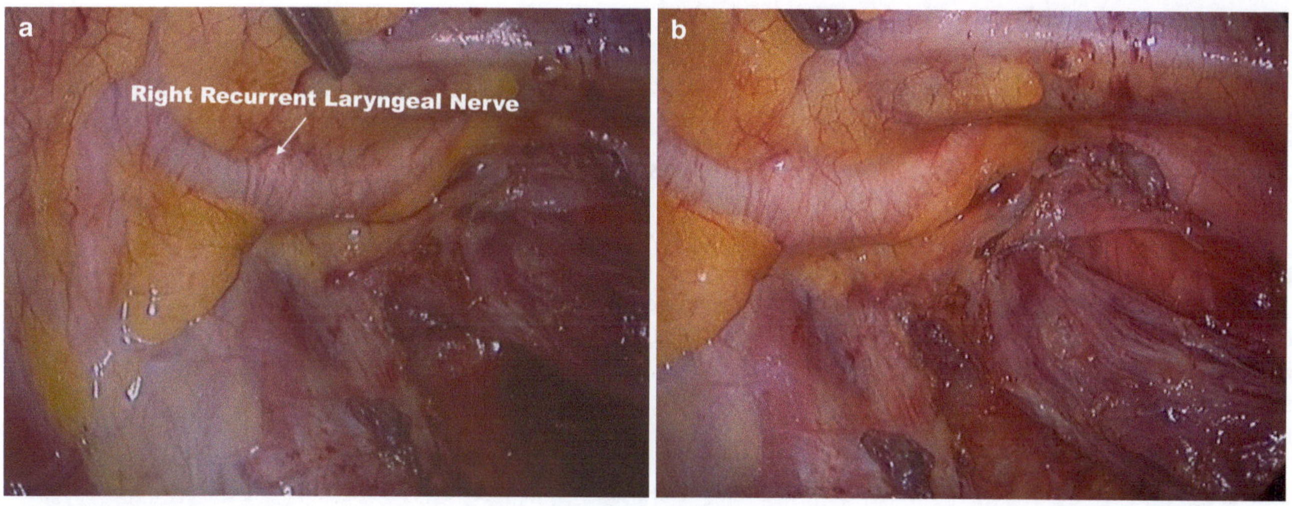

Photo 4.51 (a, b)

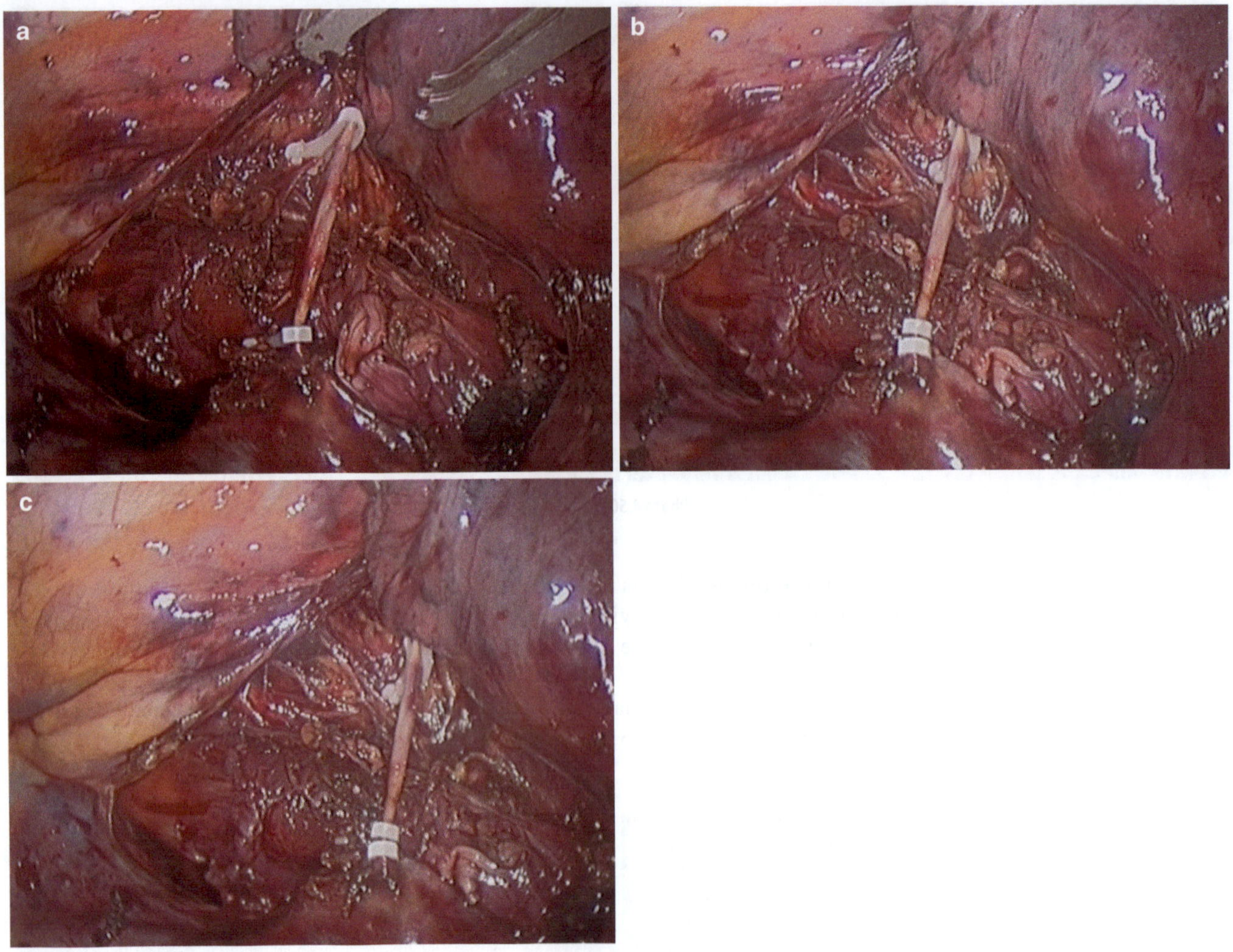

Photo 4.52 (a-c)

50. For all supra-carinal and retroazygous tumors, the azygous vein is clipped and cut for better nodal clearance (Photo 4.52a–c).

51. A window similar to that made earlier is made, and the left-hand grasper pulls the esophagus further laterally. The entire esophagus is thus separated. There are a few nodes in the paratracheal region which are dissected and cleared. If the azygous vein is preserved, care has to be taken not to pull the esophagus with a lot of force as this may lead to tearing of vein (Photo 4.53a, b).

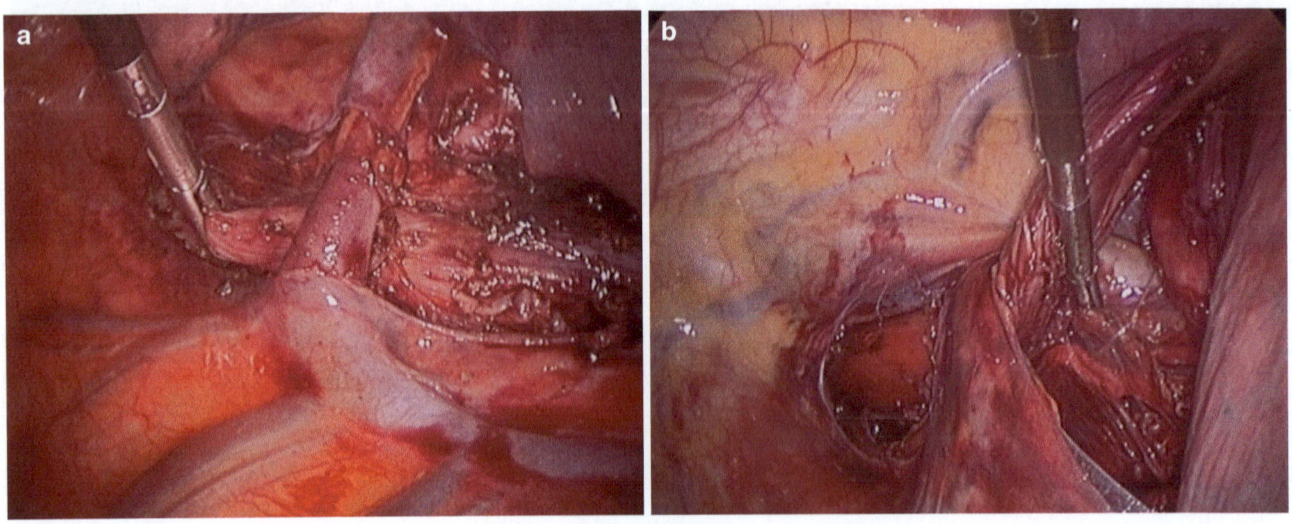

Photo 4.53 (a, b)

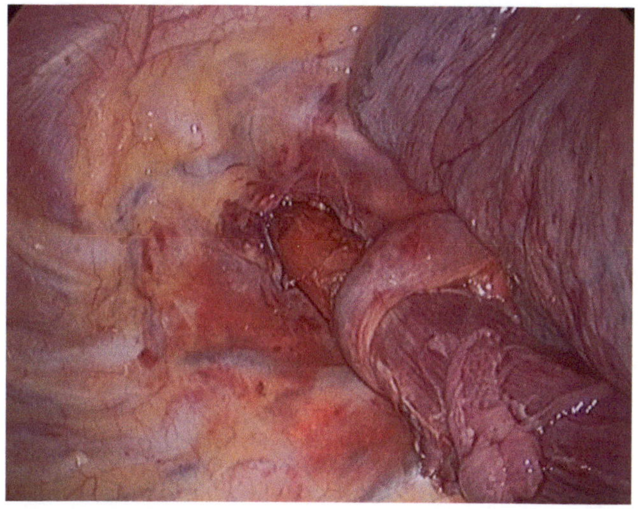

Photo 4.54

52. The esophagus is then moved craniocaudally and mediolaterally to confirm the complete esophageal mobilization (Photo 4.54).

53. A complete wash is given and the damage to the left pleura is checked. The haemostasis is confirmed and if required clips or bipolar energy is used to ensure control of bleeding (Photo 4.55a,b).

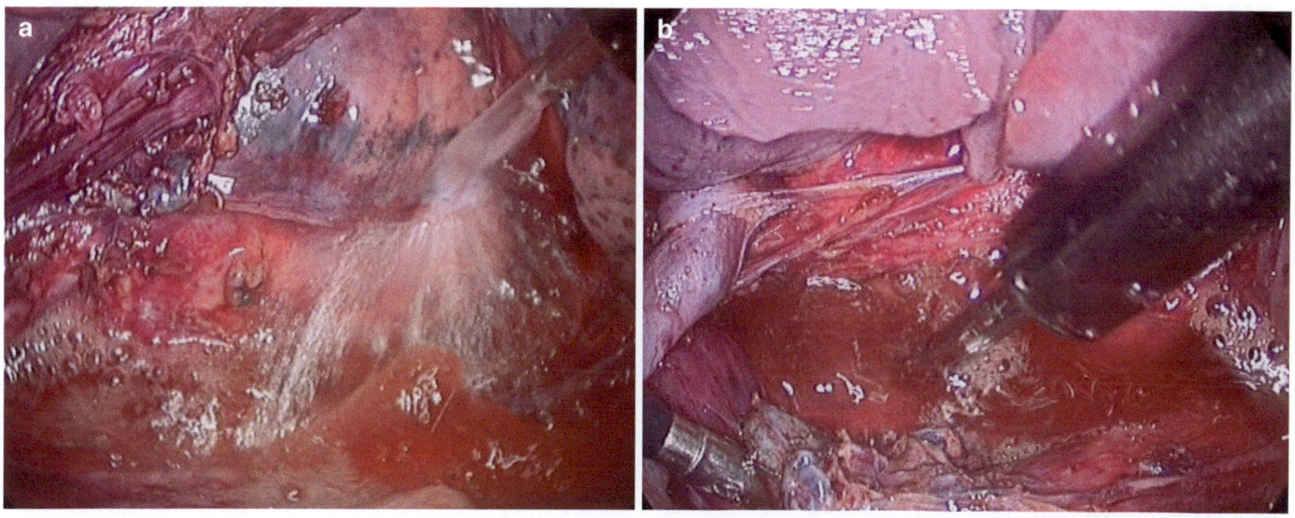

Photo 4.55 (a, b)

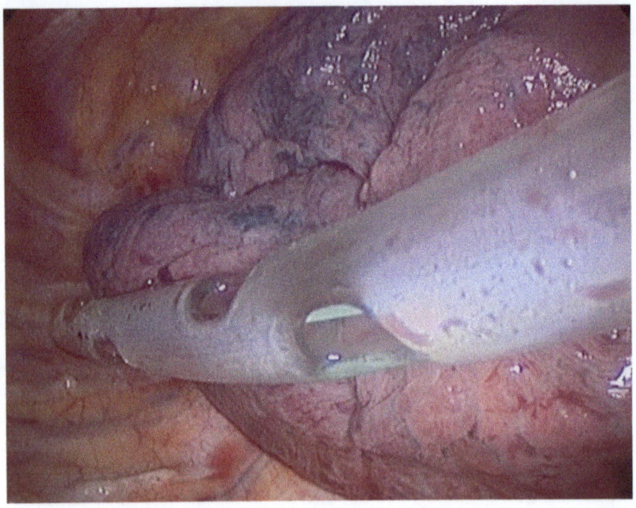

Photo 4.56

54. An intercoastal drain is inserted through the working 10 mm port, and is placed under vision with the help of the left-hand grasper. The 5 mm ports are removed under vision as the intercostal vessels many have been damaged during the insertion of the ports (Photo 4.56).

55. The lung is inflated and the camera port is removed under vision. The lung should be inflated and the intercoastal drainage tube should be open to let all the air out (Photo 4.57).

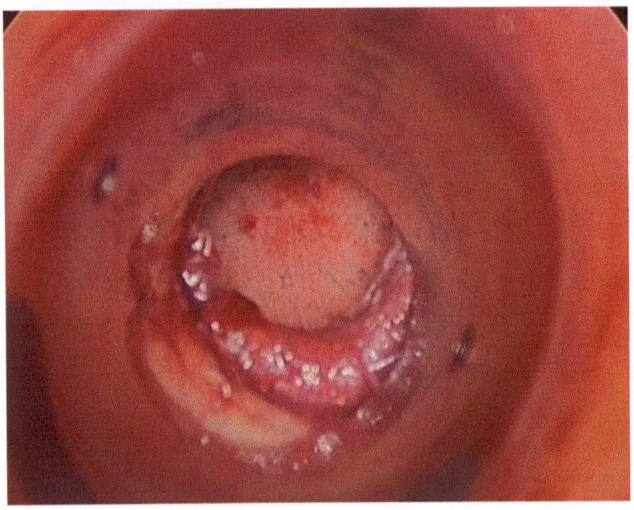

Photo 4.57

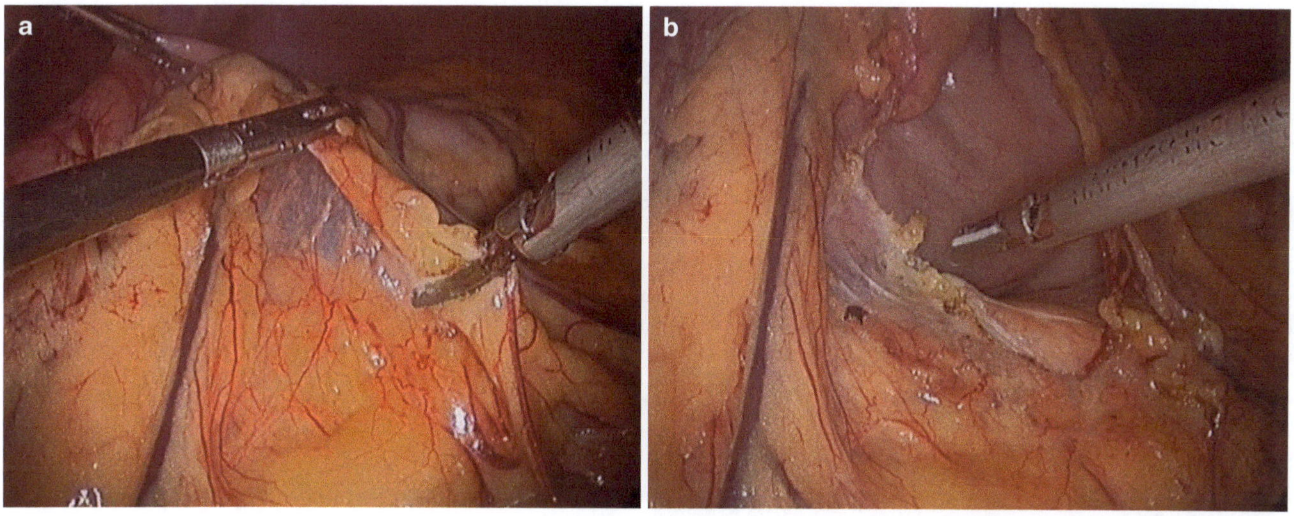

Photo 4.58 (a, b)

Mobilization of the Stomach

1. The stomach mobilization is initiated by opening the lesser sac (Photo 4.58a, b).
2. The assistant on the patients right side, pulls the stomach upward while the second assistant pulls the transverse colon downward. This maneuver facilitates the exposure of the lesser sac (Photo 4.59a, b).

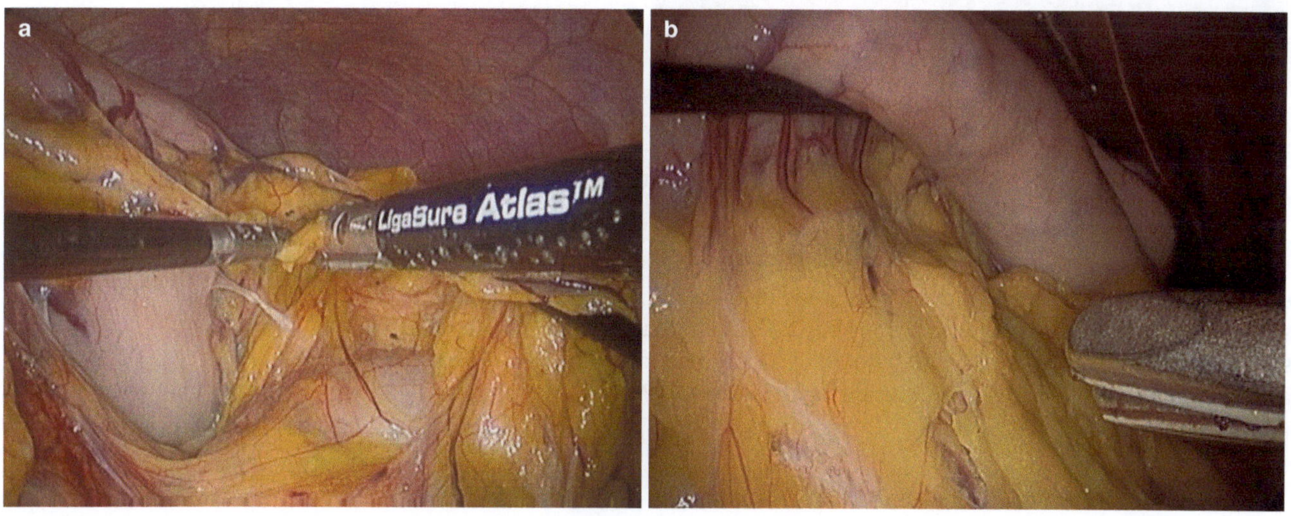

Photo 4.59 (a, b)

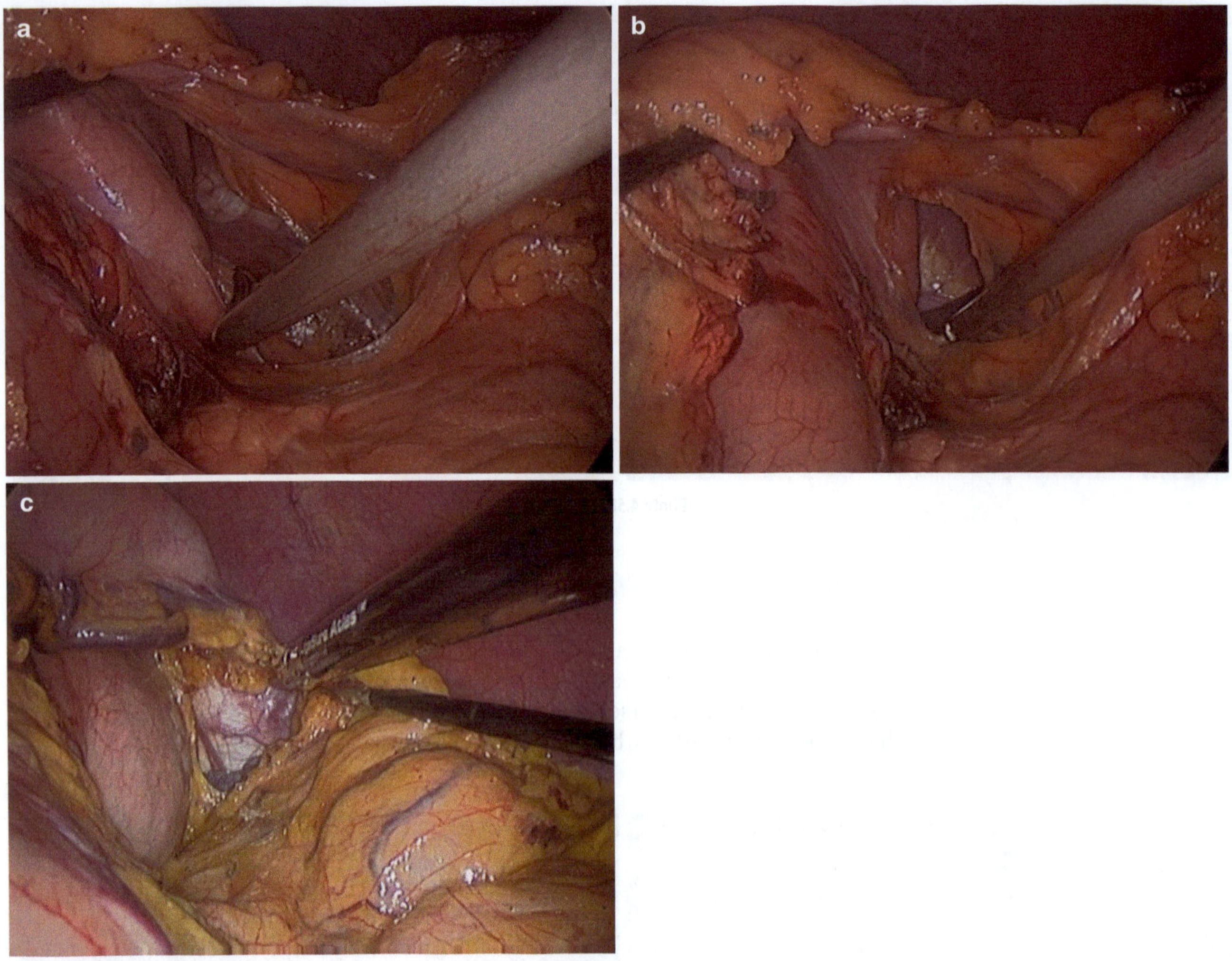

Photo 4.60 (a-c)

3. The lesser sac is opened by cutting the veins in the omentum. The opening is enlarged. The cranial assistant then inserts his instrument in the lesser sac while the second assistant pulls the omentum downward. The cut is further extended toward the short. These veins are coagulated and cut with harmonic scalpel/ligasure. The traction given by both the assistants are exaggerated with every cut (Photo 4.60a–c).

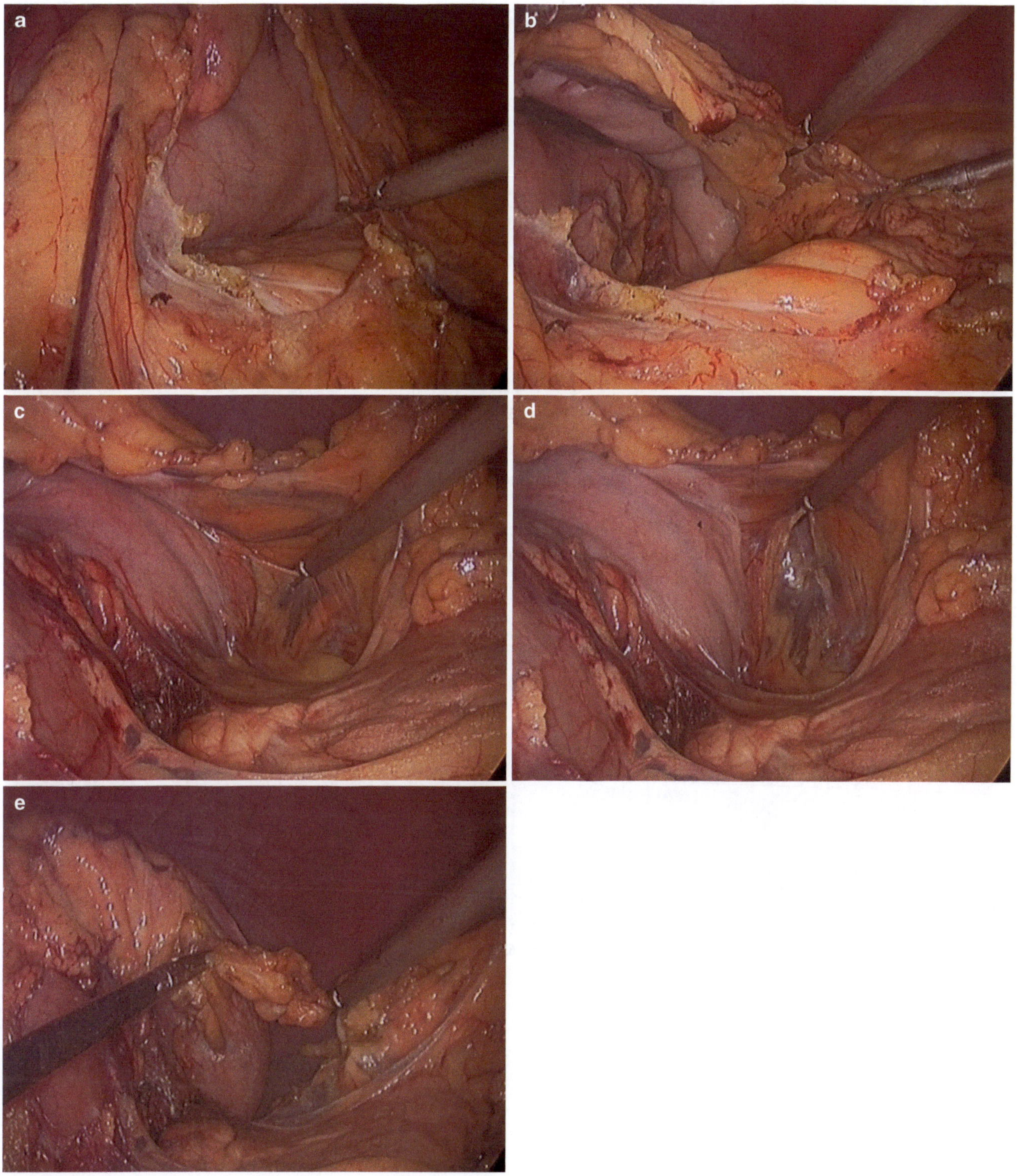

Photo 4.61 (a-e)

4. The stomach is pulled to the right and the second assistant gives light traction on the spleen. The short gastric vessels are thus stretched and well seen. These are coagulated and cut slowly. All the short gastric vessels are cut till the spleen is completely freed (Photo 4.61a–e).

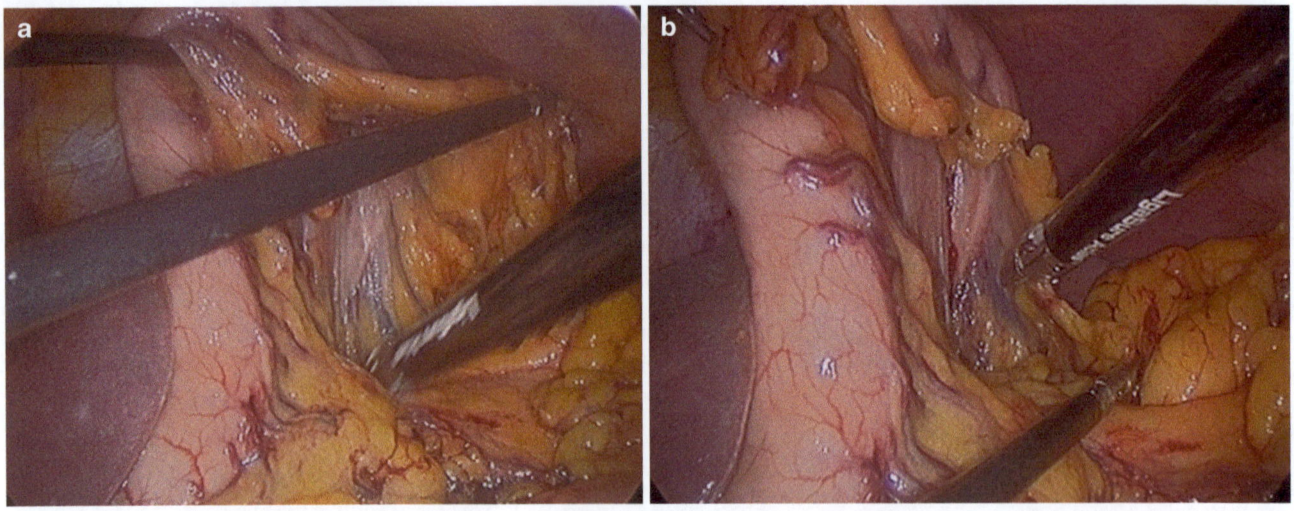

Photo 4.62 (a, b)

5. The posterior short gastric is seen at this stage and should be coagulated and cut (Photo 4.62a, b).

6. The entire stomach is then retracted on the right side. This exposes the left crus and the peritoneum over the crus is cut. Small branches of phrenic artery may be encountered here. This completes the dissection on the fundic side (Photo 4.63a, b).

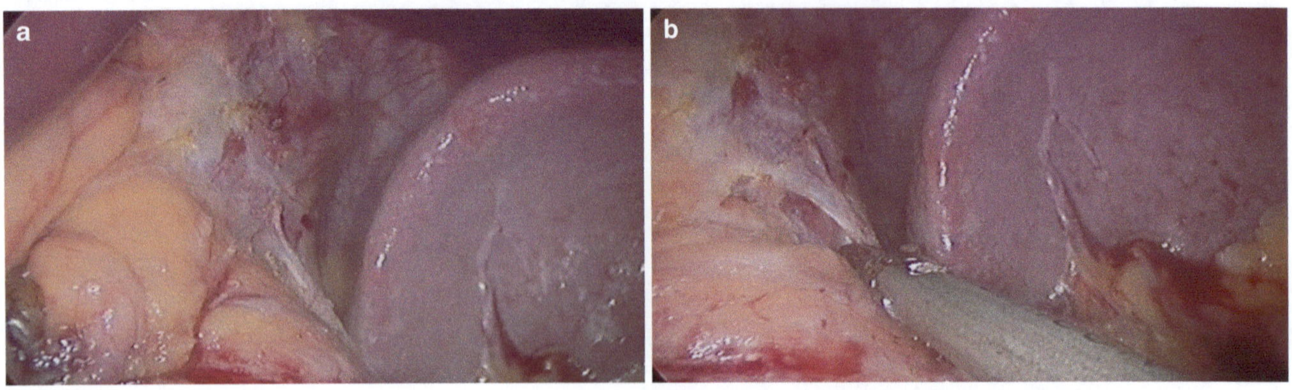

Photo 4.63 (a, b)

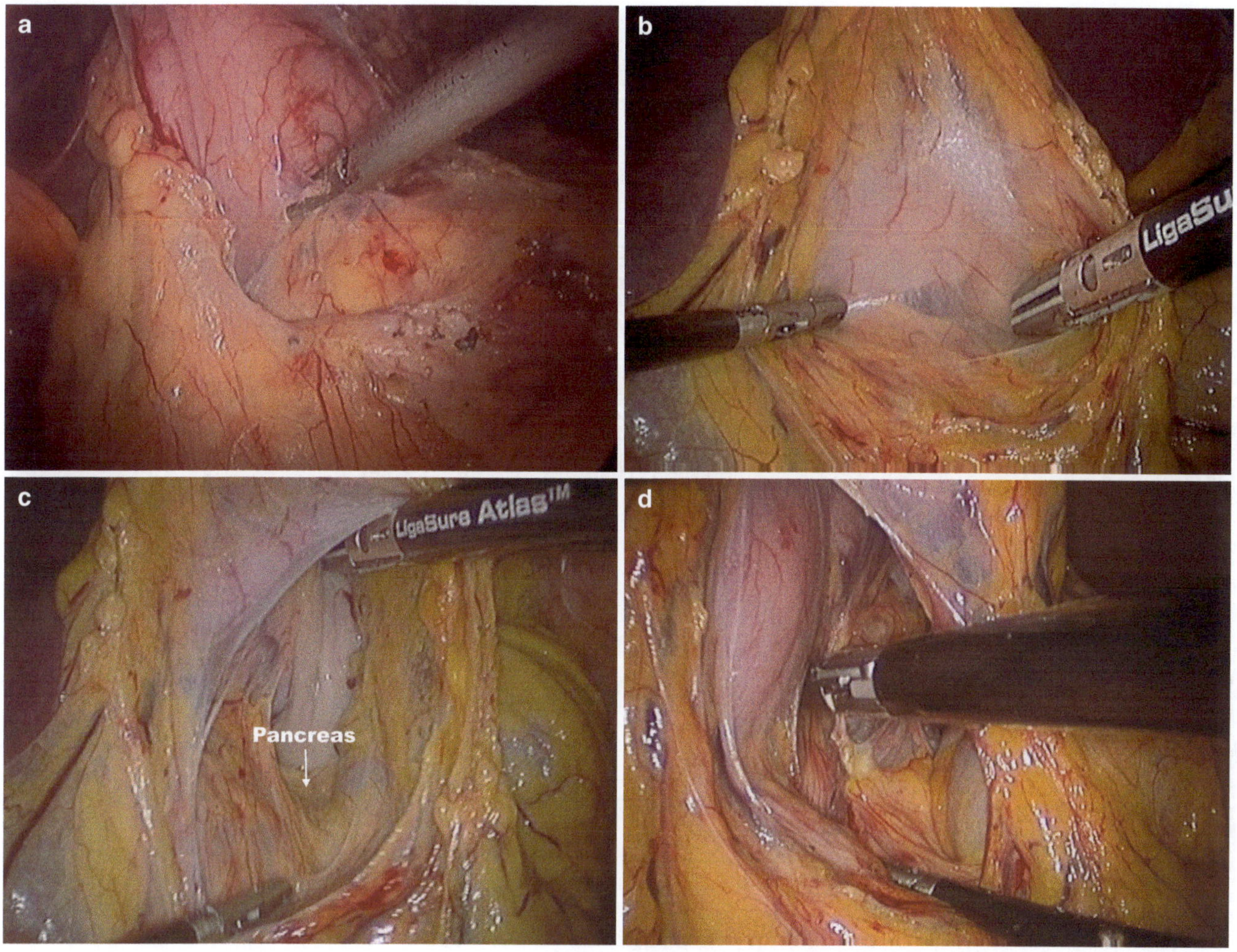

Photo 4.64 (a-d)

7. The stomach is then lifted cranially and the posterior congenital adhesions of the stomach are identified. These have to be cut to expose the pancreas (Photo 4.64a–d).
8. The stomach is completely separated from the pancreatic bed (Photo 4.65a, b).

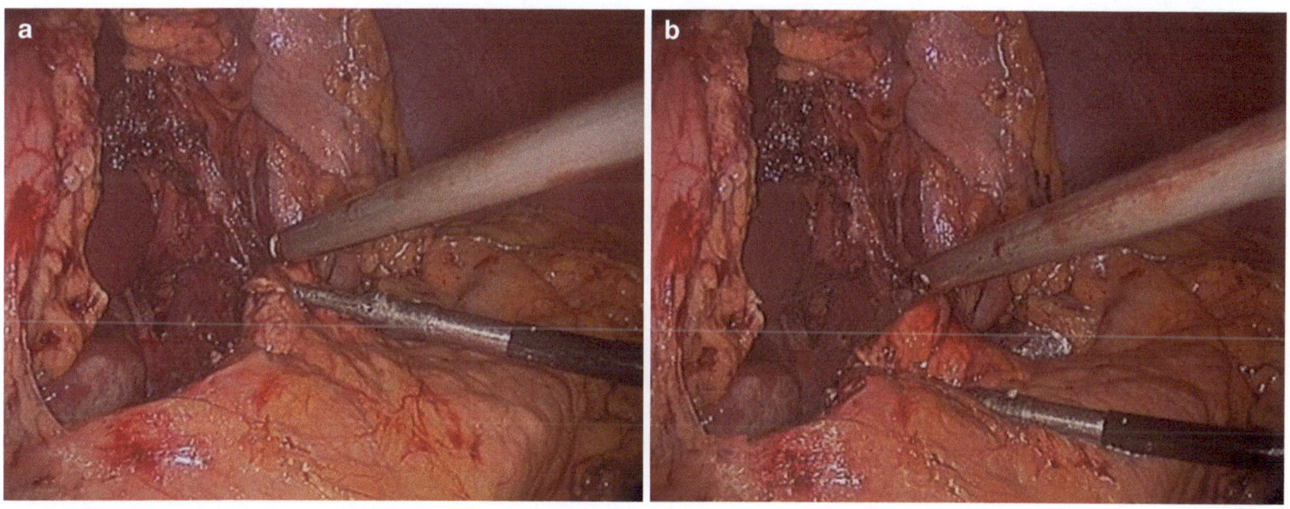

Photo 4.65 (a, b)

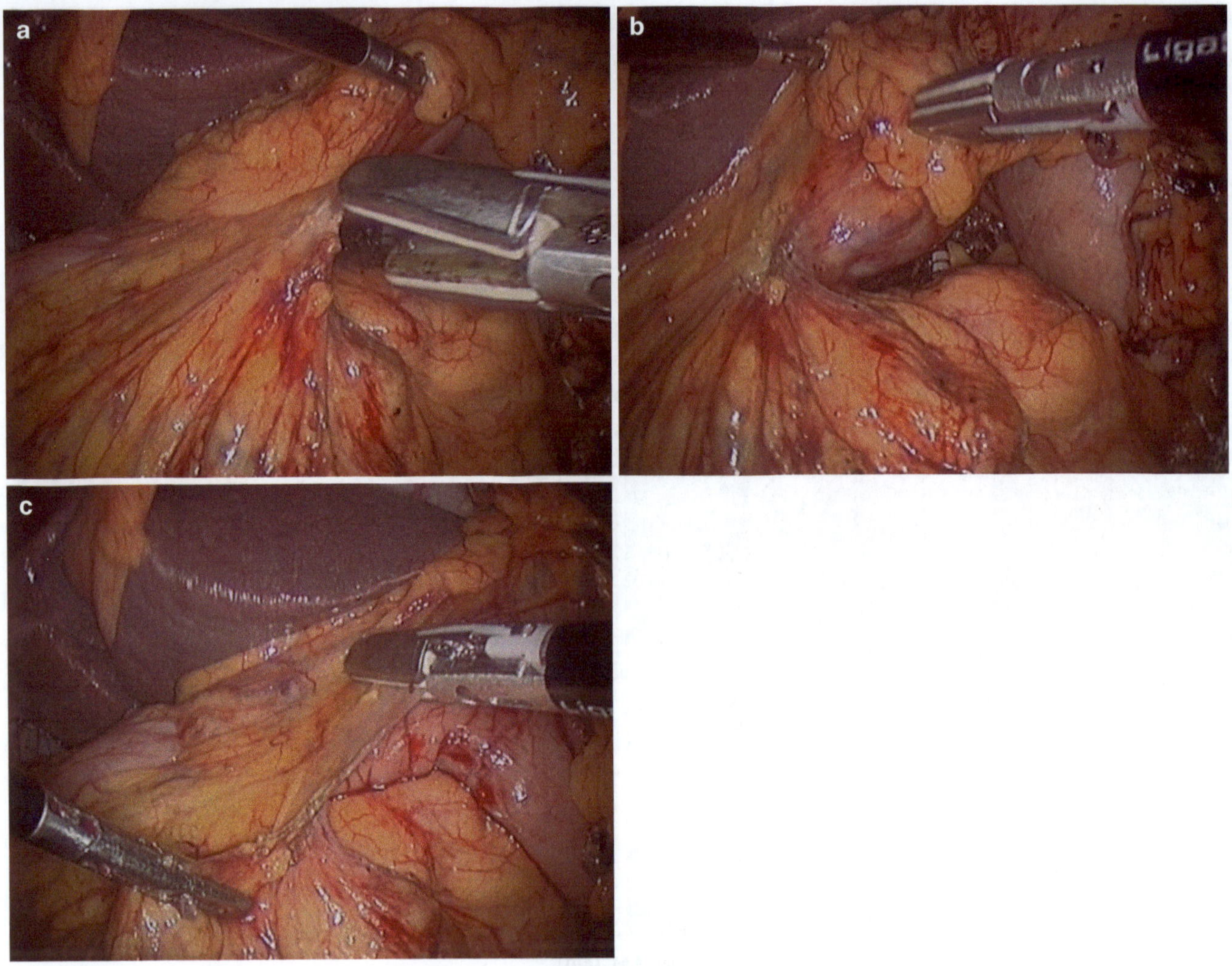

Photo 4.66 (a-c)

9. The cut in the lesser sac is then extended to the right. The cranial assistant pulls the stomach upward. The second assistant pulls the transverse colon downward. One should focus on the transverse colon and cut all the vessels in the lesser sac. Slowly, the transverse colon goes down and the head of the pancreas is exposed (Photo 4.66a–c).

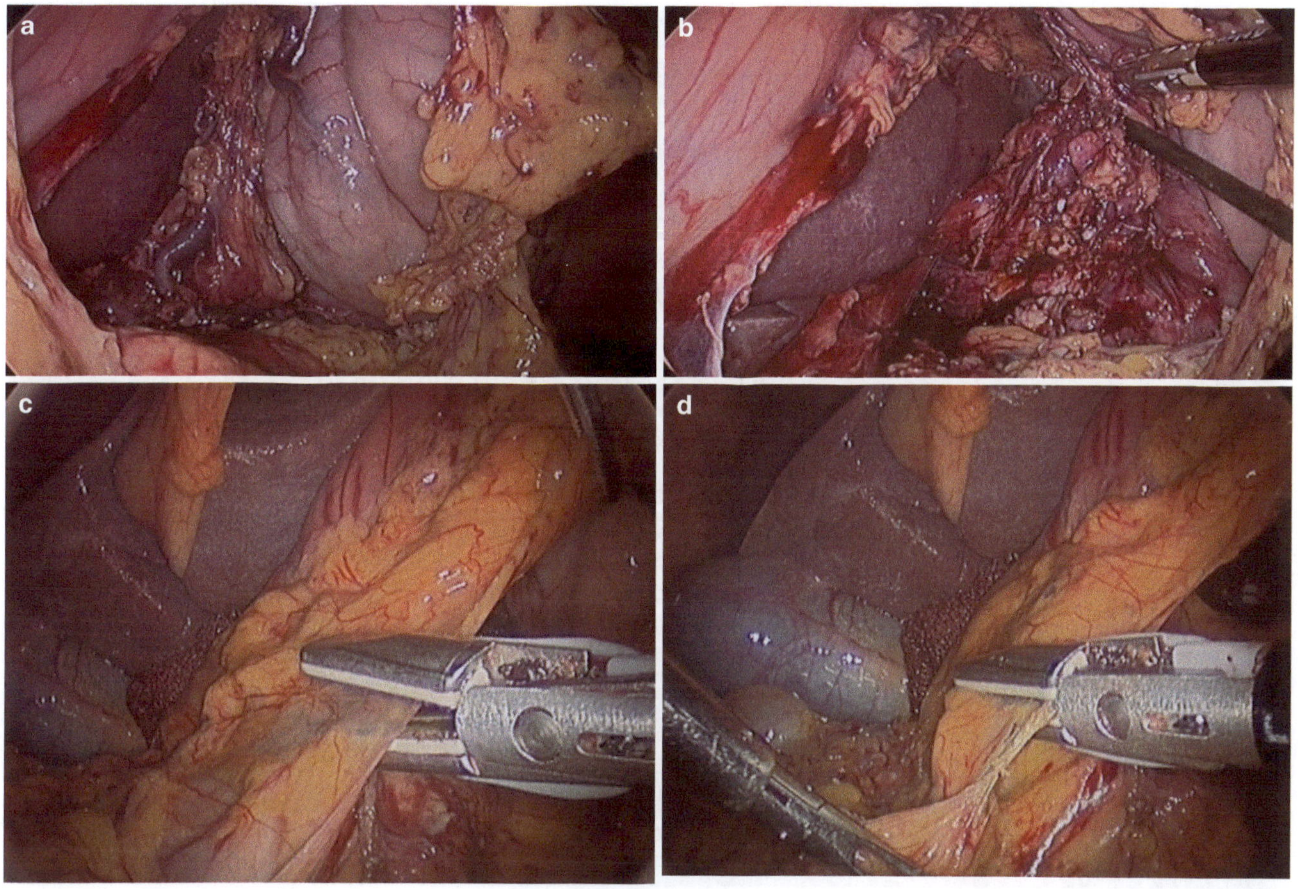

Photo 4.67 (a-d)

10. The right gastroepiploic vessels are not exposed and are always to be protected from injury. The posterior congenital adhesions are further cut till a window is made and liver can be visualized from behind the stomach (Photo 4.67a–d).

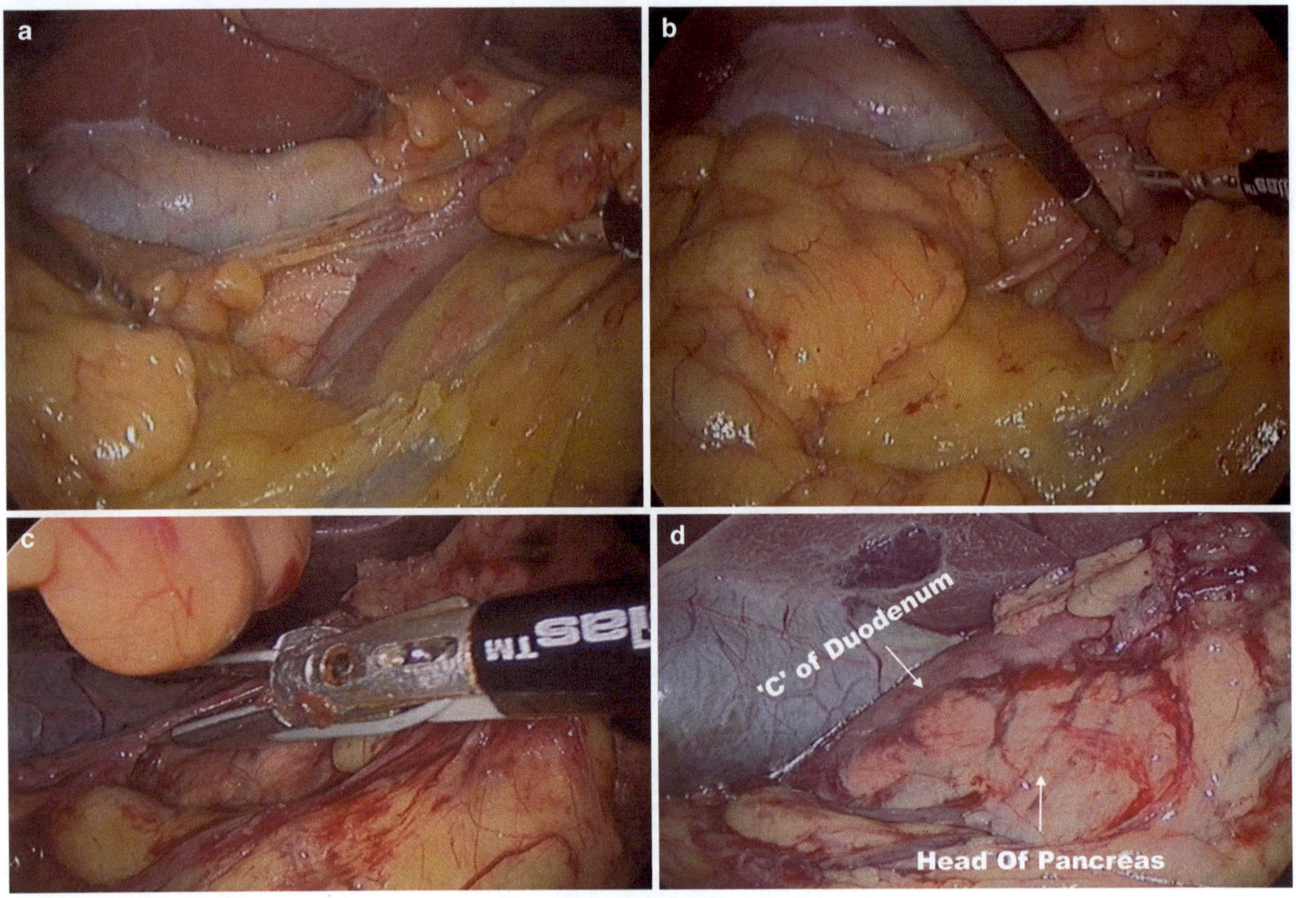

Photo 4.68 (a-d)

11. The transverse colon mobilization is continued till the hepatic flexure is reached. This exposes the second portion of duodenum. This is the end point of dissection and one need not kockerize the duodenum (Photo 4.68a–d).

12. The left gastric artery and vein (pedicle) have to be cut to complete the gastric mobilization. The pedicle can be approached by pulling the stomach cranially or from the right side. The nodes along the celiac axis are dissected and removed along with the pedicle (Photo 4.69a–k).

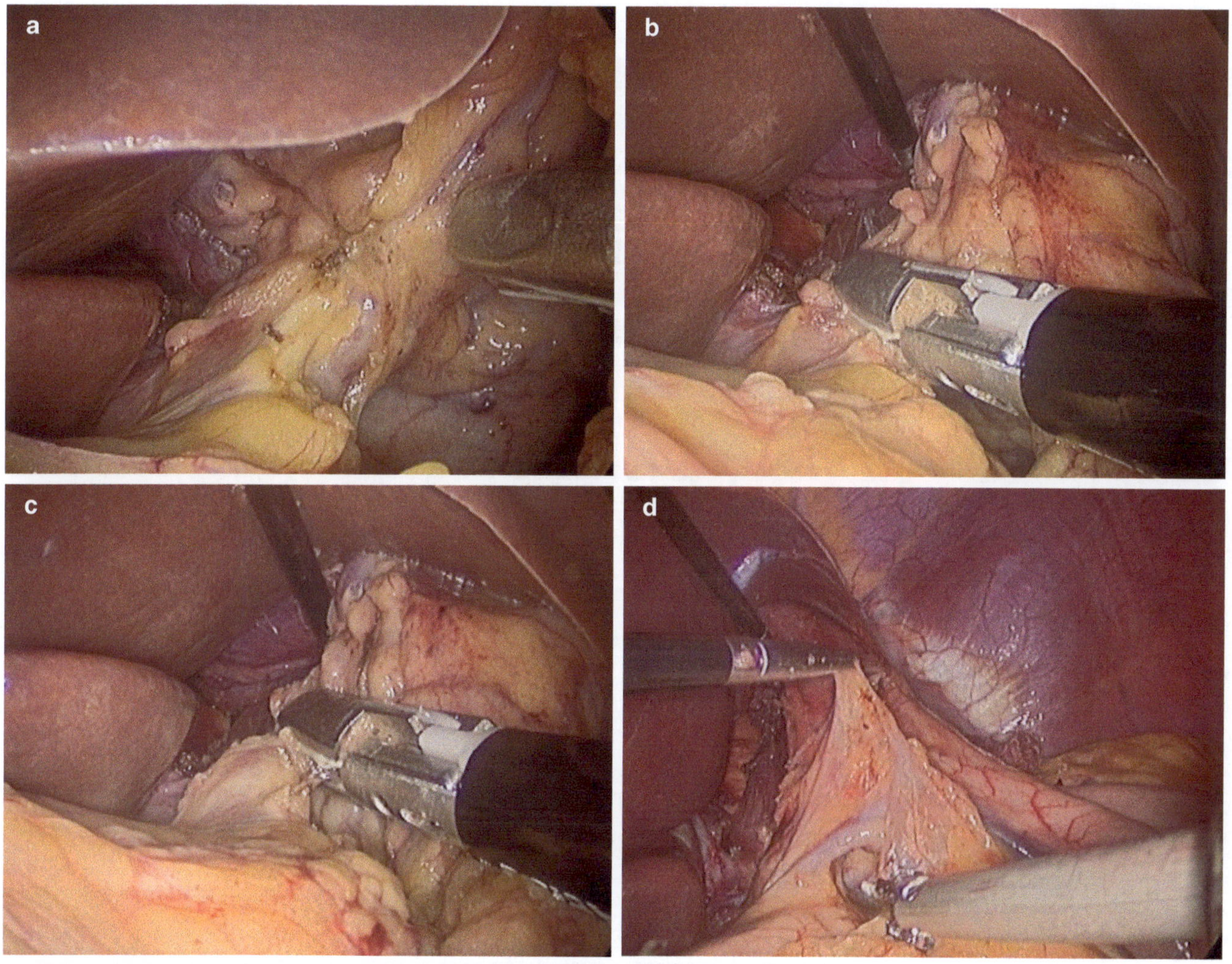

Photo 4.69 (a-d)

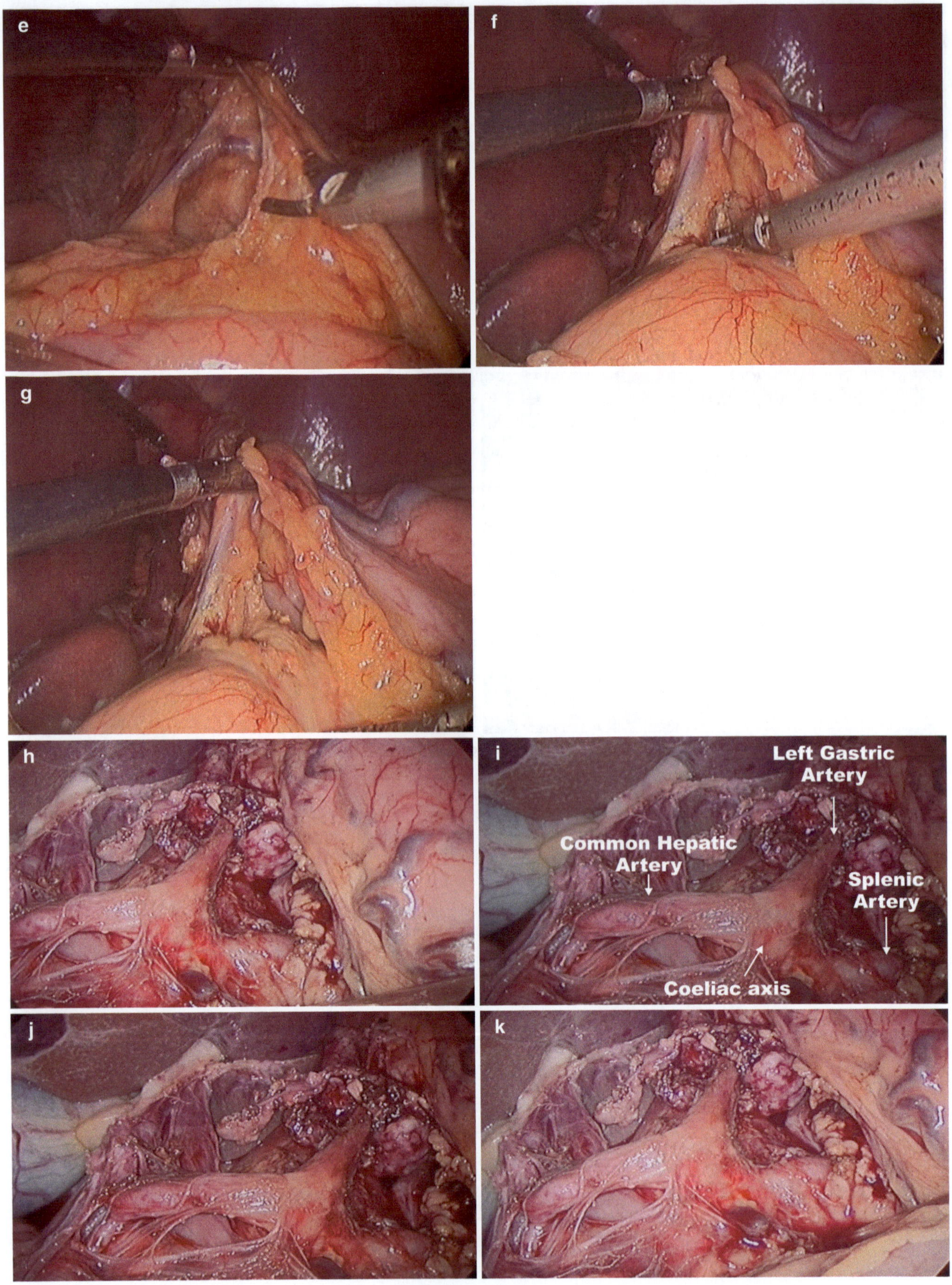

Photo4.69 (Continued)

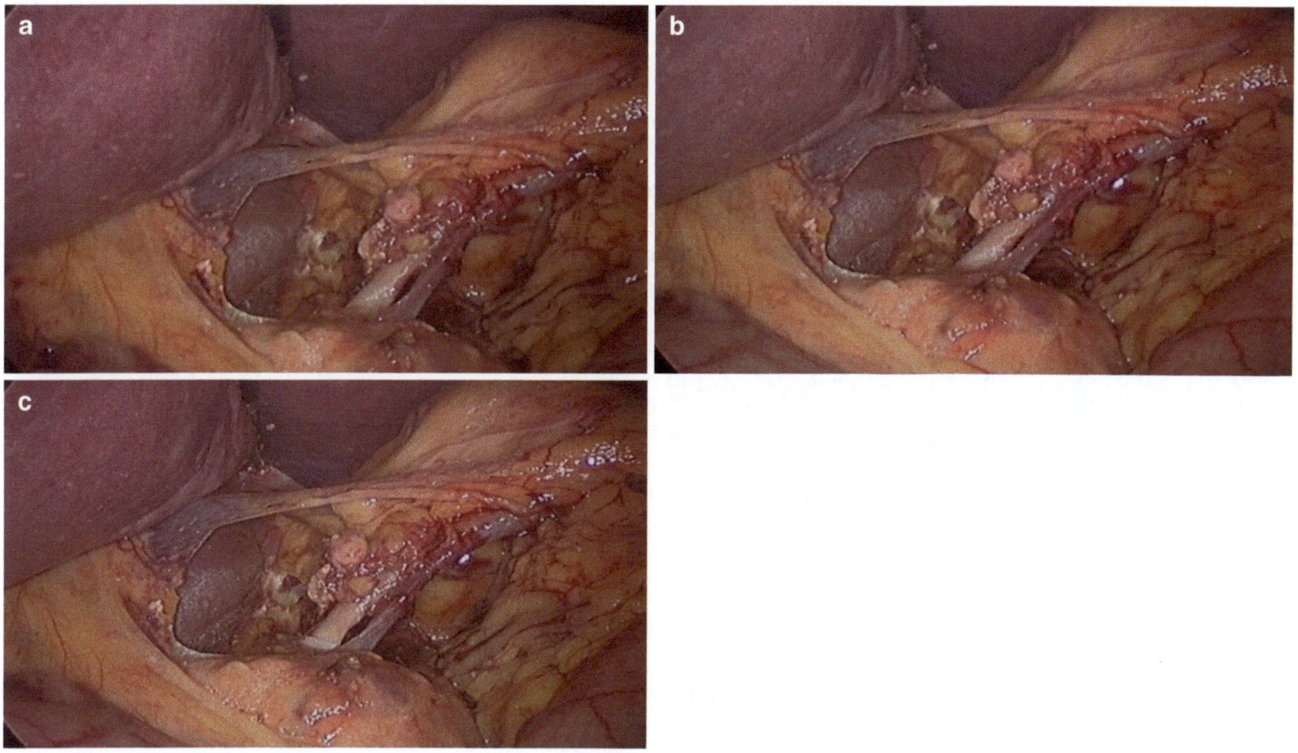

Photo 4.70 (a-c)

13. The left gastric vein and artery is clipped and cut (Photo 4.70a–c).
14. The stomach can be freed further by cutting the peritoneum over the right crus (Photo 4.71a, b).

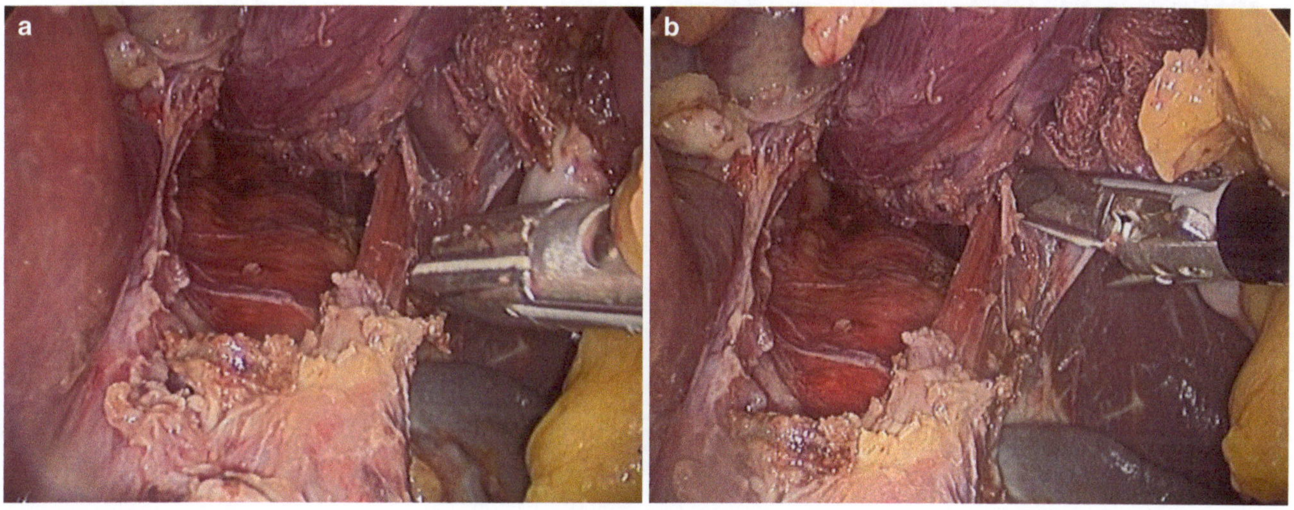

Photo 4.71 (a, b)

15. Hiatal dissection is as described in the chapter of laparoscopic transhiatal esophagectomy (Chap. 5).

Dissection of Cervical Esophagus in Neck

1. A left transverse supra-clavicular incision is taken, extending just beyond the lateral border of the left sternocleidomastoid muscle (Photo 4.72).
2. The platysma and the omohyoid muscles are cut to expose the internal jugular vein (Photo 4.73).

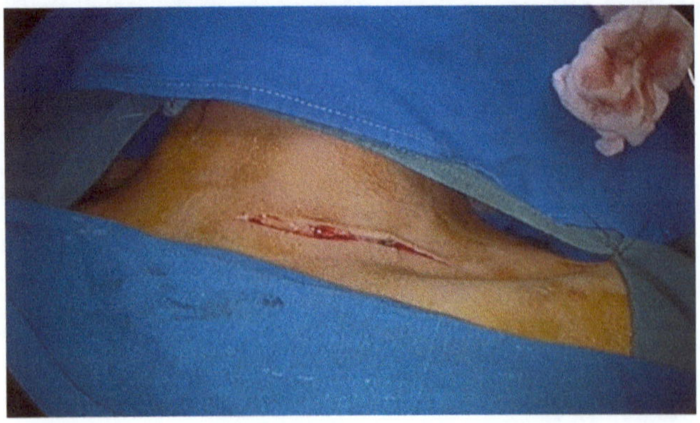

Photo 4.72

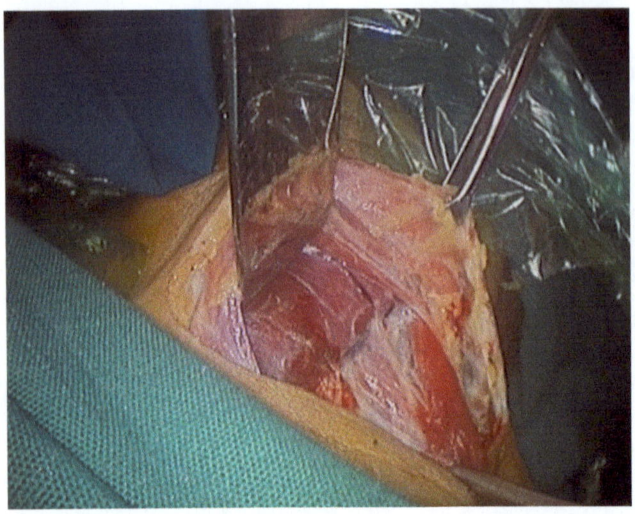

Photo 4.73

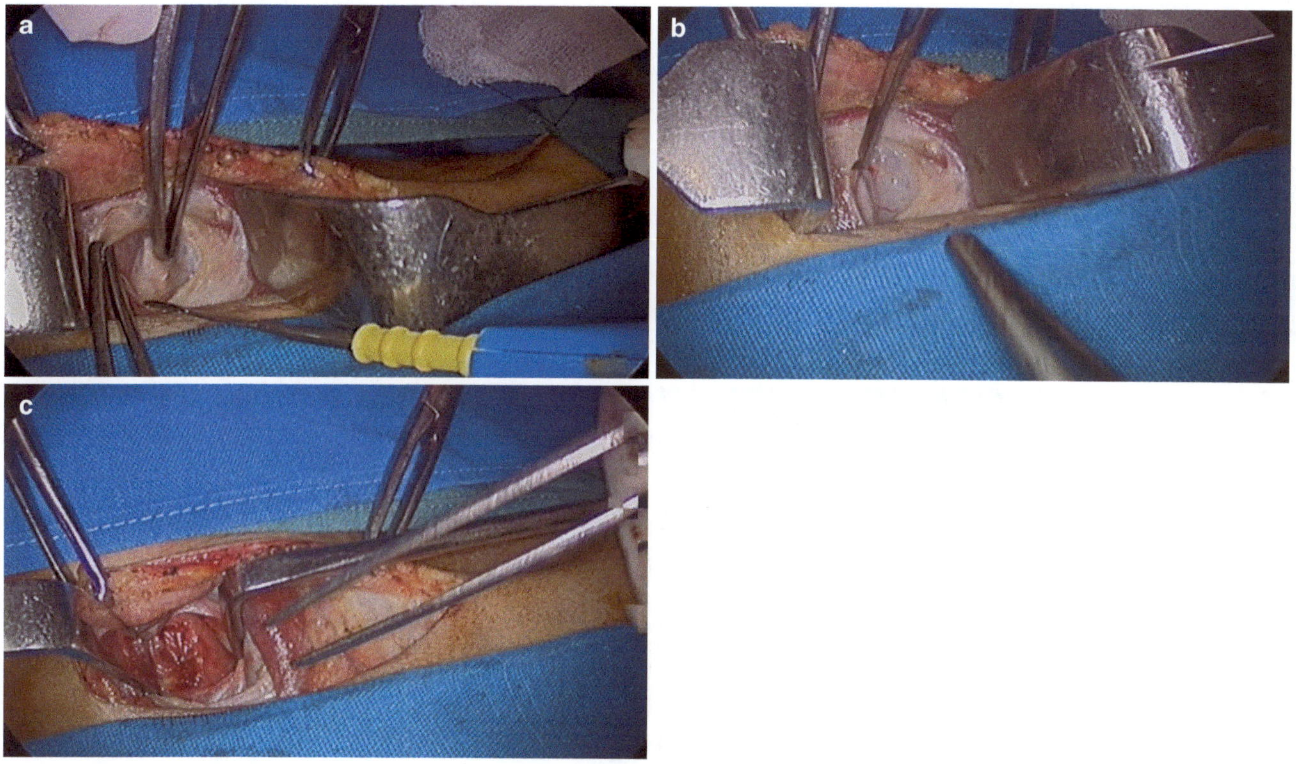

Photo 4.74 (a-c)

3. A plane is created between the two heads of sternocledomastoid (Photo 4.74a–c).
4. The esophagus is then lifted from the bed (Photo 4.75a, b).
5. Two lateral stay sutures are placed on the proximal esophagus (Photo 4.76a, b).

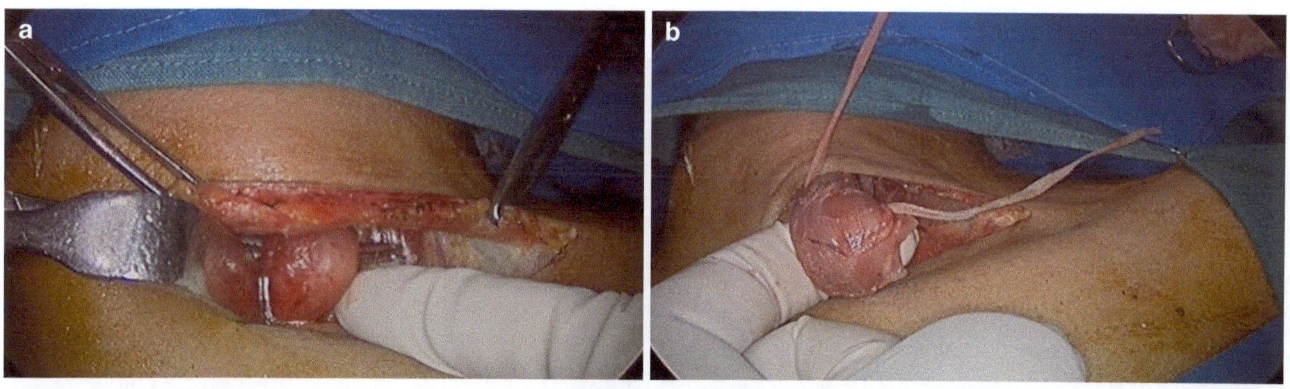

Photo 4.75 (a, b)

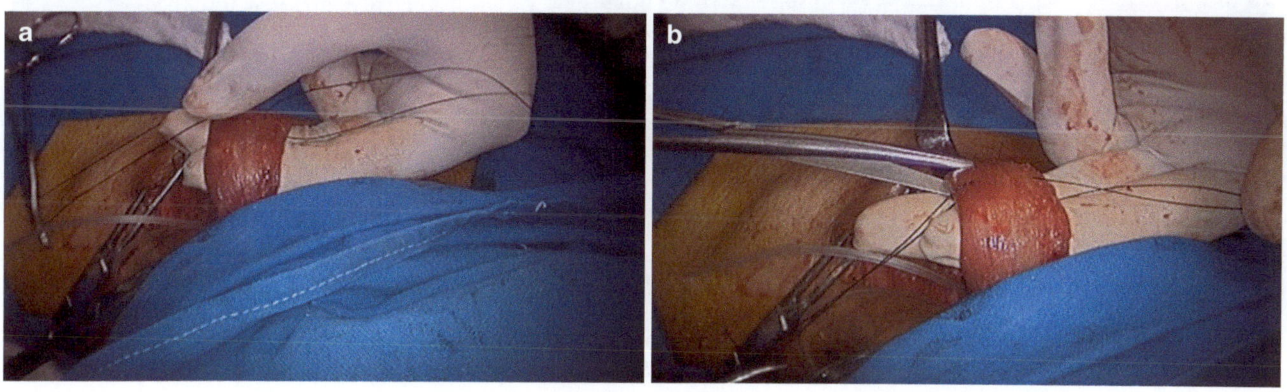

Photo 4.76 (a, b)

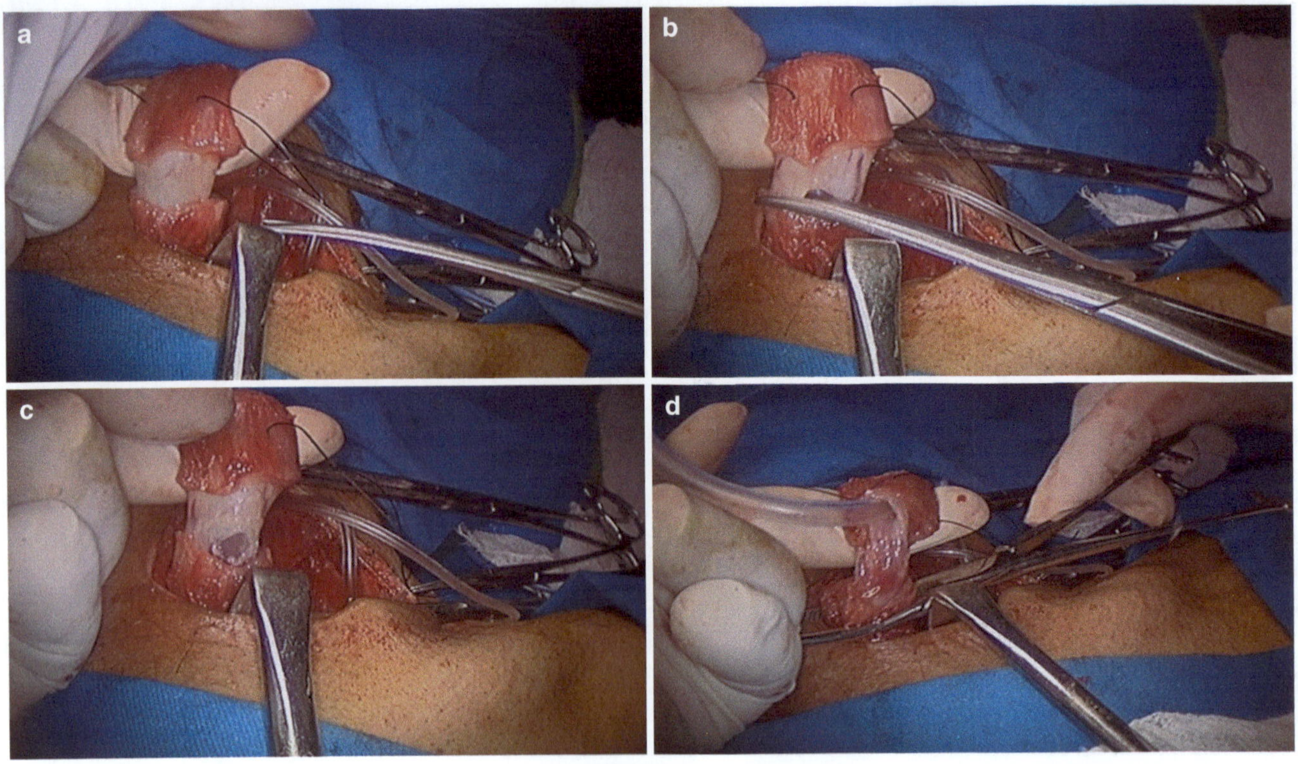

Photo 4.77 (a-d)

6. On the proximal end, the mucosal and sumucosal level of transection is kept 2–3 mm distal to the transection of the muscle layers (Photo 4.77a–d).

7. The distal cut end of the esophagus is tied and a Levine tube is transfixed to it (Photo 4.78a–d).

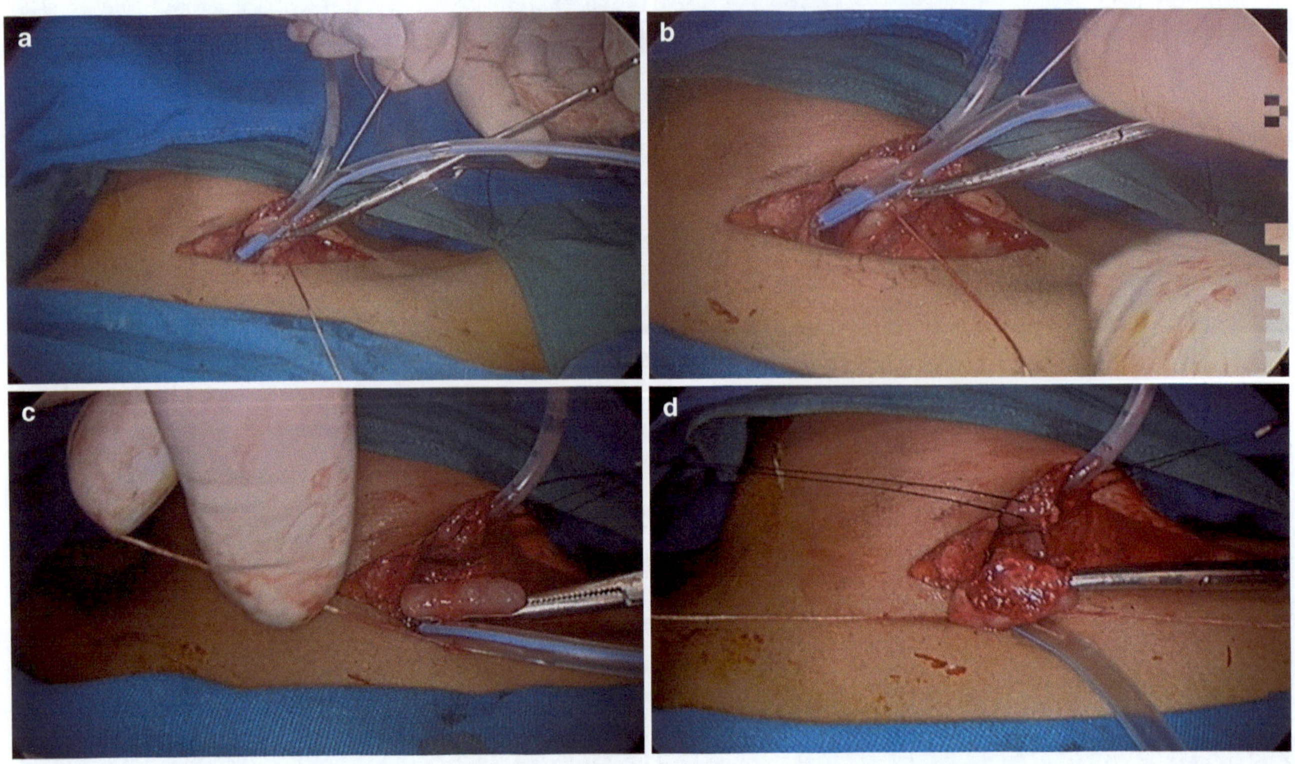

Photo 4.78 (a-d)

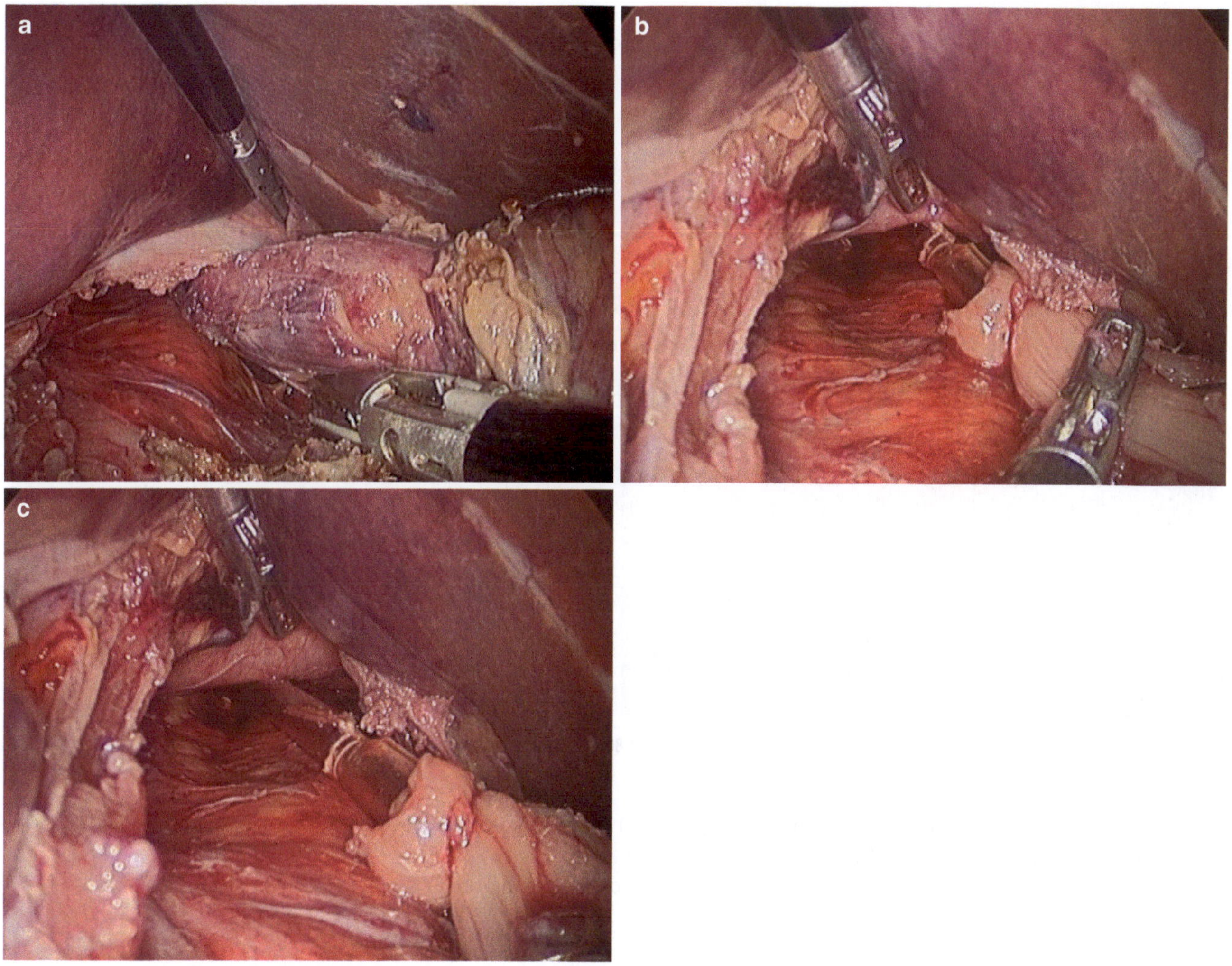

Photo 4.79 (a-c)

Specimen Retrieval and Preparation of Gastric Tube

1. The esophagus is pulled into the abdominal cavity (Photo 4.79a–c).

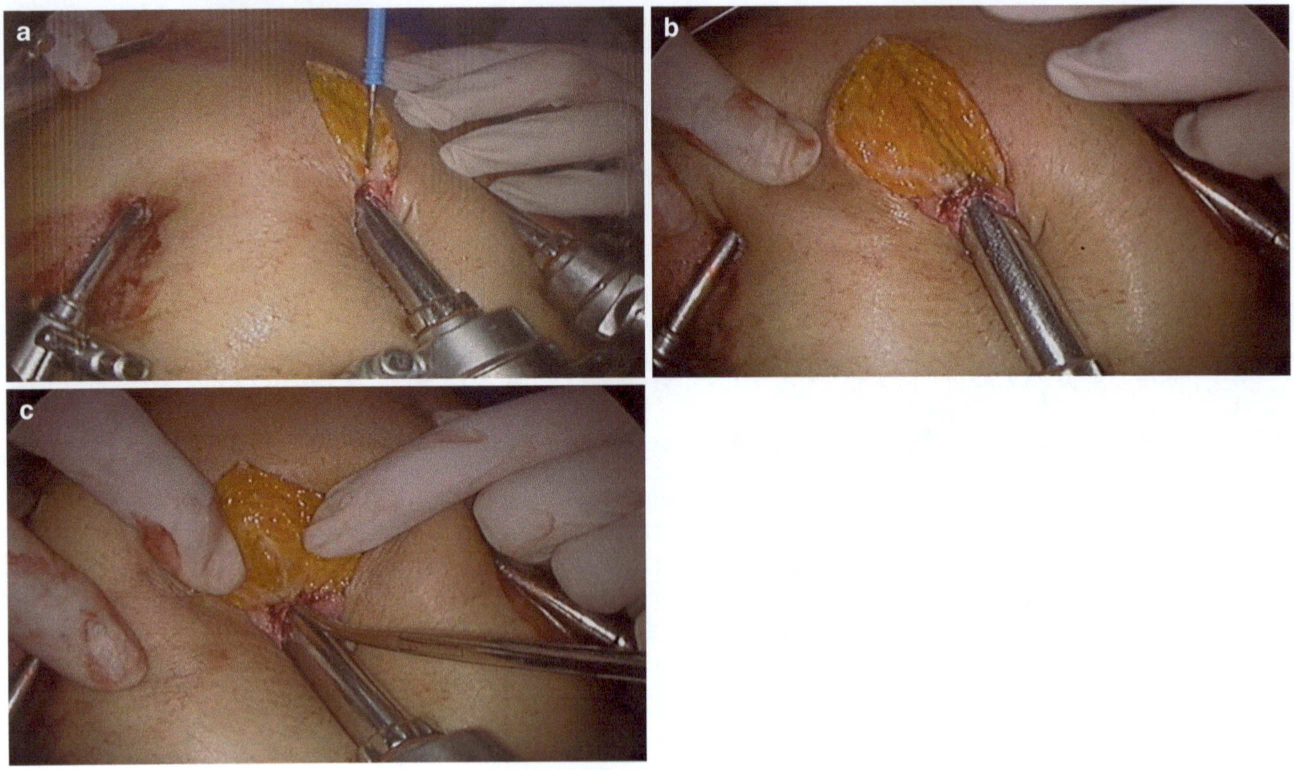

Photo 4.80 (a-c)

2. A small midline incision (usually 5 cm in thin patients) is used to deliver the specimen and the stomach outside the abdomen (Photo 4.80a–c).

3. A stomach tube of 5–6 cm width is prepared extracorporeally, using linear staplers (Photo 4.81a–g).

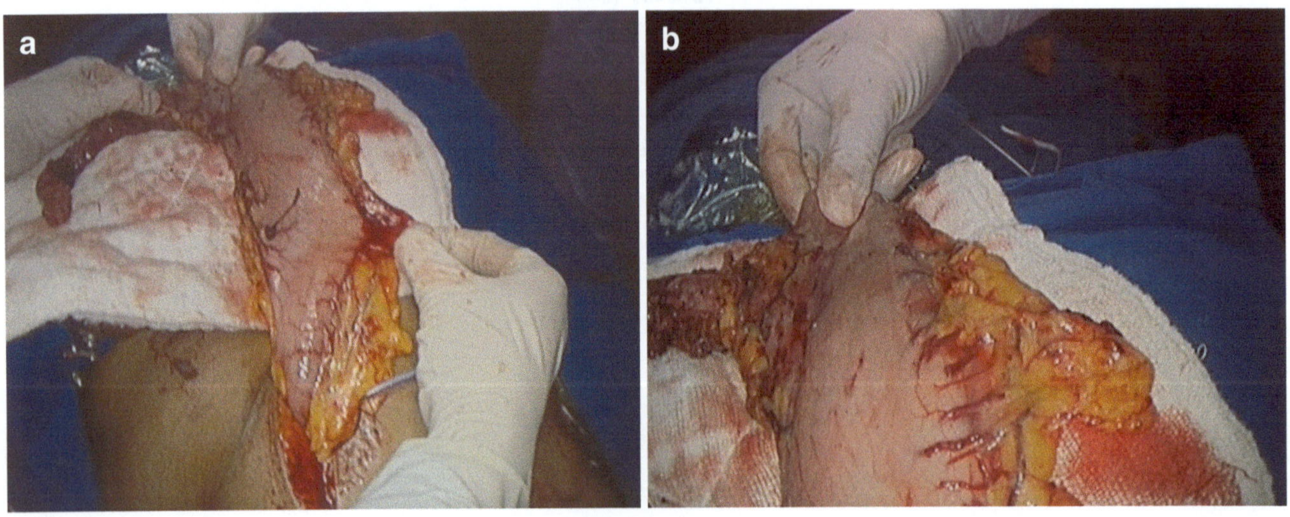

Photo 4.81 (a-g)

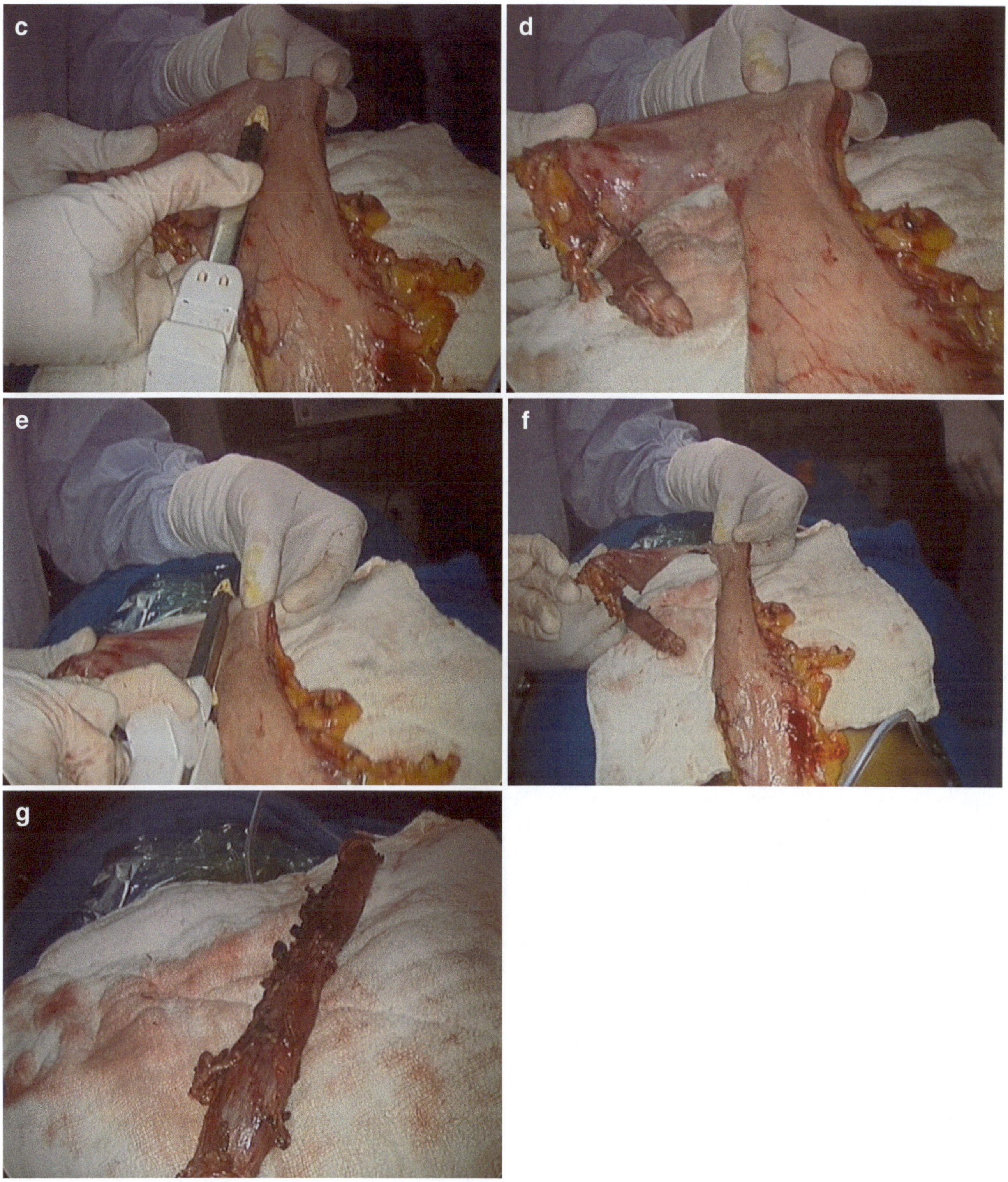

Photo 4.81 (Continued)

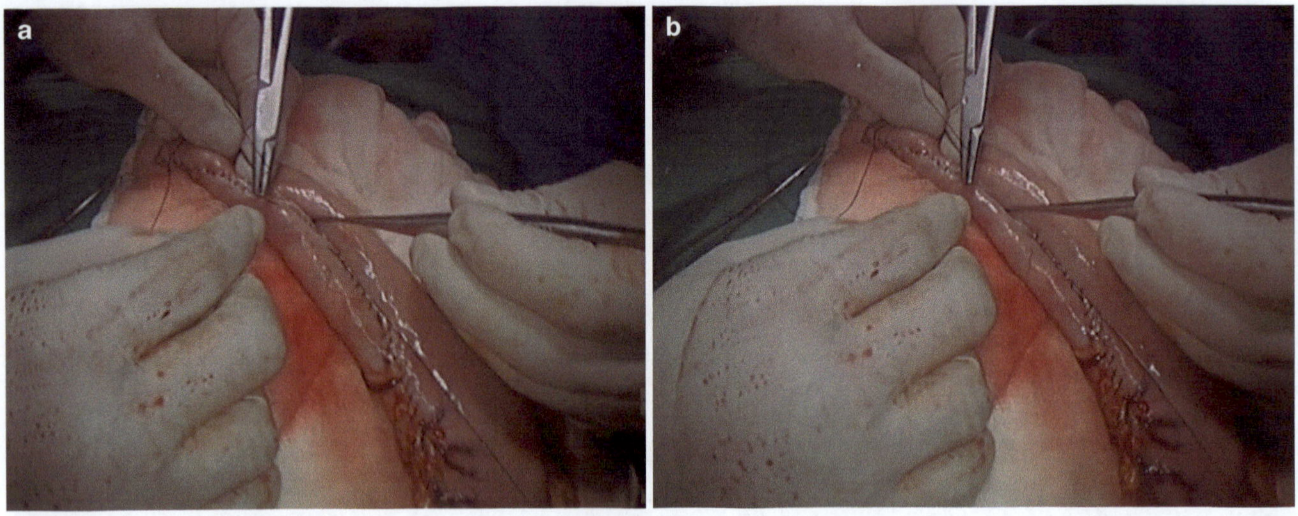

Photo 4.82 (a, b)

4. The staple-line is reinforced by continuous 3:0 running sutures (silk or PDS) (Photo 4.82a, b).

5. The Levine tube is transfixed to the stomach tube on its anterior wall. The conduit is thus pulled into the neck (Photo 4.83a, b).

6. A feeding jejunostomy is performed in all patients (Photo 4.84).

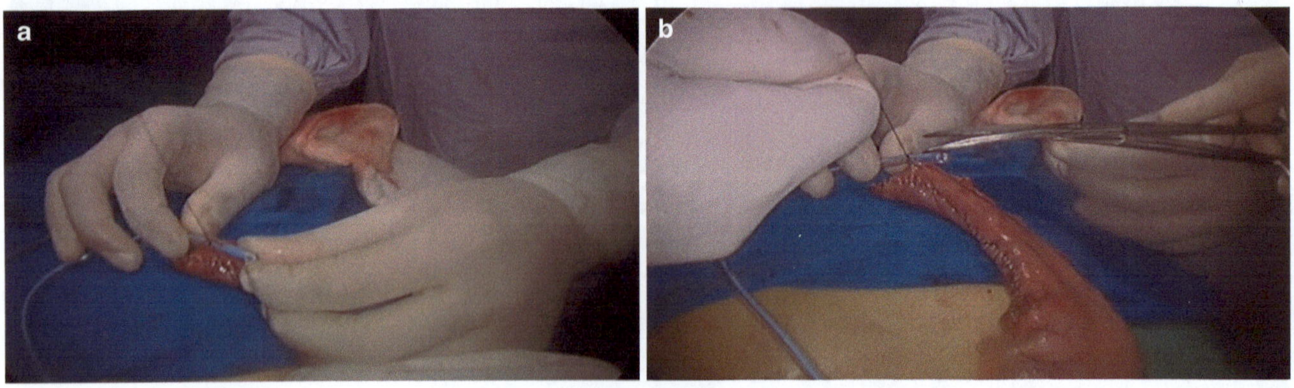

Photo 4.83 (a, b)

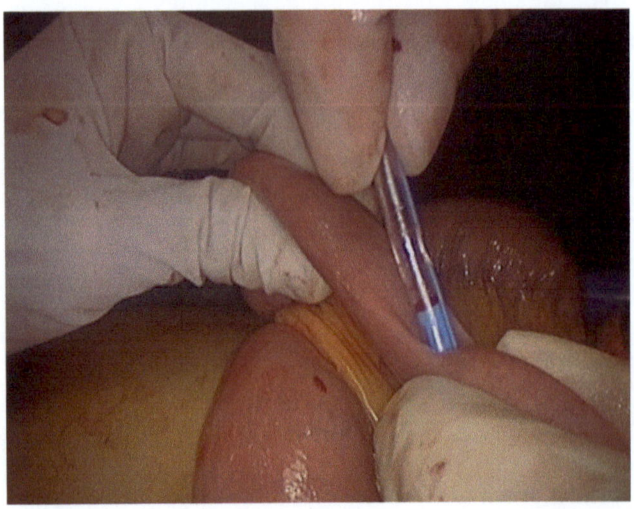

Photo 4.84

Esophago-Gastric Anastomoses

1. The esophagus is anastomosed to the posterior wall near the apex of the gastric conduit to create an inverted ink-bottle effect (Photo 4.85a, b).
2. A posterior layer of seromuscular interrupted 3:0 silk sutures are taken (Photo 4.86a, b).
3. An opening is made on the stomach wall with a diathermy (Photo 4.87a, b).

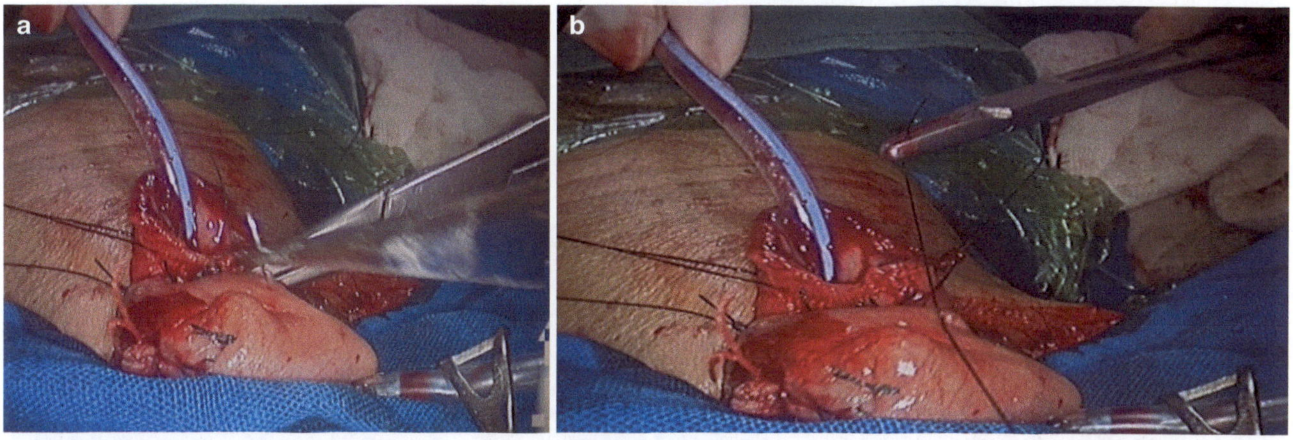

Photo 4.85 (a, b)

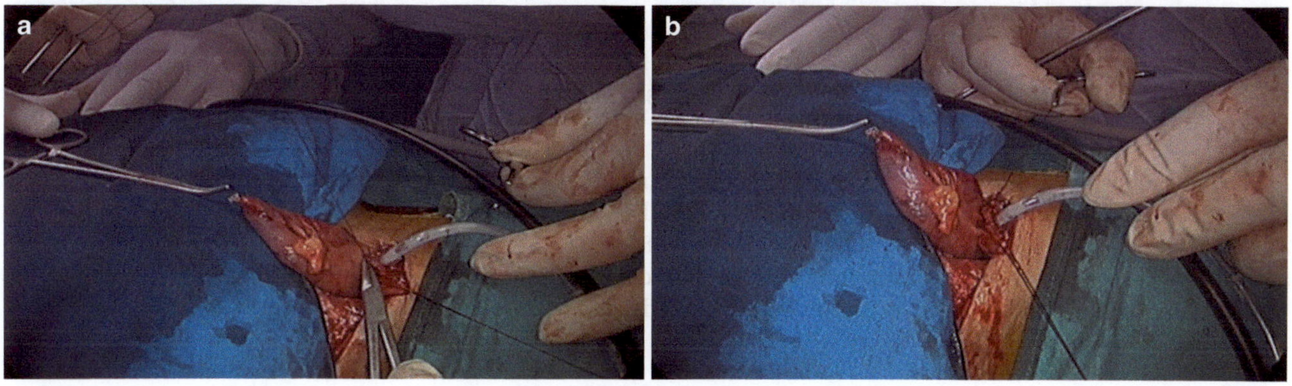

Photo 4.86 (a, b)

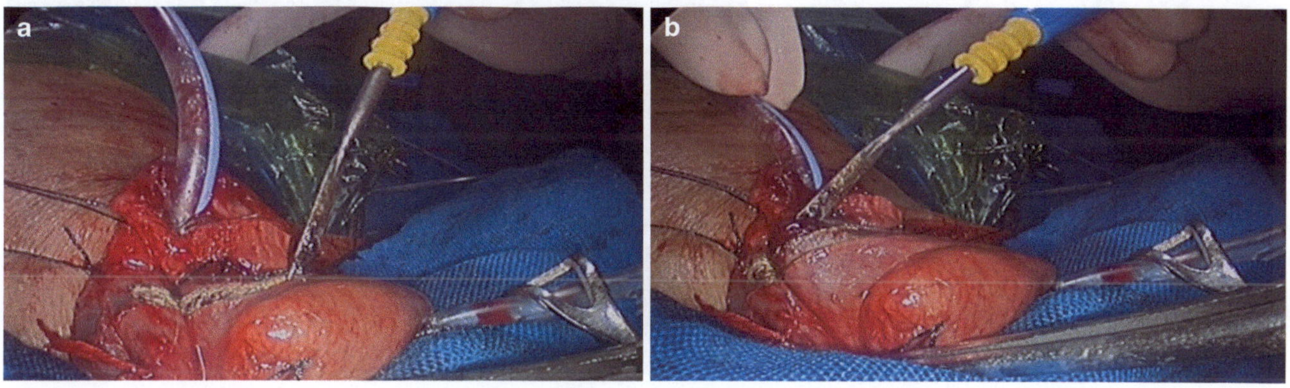

Photo 4.87 (a, b)

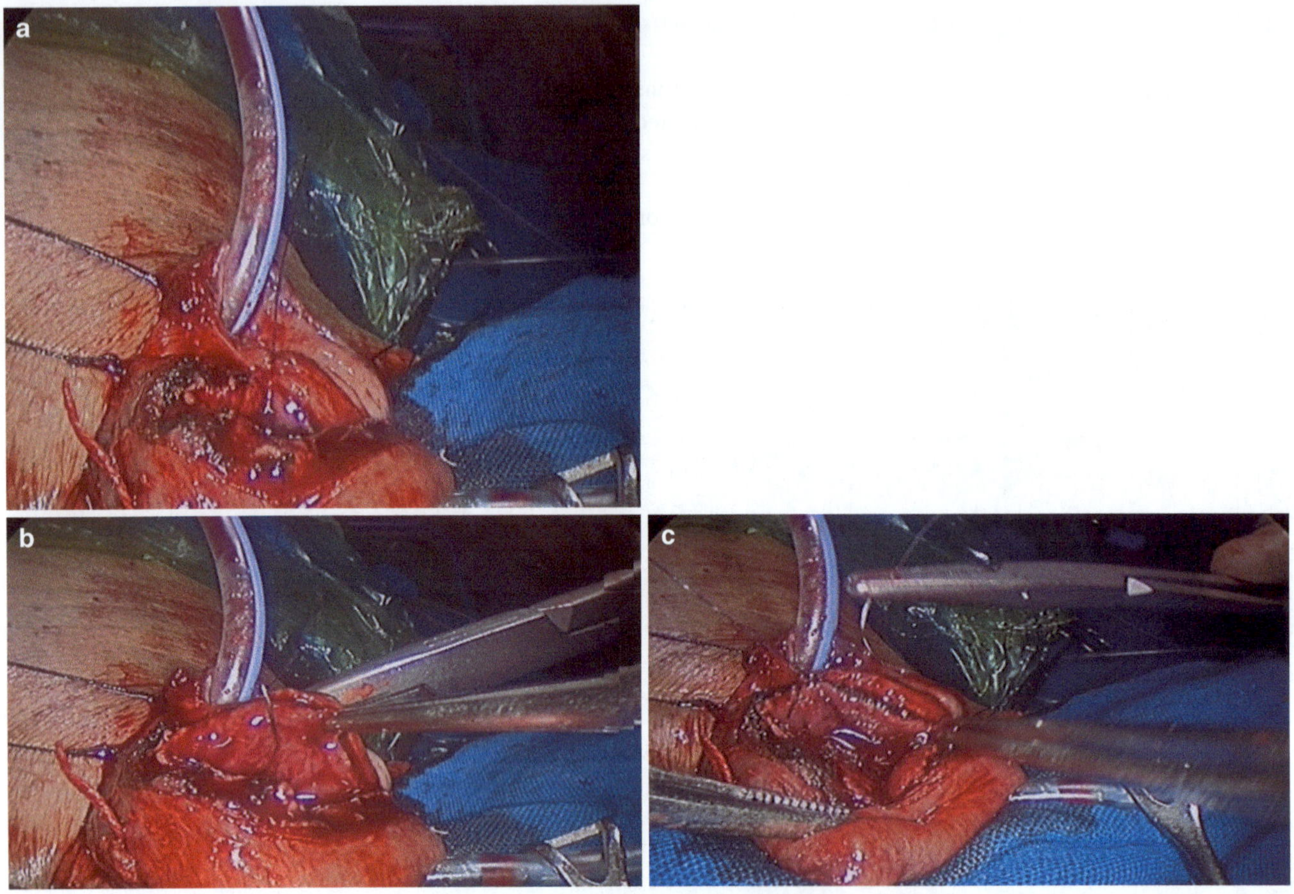

Photo 4.88 (a-c)

4. Continuous full-thickness sutures of 4:0 PDS/Vicryl are taken. This is the second layer and includes the full thickness of the posterior wall of the stomach and full-thickness of the posterior wall of the esophagus (Photo 4.88a–c).

5. A nasogastric tube is passed across the anastomosis and the second layer is continued anteriorly as the third layer. A fourth layer of interrupted 3:0 silk/PDS seromuscular sutures completes the anastomosis (Photo 4.89a, b).

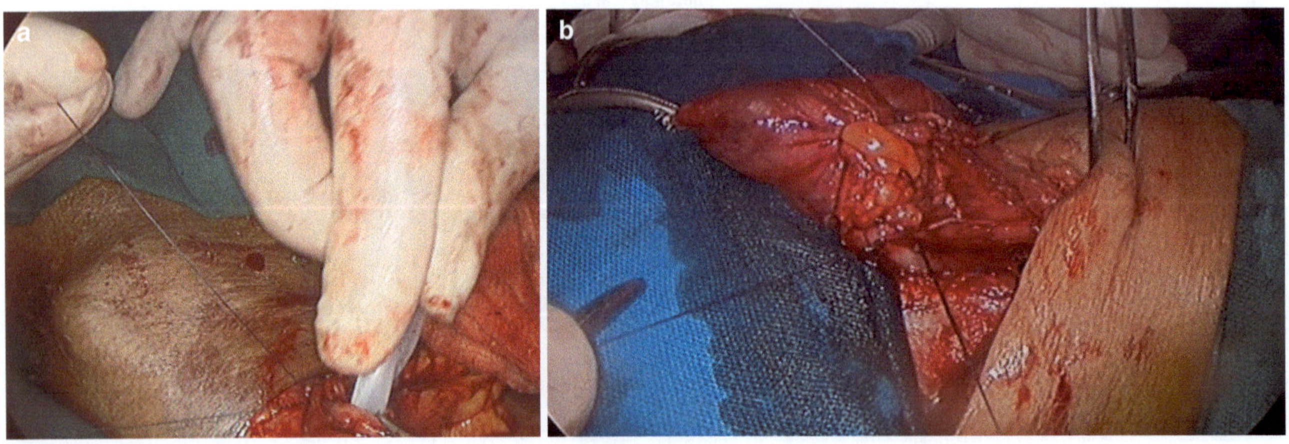

Photo 4.89 (a, b)

Complications and Their Management

(a) Thoracoscopic Part

A left pleural tear is relieved by inserting an intercostal drainage tube in the left second or third intercostal space. It is difficult to insert it because of the position of the patient.

Excessive stretching of the azygous vein can cause the vein to tear and so the vein should not be excessively stretched. Metal clips on the azygous can slip; hence, preferably vascular locking clips should be used. In case of injury, the vein should be promptly grasped with the left-hand grasper and clipped through the right-hand working port.

The direct aortic branches should be clipped and not taken with bipolar or any other energy source. Metal clips are not used for the direct branches of the aorta in the thorax, since they can slip due to the respiratory movements.

The thoracic duct should be identified and injury to it avoided. If clear lymphatic fluid is seen oozing out, the duct injury should be identified and the duct clipped.

Bleeding near the hilar regions and carina is common and is controlled best by bipolar and packing with a gauze strip for some time.

Injury to the recurrent laryngeal nerves is to be guarded against near the aortic arch and the tracheo-esophageal groove.

The posterior wall of trachea is membranous and dissecting near it is done with extreme caution. Use of energy sources should be completely restricted near the nerves, the membranous trachea or very close to the bronchi.

Lung injury commonly occurs if the lung is not completely deflated during insertion of the first port or in the presence of adhesions. If adhesions are suspected in advance, then a finger can be inserted through a small incision and the adhesions separated before inserting the port. Small lung injuries usually stop bleeding due to the pressure applied when retracting the lung upward.

If for any reason conversion to open thoracotomy is deemed necessary, it can be done without changing the position of the patient and is thus performed expeditiously in an emergency. This is as opposed to the prone position for thoracoscopic esophagectomy, where the patient needs to be turned for an emergency thoracotomy. We do not find difficulty in exposure during thoracoscopic esophagectomy in the lateral position, provided the right lung is completely deflated by the anesthetist. Moreover, the thoracoscopic anatomy is easier to understand for surgeons who are used to performing this surgery by the open technique. Our experience is, that dissections above the level of the arch of aorta are always more difficult in the prone position as compared to the lateral position. Hence we find the lateral approach to be preferable in supra-carinal growths.

(b) Laparoscopic Part

It is better to remain cautiously away from the splenic hilum when sealing the short-gastric vessels. They should thus be taken close to the stomach wall, since bleeding at the splenic hilum is often difficult to control laparoscopically. Clips are used judiciously in this area when required.

(c) Neck Dissection

The orientation of the stomach conduit is always checked to avoid twisting.

Care is taken during mobilization of the esophagus in the neck not to injure the left recurrent laryngeal nerve in the tracheo-esophageal groove. The posterior wall of the trachea is membranous and extreme care is taken not to tear it during the mobilization of the esophagus in the upper mediastinum.

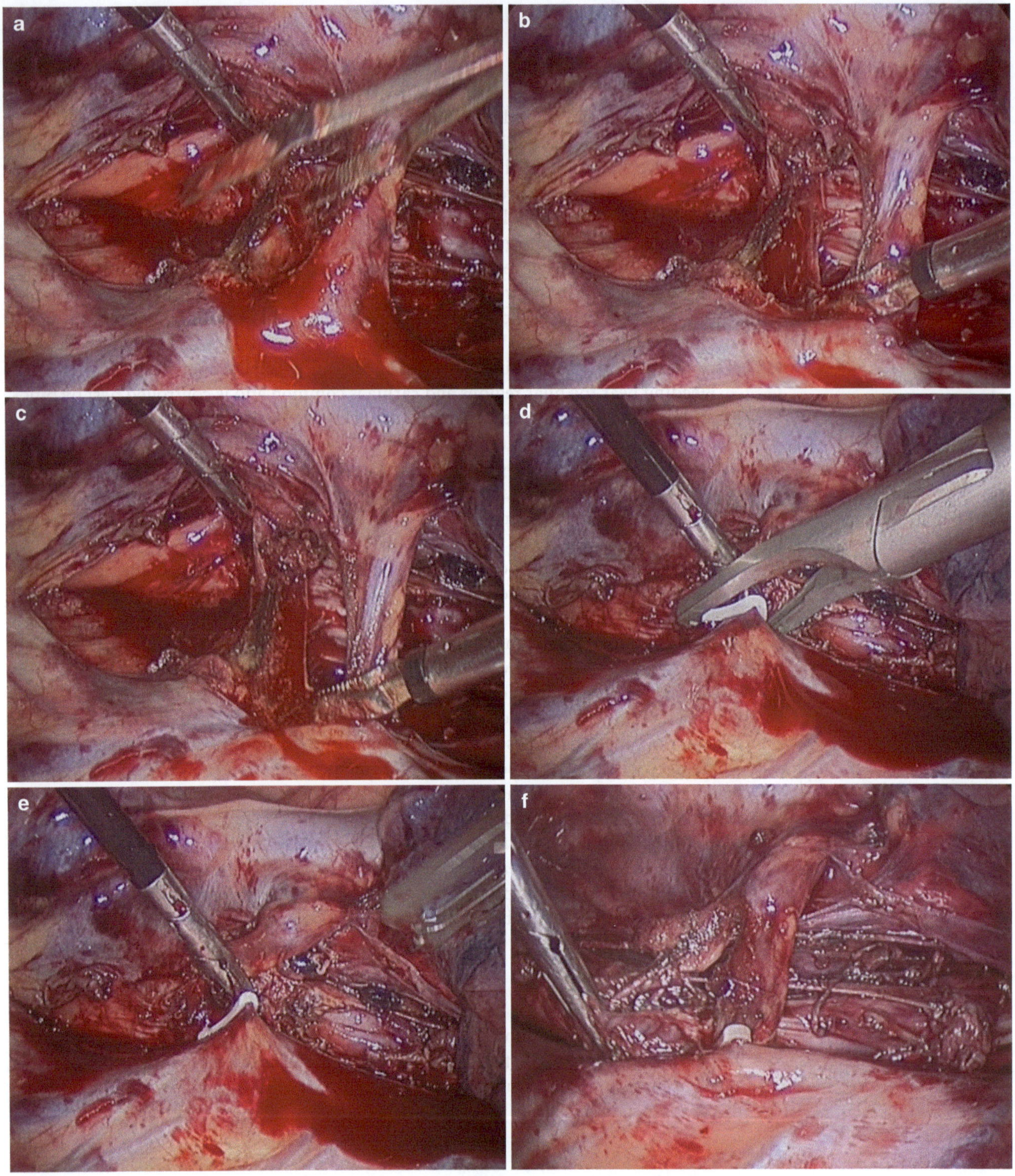

Photo 4.90 (a-f)

Photos of Some Complications

1. *Minor azygous vein bleed:* During nodal clearance at the level of azygous vein, minor bleeding from the azygous vein may take place. It should be identified before major vein injury. Keep the left hand free and compress the azygous vein. A hemoclip may then be applied to stop the bleeding (Photo 4.90a–f).

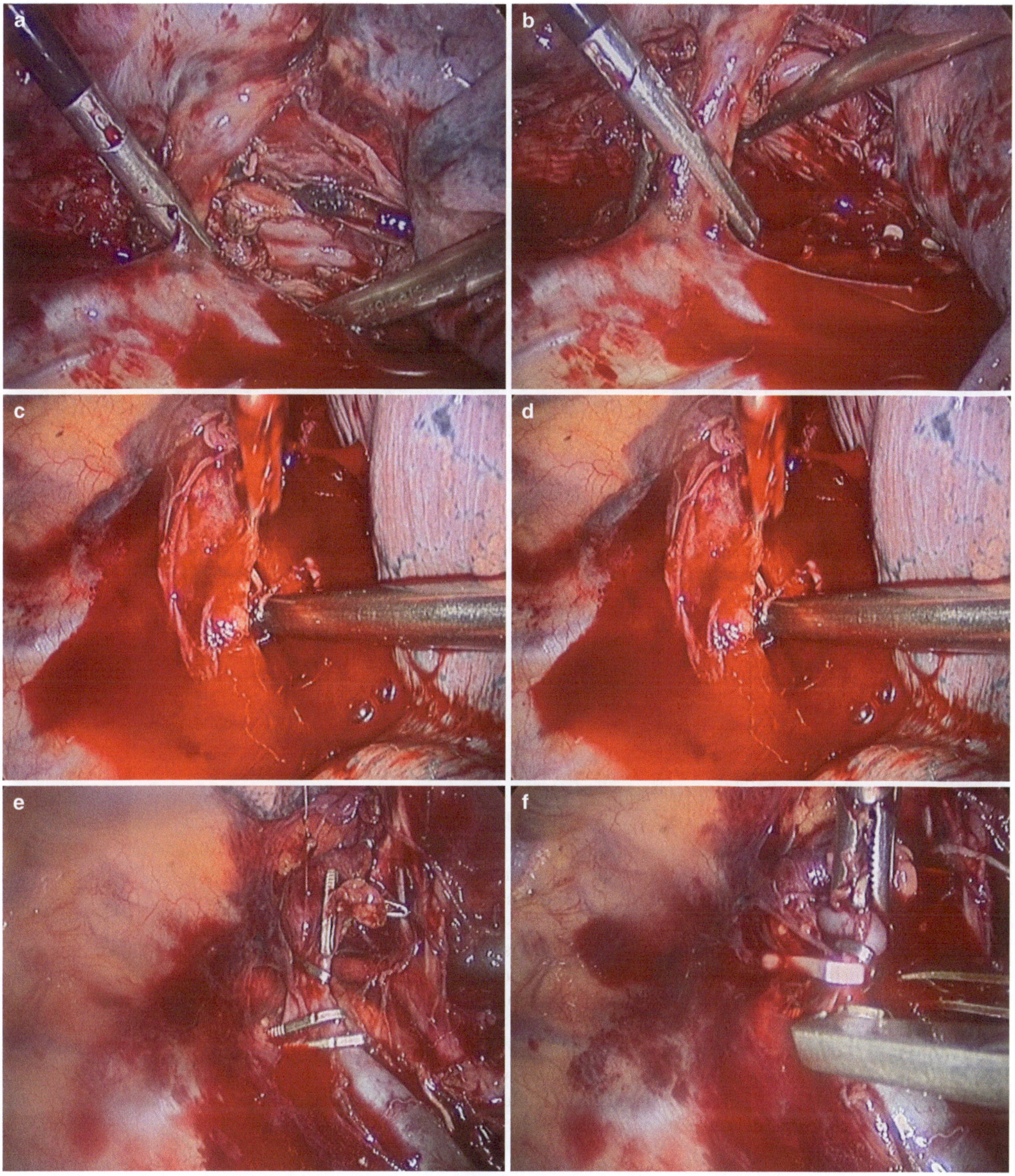

Photo 4.91 (a-f)

2. *Major azygous vein bleed:* The underlying tumor may lead to stretching of the azygous vein making it vulnerable for injury. The left-hand grasper should compress the vein. One additional port may be inserted for sucking the blood. Temporary control of hemorrhage is done by application of metal clips. Finally the azygous vein is clipped with hemolok clips (Photo 4.91a–f).

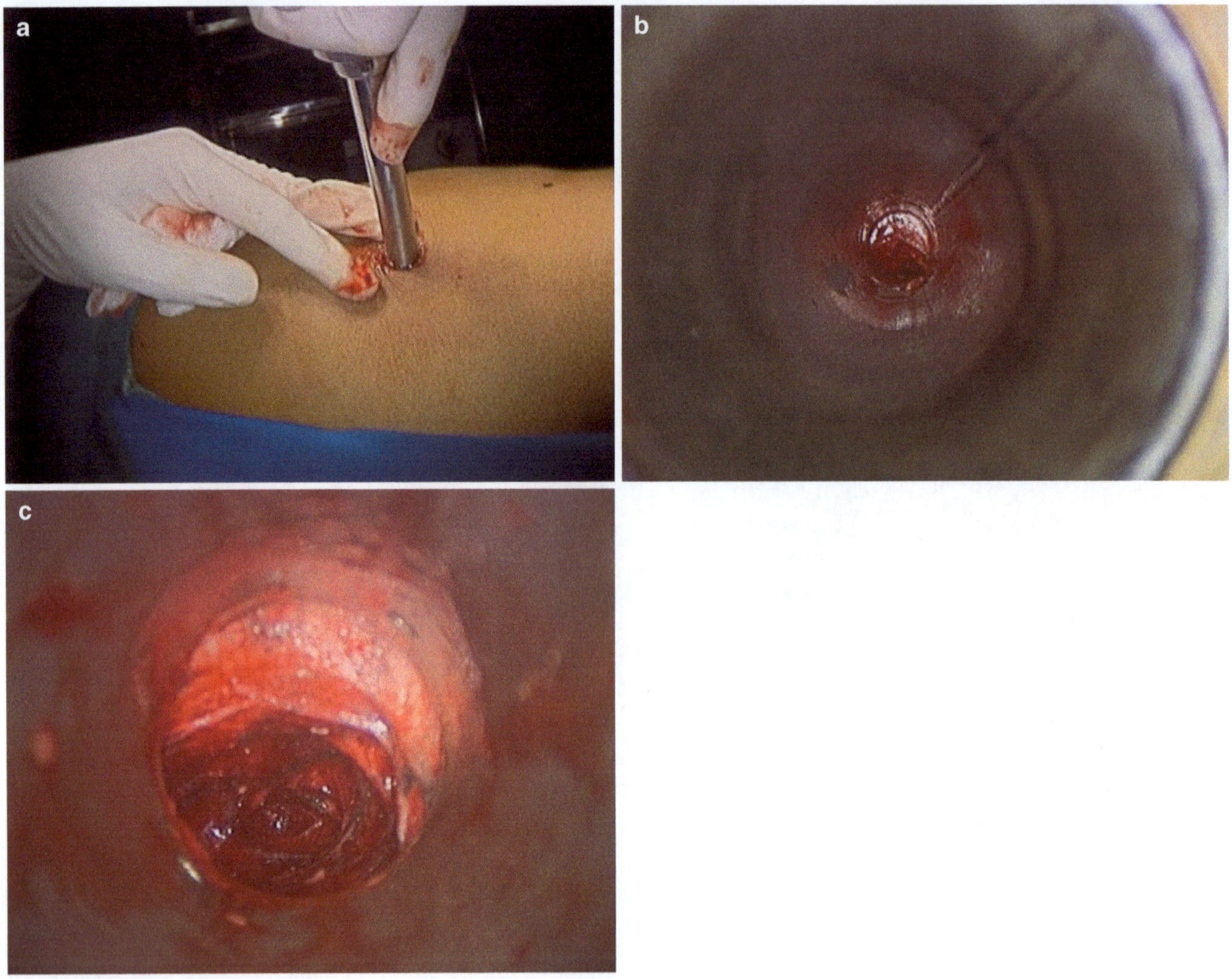

Photo 4.92 (a-c)

3. *Lung injury:* The lung is prone to injury during the insertion of primary trocar. This is likely to happen when lung is not collapsed. Before insufflation one can notice the trocar entry into the lung. Withdraw the trocar and ask the anesthetist to collapse the lung. Insufflate CO_2 and look for injury. Usually the injury is minor and is due to entry into the lung parenchyma. The bleeding can be stopped by using bipolar forceps. Major vascular or bronchial injuries are unknown in lateral position as the first trocar entry is in the posterior axillary line (Photo 4.92a–c).

4. *Thoracic duct injury:* The thoracic duct is usually very well-identified. Sometimes it gets lifted along with the tumor and may be seen as a shiny tubular/beaded structure. On its identification it is usually better to clip the duct. At the end of surgery one should reexamine the entire thoracic duct area. If any lymph is seen oozing, it is advisable to clip the duct again (Photo 4.93a, b).

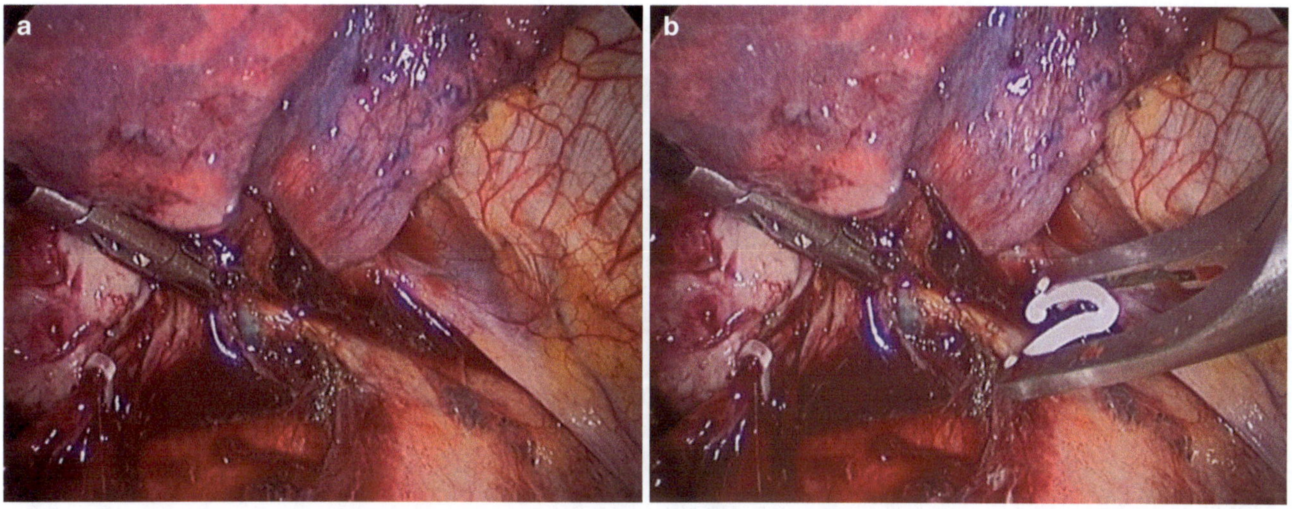

Photo 4.93 (a, b)

5. *Liver injury:* The liver injury is due to the retraction by the grasper. This is common in patients with a large, floppy left lobe. The parenchymal injury can be identified. One can compress the liver with the use of gauze, or the bleeding can be stopped using bipolar energy source (Photo 4.94a–c).

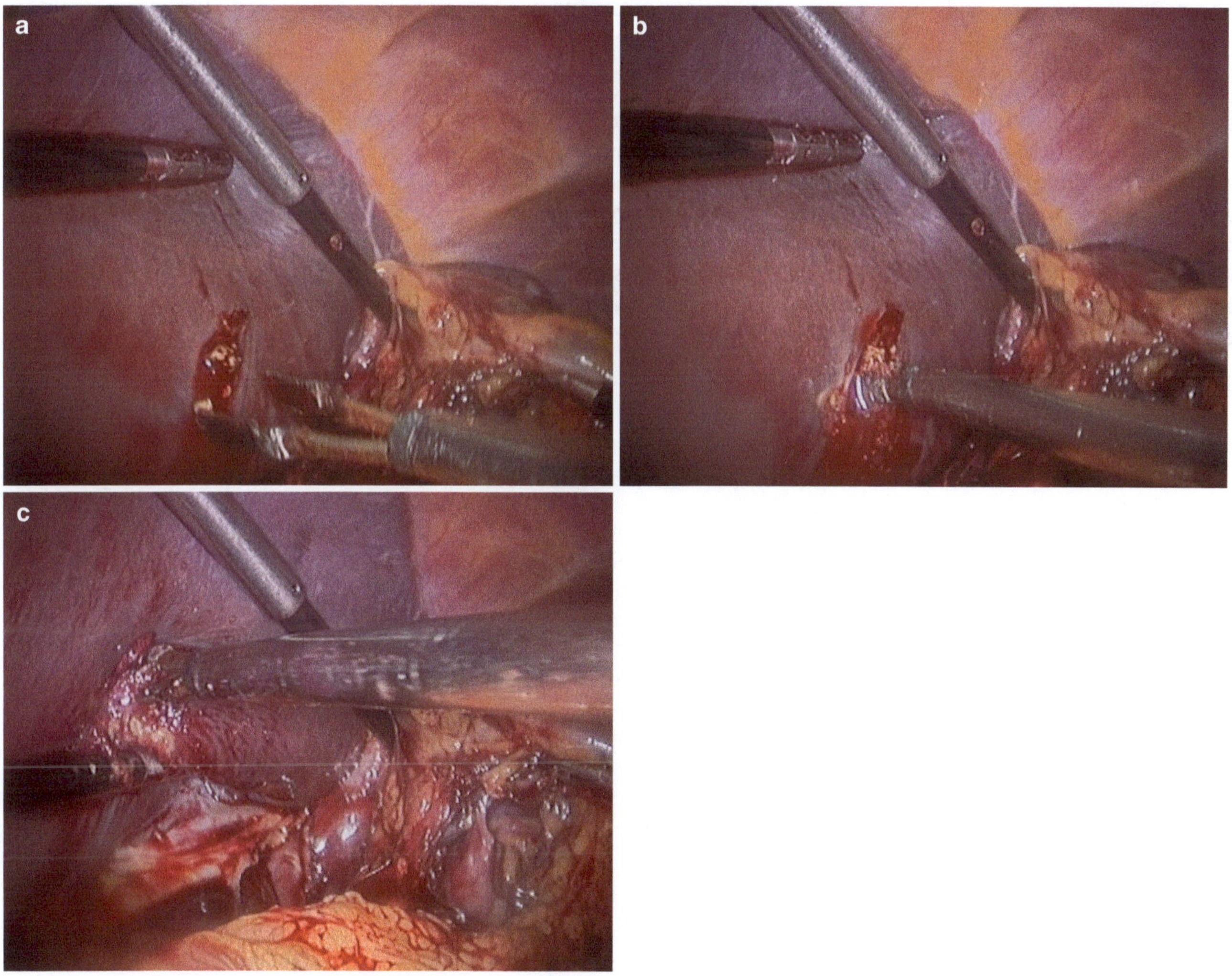

Photo 4.94 (a-c)

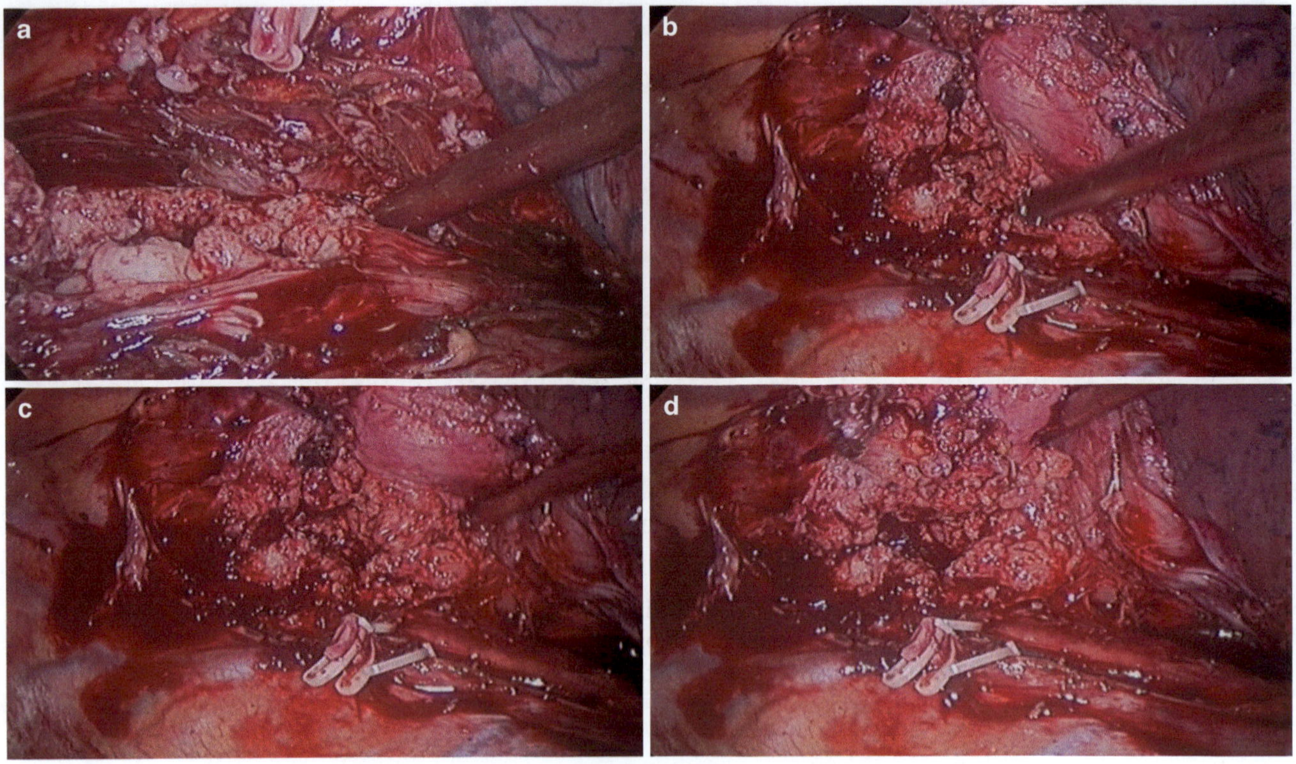

Photo 4.95 (a-d)

6. *Entry in to the tumor:* Large tumors have to be handled carefully especially in those patients who have received anterior chemotherapy or radiotherapy. This injury takes place when one tries to lift the esophagus from its bed. The entire tumour which has been spilled, as well as the saliva, should be aspirated and removed with a suction canula. Then an attempt must be made to complete the dissection of the entire esophagus. Then, try and complete the entire esophageal dissection. The ruptured esophagus should then be removed transthoracic by putting it into the endobag. One should avoid thoracoscopic esophagectomy in large, lengthy, bulky tumors. Over enthusiastic approach may lead to esophageal rupture/perforation (Photo 4.95a–d).

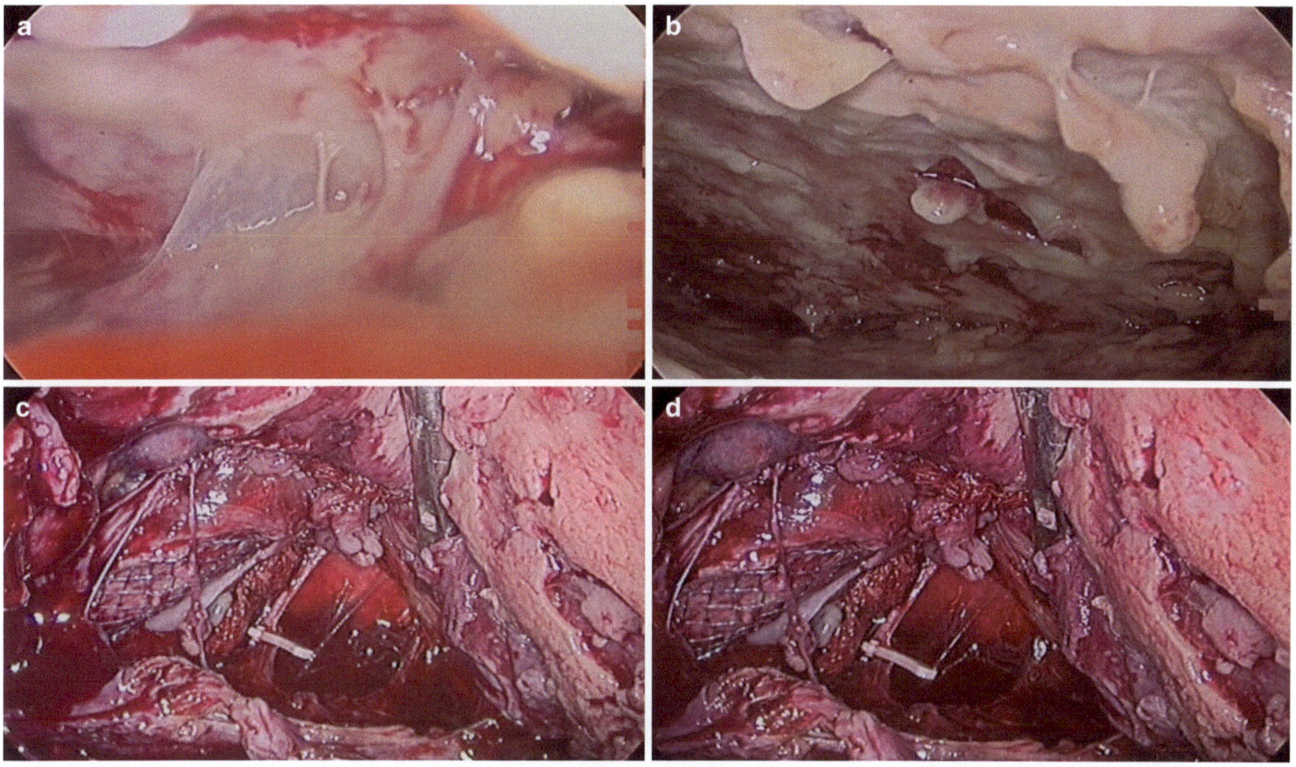

Photo 4.96 (a-d)

7. *Thoracoscopy in post-stenting patient with esophageal rupture:* esophageal ruptures following esophageal biopsies are known. But sometimes a perforation may take place following stenting. We have swhown a few pictures of one such patient who had esophageal perforation following stenting. The stent can be seen in the mediastinum along with esophageal perforation (Photo 4.96a–d).

5

Laparoscopic Transhiatal Esophagectomy

Shailesh Puntambekar, Rajan B. Jagad, and Anjali M. Patil

Introduction

Transhiatal esophagectomy is essentially performed for cancers of the lower one third of esophagus or tumors at the gastro-esophageal junction.

Laparoscopic transhiatal esophagectomy has converted an essentially blind procedure in to a directly visualized procedure wherein every step can be well demonstrated. The magnification helps to achieve the precise planes of dissection with minimal chances of damaging the pleura. During preparation of the conduit, there is less handling of the stomach, so a laparoscopically mobilized stomach tube is better vascularized.

CO_2 insufflation facilitates mediastinal dissection; the direct branches of the aorta to the esophagus are clearly identified and clipped. Therefore the chances of bleeding are minimized. The thoracic duct is also clipped, hence chylous leaks are minimized.

The precise dissection and minimal blood loss helps lower the morbidity. This procedure has no effect on either the total hospital stay or commencement of oral feeds.

Indications of Laparoscopic Transhiatal Esophagectomy (THE)

1. Cancers of the lower one third of the esophagus
2. Cancers of the upper one third of the esophagus
3. Post-cricoid cancers(requiring laryngo-pharyngectomy with gastric pull-up)
4. Lower-middle one-third tumors with poor PFTs (pulmonary function tests)
5. Cardio-esophageal tumors

Contraindications

1. Cancers of the middle one third of the esophagus
2. Heavy nodal burden in the mediastinum

Investigations

Chest radiograph, barium swallow studies, endoscopic biopsy, and computed tomography (CT scan) are routinely done. Positron emission tomography (PET), MRI, EUS, and bronchoscopy may be required in addition. CT or EUS can determine the anatomic location and enlargement of the mediastinal, perigastric, or celiac lymph nodes.

Routine blood chemistry and medical evaluation for pulmonary and cardiac status is done. Nutritional assessment and perioperative preparation are important since a major cause of mortality is malnutrition and the majority of patients are nutritionally debilitated. The pulmonary function tests (PFTs) are also performed.

Preoperative Preparation

Patients are admitted at least 2 days prior to surgery.

Respiratory exercises in the form of incentive spirometry are begun 2 days prior to surgery. A central venous access is taken. Intravenous antibiotics are started a day prior to the surgery.

Anesthesia

A combination of regional (epidural) and general anesthesia is used. Hypotensive anesthesia is an important part of the procedure and helps to minimize blood loss.

Patient, Port, and Surgeon Positions

The patient is placed in a Modified Lloyd Davis position with neck extension.

For the laparoscopic part, the operating surgeon stands in the space between the legs of the patient. The camera assistant is on the left of the operating surgeon. The first assistant surgeon stands on the right side of the patient. A second assistant stands on the left of the patient. A second monitor is placed on the right of the patient for the assistant to view.

A Verress needle is introduced through the Palmer's point to create pneumoperitoneum.

- A primary, 11-mm port is inserted at the junction of the upper two third and lower one third of the line joining the xiphisternum to the umbilicus. This is the camera port.
- An 11-mm working port is inserted in the left and a 6-mm working port is inserted on the right of the camera port.
- The working ports are inserted in the right pararectal area in the midclavicular line.
- The distance between the working and the camera port should be at least equal to the combined breadth of four fingers. The working port should form a triangle on front of the camera port.
- A 6-mm port is inserted in the epigastrium. A blunt grasper passed through this port is used to retract the left lobe of the liver.
- Another 6-mm port is placed on the left in anterior axillary line at the level of the umbilicus. This is used by the second assistant on the left side. This is used mainly to retract the stomach or to lift it up. The patient is given a 15° head-up position before starting the procedure. (See photos 5.1 to 5.3)

Procedure

The procedure starts by cutting the gastrohepatic omentum in its avascular part and identifying the right crus of diaphragm. This can be visualized by retracting the left lobe of liver with an atraumatic grasper, inserted through the 5-mm port at the xiphisternum. This instrument is used like a stick, the tip supported against the diaphragm and the shaft lifting the liver. The esophageal mobilization is done prior to the stomach mobilization, so that the stomach acts as a natural retractor and steadies the esophagus during dissection. The assistant on the left pulls the stomach downward and to left, stretching the peritoneum over the right crus.

Defining the Hiatus

The peritoneum over the right crus is incised using a harmonic scalpel. The retro-esophageal plane is entered by blunt dissection. The pneumoperitoneum helps to open this space further. The peritoneal cut over the right crus is extended upward, toward the apex of hiatus thus completely exposing the right crural fibers.

The next step is to identify the posterior vagus. Once the vagus is identified the dissection should continue posterior to the vagus and not between the vagus and esophagus. Dissection between the vagus and esophagus can lead to troublesome bleeding. The left-hand grasper lifts up the esophagus along with the vagus and the dissection posterior to the vagus is continued till the left crural fibers are visualized. The posterior window is enlarged till the dome of the diaphragm is seen. The esophagus is continuously retracted anteriorly and caudally with the left-hand grasper during this dissection. This traction is further enhanced by the second assistant on the left, by pulling on the fundus of the stomach.

The dissection then proceeds to the right side of the esophagus. The right pleural reflection can be seen at this stage. The pleura is gently reflected off the esophagus. This dissection is better done with the left-hand grasper, or using the tip of a suction catheter, carefully pushing the pleura away as far as possible.

CO_2 insufflation aids this dissection. Inadvertent pleural injury is managed by insertion of an ICD tube. However, a pleural injury at this stage can be extremely troublesome, since it leads to continuous loss of pneumoperitoneum.

Once the right pleura and hiatus are defined, intra-hiatal dissection is started.

Posterior Dissection

The esophagus is retracted anteriorly by the left-hand grasper along with the posterior vagus which is now clearly defined. Dissection is begun between the aorta and esophagus, again remaining behind the nerve. The paraesophageal nodes are removed with the esophagus. The entire fibro-fatty tissue over the aorta is also removed. The posterior dissection is done either with the harmonic shears or with the suction canula. The direction of the dissection should be from the aorta toward the esophagus, sweeping all the tissues toward the esophagus.

A few direct branches of the aorta supplying the esophagus are seen as vertical strands. It is better to use clips to seal these vessels before cutting them, since these are direct aortic branches, and are under high pressure. The use of bipolar or harmonic is not recommended for this purpose. Dissection is continued proximally behind the esophagus. This is again facilitated by the CO_2 gas which enters the planes of dissection.

Dissection on the Right Side

Once the esophagus is completely mobilized on the posterior aspect, the same plane of dissection is used to push the right wall of esophagus further away from the pleura. During this dissection, the esophagus is retracted to the left side with a grasper to further dissect the plane on the right side, proceeding cranially.

The upper limit of dissection is the right main bronchus which is better palpated than visualized. The hemiazygous may be seen at this stage to the right of the esophagus. The azygous vein is not seen, as it lies above the right main bronchus. Dissection above the level of carina is not possible due to the presence of the aortic arch, which limits the dissection. The posterior vagus is cut at the level of right main bronchus. The esophagus can be pulled further to the left and the dissection continued further cranially on the right side. The traction on the esophagus toward the left is accomplished with the left-hand grasper but can also be maintained by the assistant on the left by pulling the cardio-esophageal junction.

Anterior Dissection

The esophagus is pulled caudally and posteriorly with the left hand. The anterior dissection, between the heart and esophagus, is the easiest part of dissection, as no major vascular structures are encountered here. The pericardium is a tough structure and is rarely involved by the disease. The dissection can often be achieved with blunt tipped instrument such as a suction cannula. The anterior space can be opened further by placing the assistant's grasper at the apex of hiatus for retraction. The carina is the upper limit of this dissection.

Left Sided Dissection

Once the right-sided, posterior, and anterior dissections are completed, the esophagus becomes mobile and thereby manipulation becomes more difficult. The left-sided dissection is commenced. The first assistant's grasper holds the left crus and pushes it to the left, to widen this space. The fundus and the entire stomach are rolled to the right side by the second assistant on the left. This exposes the cardio-esophageal junction on the left side and the peritoneum overlying it is cut. The left pleura is closely adherent here and care has to be taken to protect it from damage. Once the pleura is seen it is carefully reflected away from the esophagus by using the right-hand grasper, while the left hand pulls the esophagus.

The anterior vagus can be seen on the left side of the esophagus and is again an important landmark for dissection. The plane of dissection lies between the vagus and the left pleura and not between esophagus and vagus. By pulling on the vagus, sufficient traction can be applied facilitating dissection further cranially. Thus the vagus should not be cut early in the dissection. At this stage all paraesophageal nodes are removed with the esophagus. The dissection is done either with harmonic shears or with a suction canula. The cranial limit of dissection is the left main bronchus. The anterior vagus is cut at this level.

The esophagus is pushed to the right side and the sign of completed dissection is the visualization of descending aorta from the left side of esophagus. The esophagus is then pulled caudally and rolled to check that it is free all around its circumference.

Nodal Dissection

The nodal dissection at the coeliac axis is performed using the bipolar forceps or the Harmonic Ace (Ethicon Endo-surgery Inc. Cincinnati, OH). Nodes around the base of the left gastric vessels are dissected to delineate the left gastric artery and vein separately. The left gastric vein is clipped and cut. The common hepatic artery and the splenic artery are identified. The loose areolar tissue and nodes along the common hepatic artery are dissected and taken medially, along with the gastric nodes. The small vessels supplying the nodes may bleed, but the bleeding usually stops once the node has been completely removed. The nodes along the splenic artery are removed. For this, the assistant on the left side has to gently depress the cranial part of the head of pancreas. This helps the camera to reach the coeliac axis and show the splenic vessels well during the lymph node clearance. The para-aortic nodes in this region are cleared, again proceeding toward the hiatus. Completed nodal dissection bares the coeliac axis entirely; this is seen as the "Mercedes Benz" sign. The magnification offered by the laparoscopic approach greatly aids the lymph node dissection and improves precision.

The left gastric artery is ligated or clipped and cut. The vessels along the lesser curve are clipped at an adequate distance distally. This can also be done extracorporeally during specimen removal.

Stomach mobilization, mobilization of the esophagus in the neck, specimen retrieval and creation of the stomach tube, esophago-gastric anastomosis in the neck, and the postoperative management are the same as described for thoracoscopic esophagectomy (See Chap. 4).

Atlas of the Operative Procedure of Laparoscopic Transhiatal Esophagectomy

1. The patient is placed in Modified Lloyd Davis position with 15–20° head-up. The neck is extended and turned to the right side (Photo 5.1).

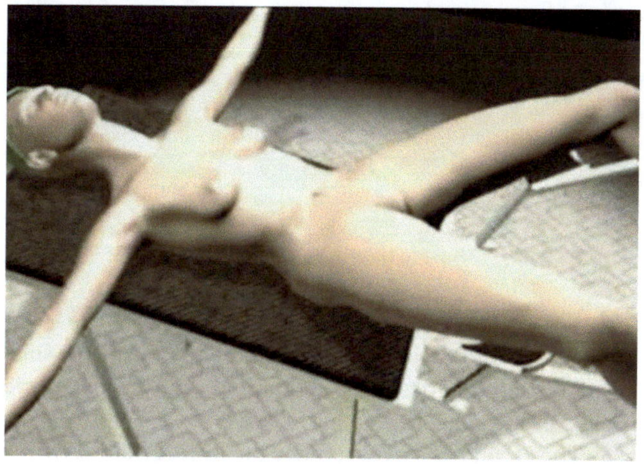

Photo 5.1

2. The surgeon stands between the legs of the patient. The camera assistant is on the left side of the surgeon and the scrub nurse is on the right side of the surgeon (Photo 5.2).

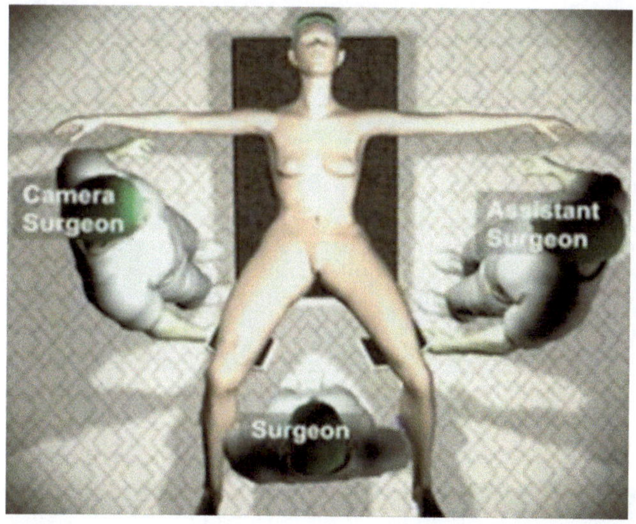

Photo 5.2

3. Port positions:
   (a) Pneumoperitoneum is created by a Verress' needle inserted through the Palmer's point or through the umbilicus.
   (b) The primary port is inserted blindly or using visiport at the junction of upper two third and lower one third of the line joining the xiphisternum and umbilicus.

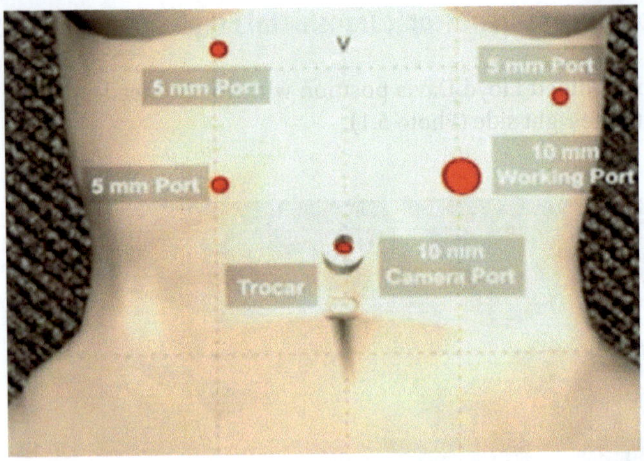

Photo 5.3

(c) Secondary ports are inserted under vision as shown (Photo 5.3).

4. An examination of the abdominal cavity is performed to assess the extent of the disease and to rule out any metastatic disease (Photo 5.4a, b).

5. The second assistant retracts the liver (Photo 5.5).

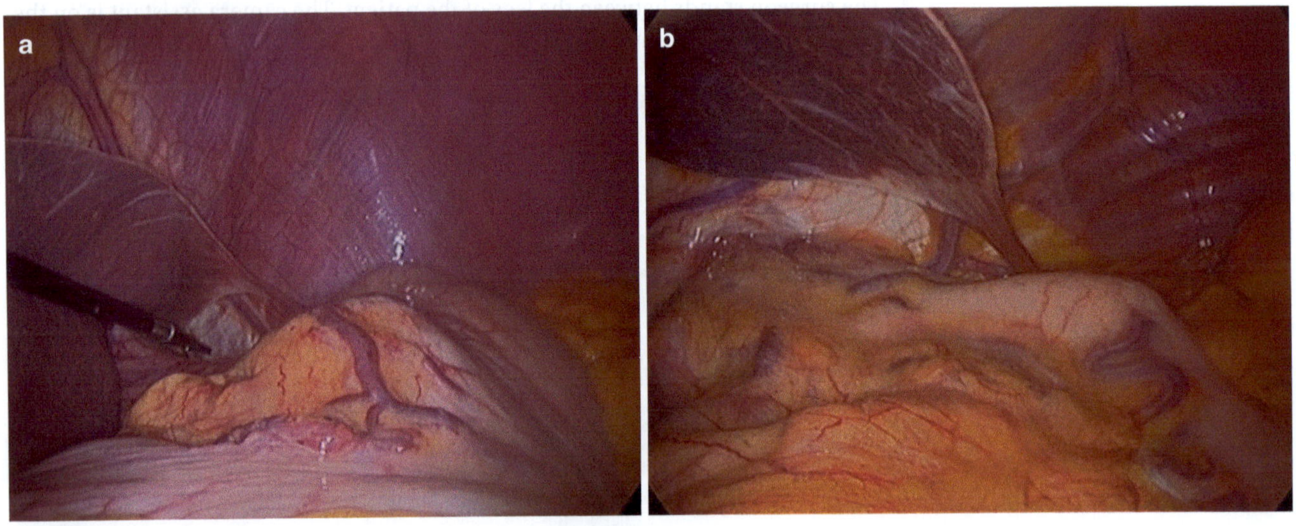

Photo 5.4 (a, b)

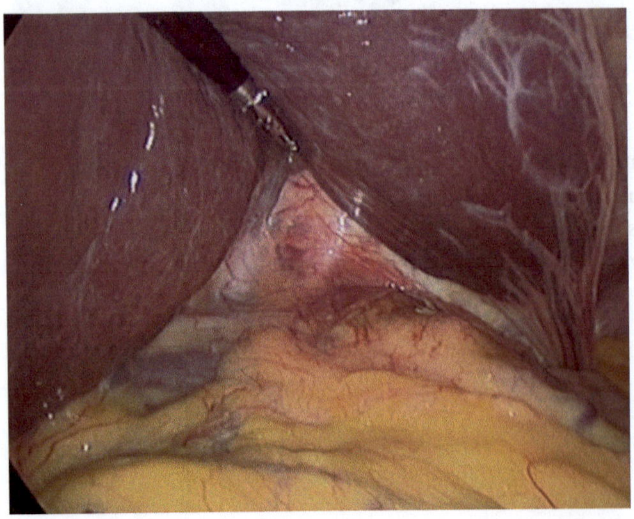

Photo 5.5

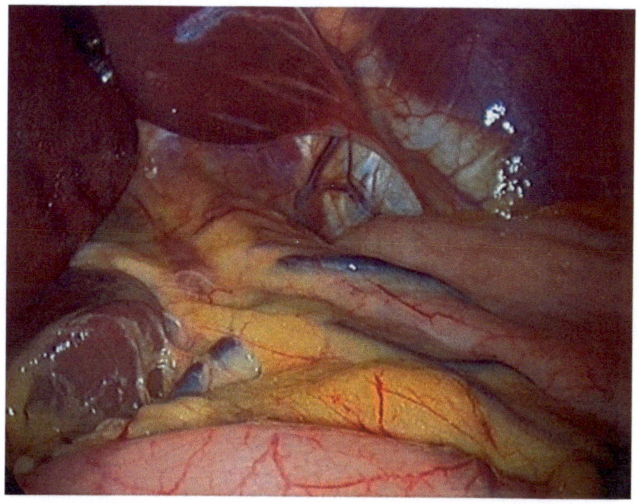

Photo 5.6

6. The first assistant retracts the stomach downward and laterally (Photo 5.6).
7. The left hand grasper is used to stretch the gastrohepatic ligament which is cut using the ACE harmonic (Photo 5.7a–c).

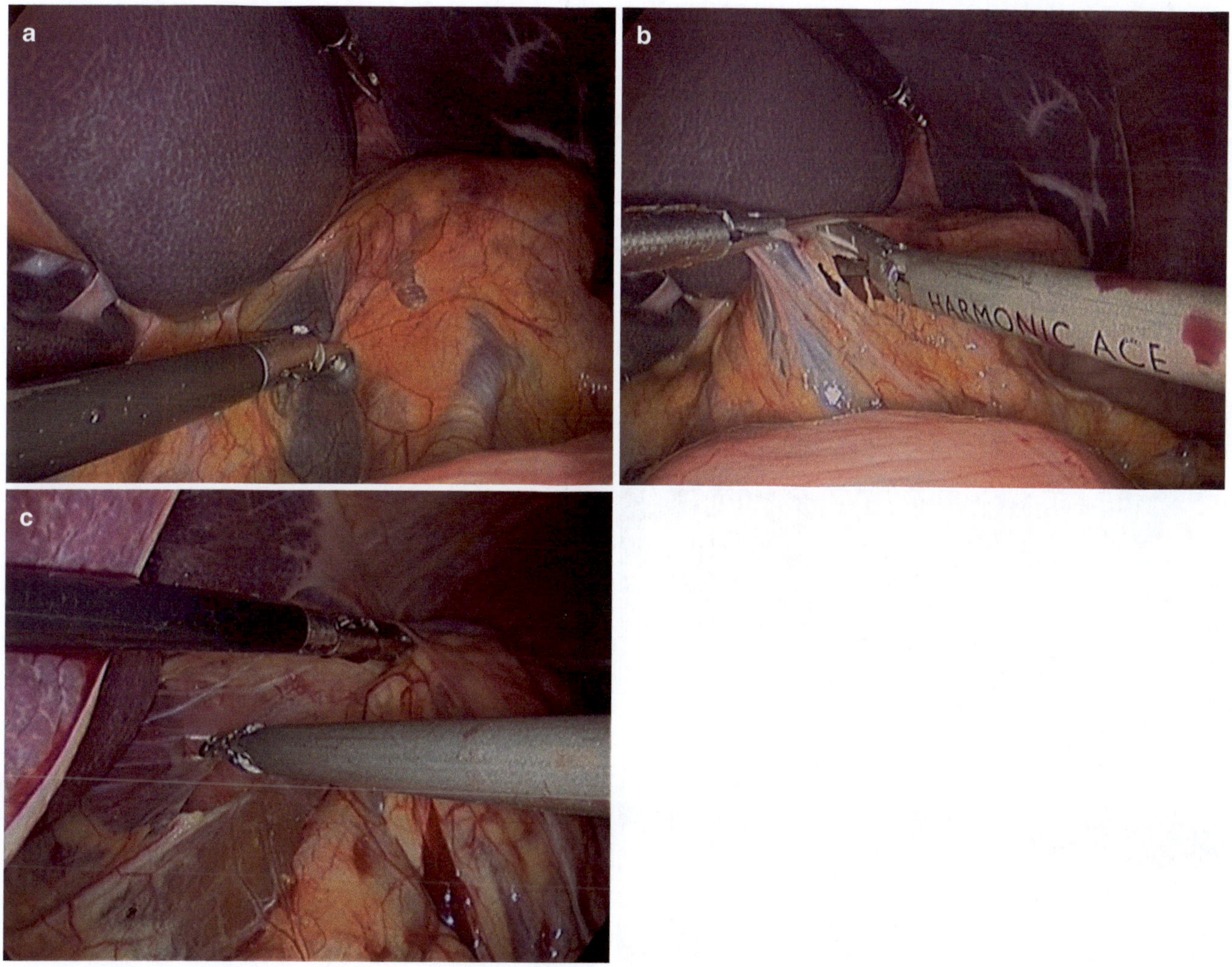

Photo 5.7 (a–c)

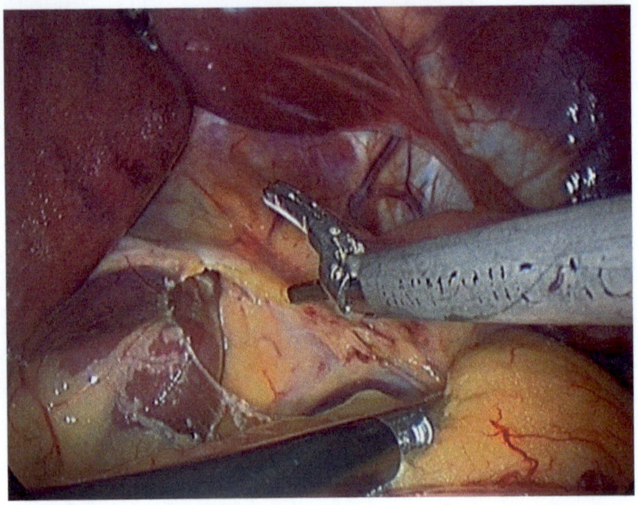

Photo 5.8

8. The cut is extended upward to the hiatus (Photo 5.8).
9. Right crus of the diaphragm is identified and the peritoneum over it is cut (Photo 5.9a–c).

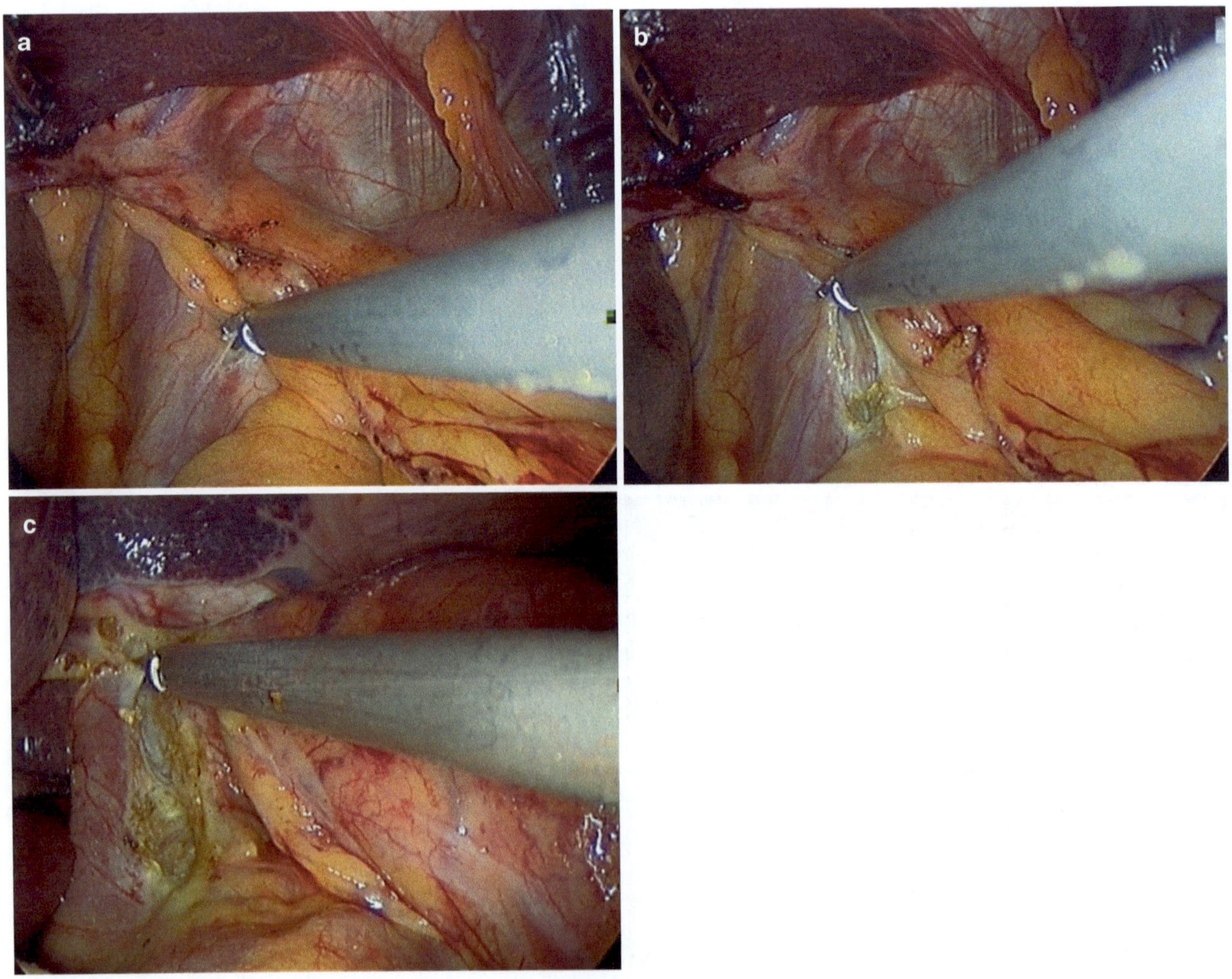

Photo 5.9 (a–c)

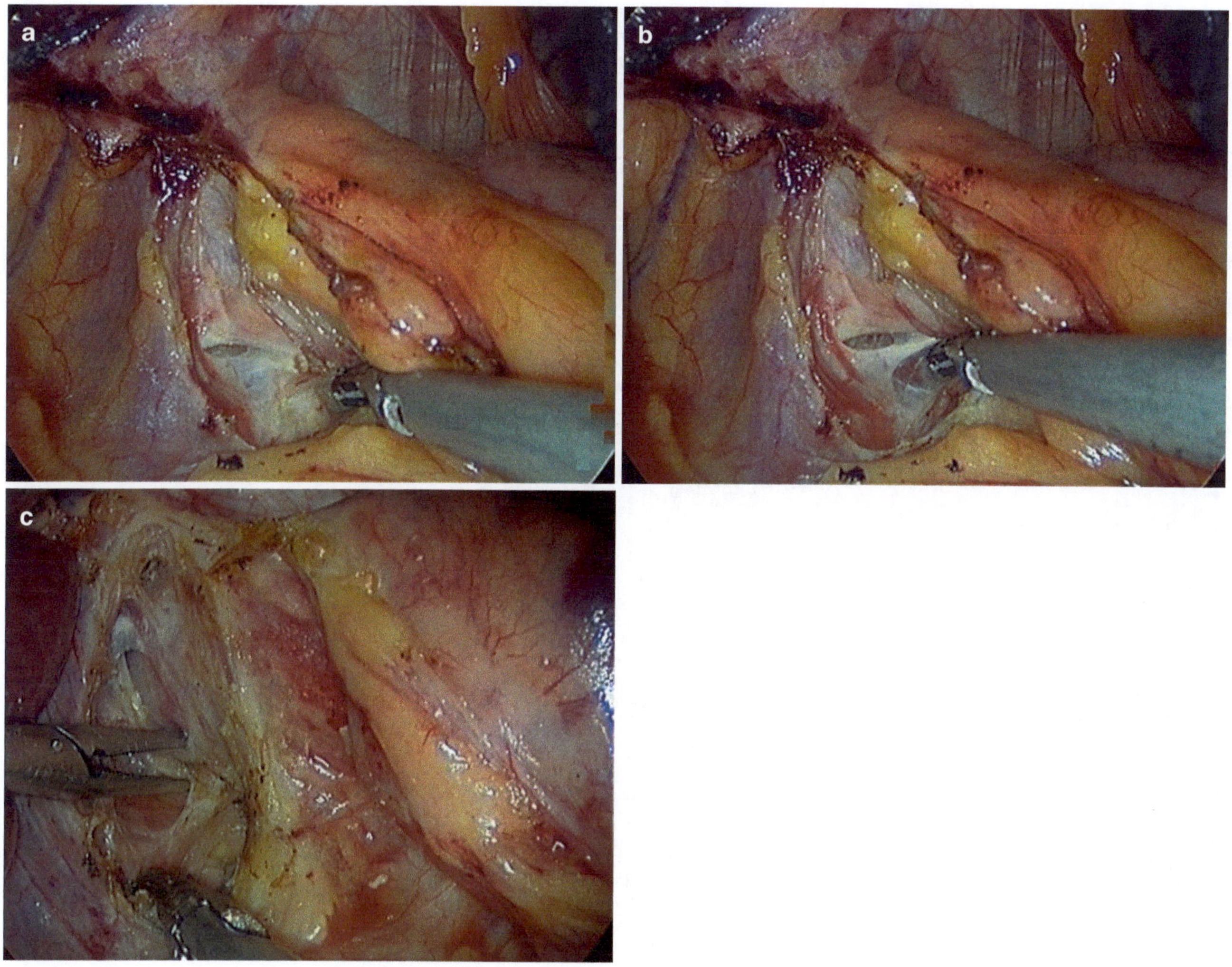

Photo 5.10 (a–c)

10. Dissection is performed medial to the right crus remaining parallel to it (Photo 5.10a–c).

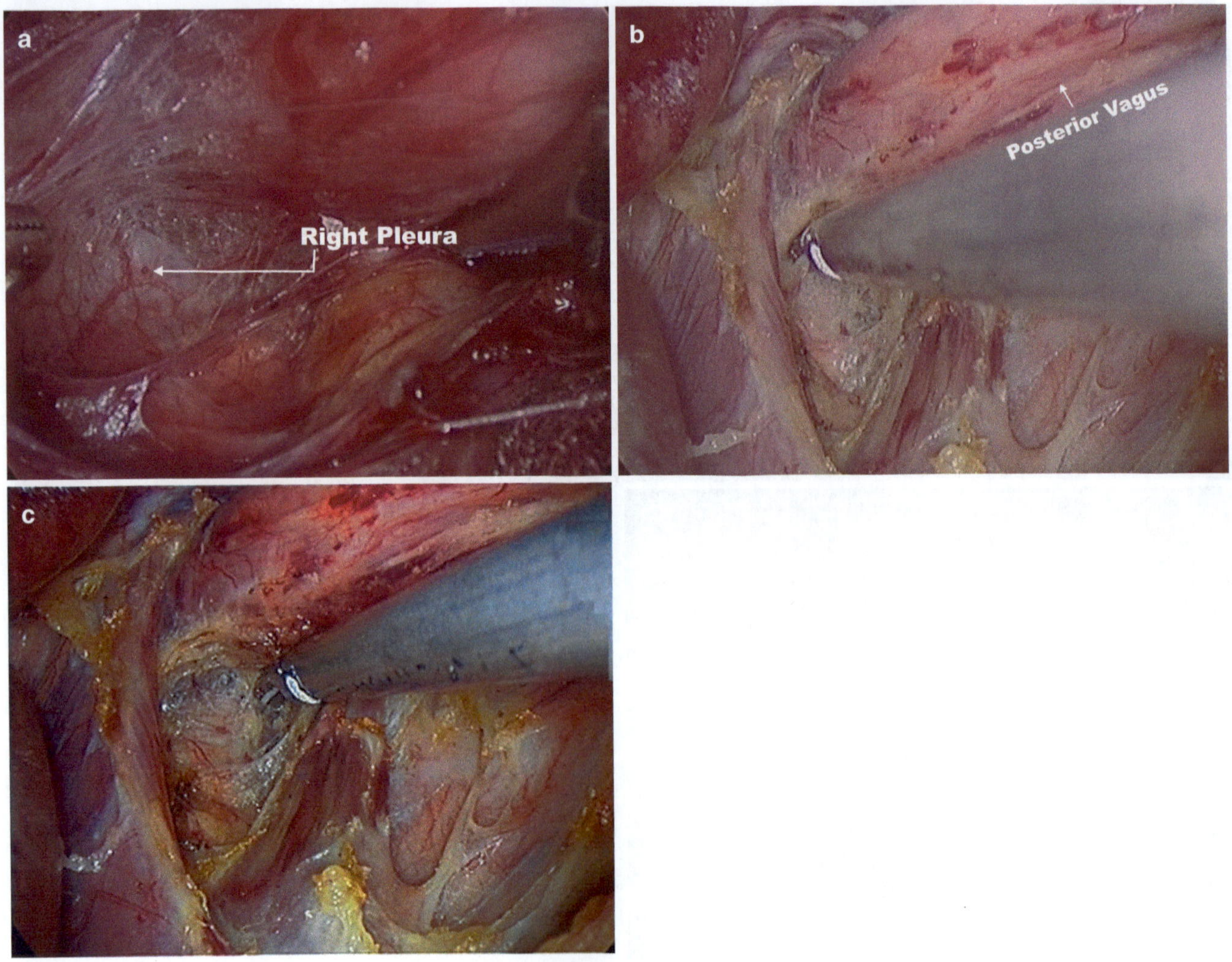

Photo 5.11 (a–c)

11. The dissection is continued posterior to the esophagus. CO_2 gas helps to open up the retroesophageal space (Photo 5.11a–c).

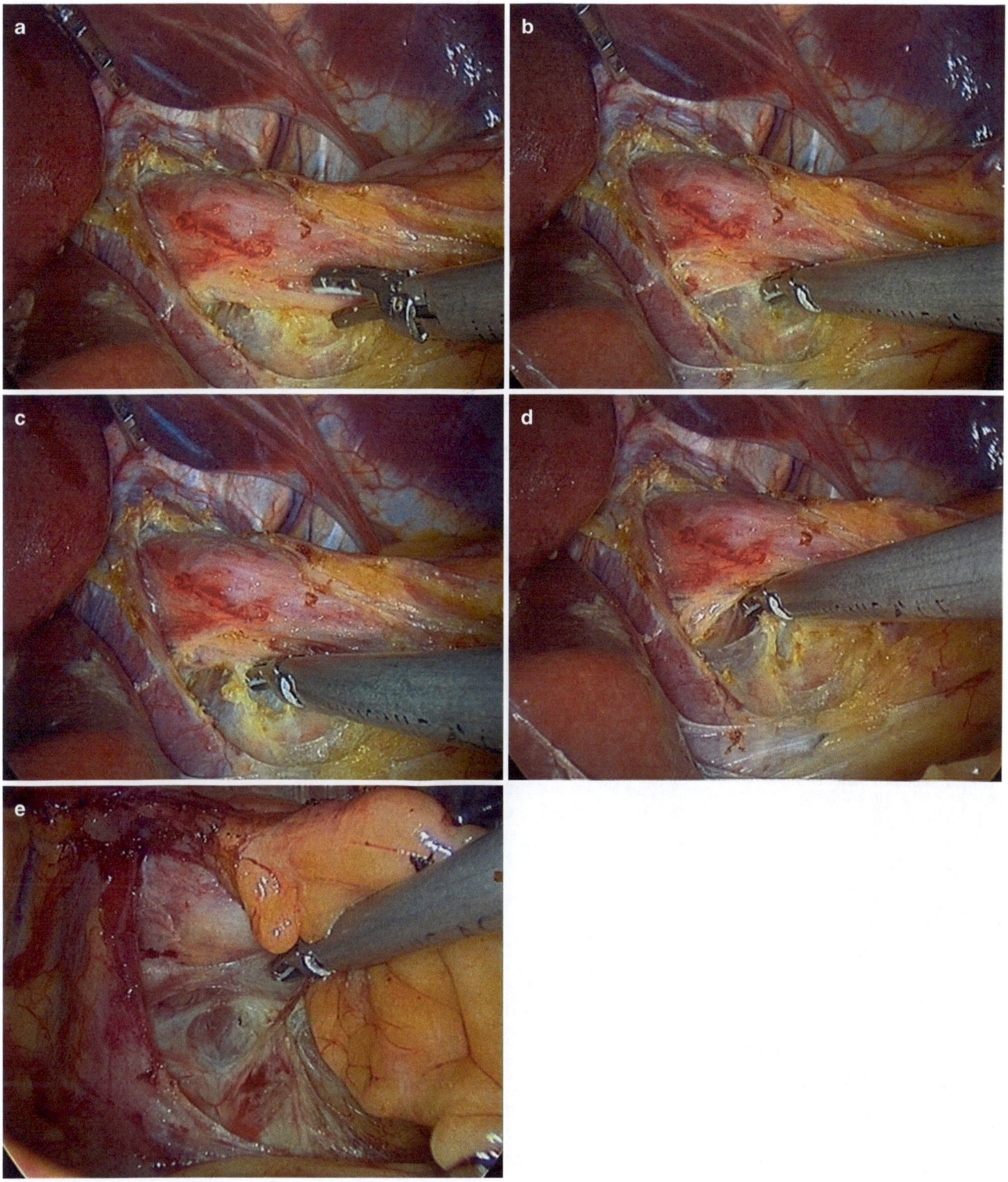

Photo 5.12 (a–e)

12. Posterior vagus is identified; dissection remains outside the posterior vagus nerve (Photo 5.12a–e).

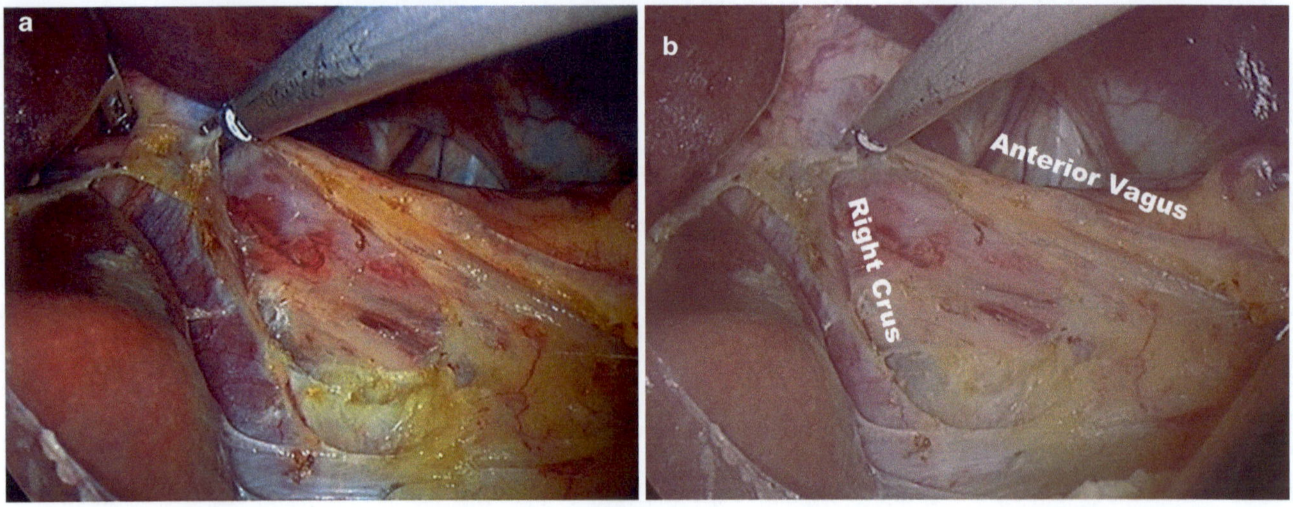

Photo 5.13 (a, b)

13. The peritoneal cut of right crus is extended upward toward the apex of hiatus (Photo 5.13a, b).

14. The assistant pulls the esophagus caudally and to the left. The operating surgeon's left hand grasper lifts the esophagus upward. This facilitates the dissection posterior to the esophagus. This dissection is continued posteriorly till the left crus is identified (Photo 5.14a–c).

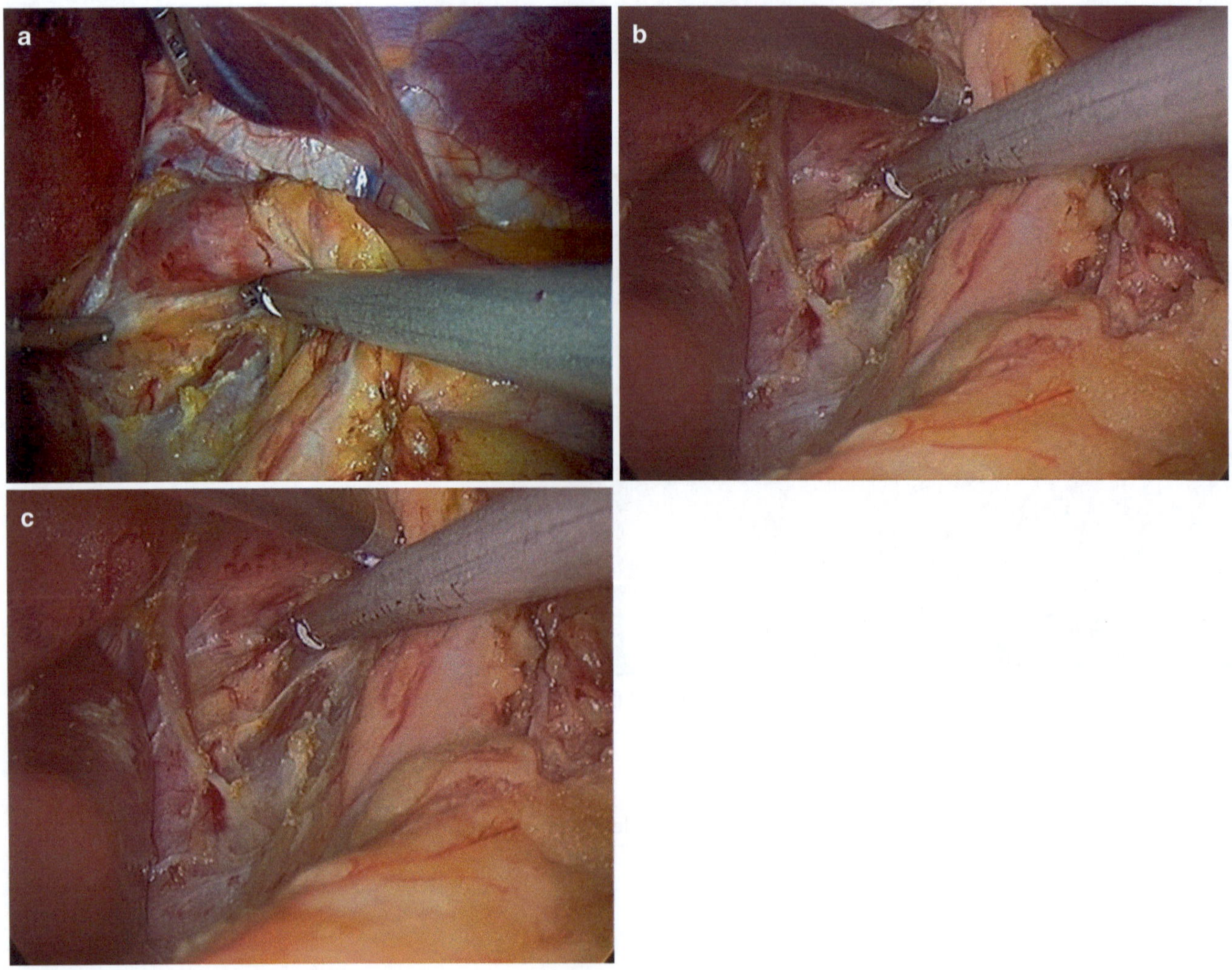

Photo 5.14 (a-c)

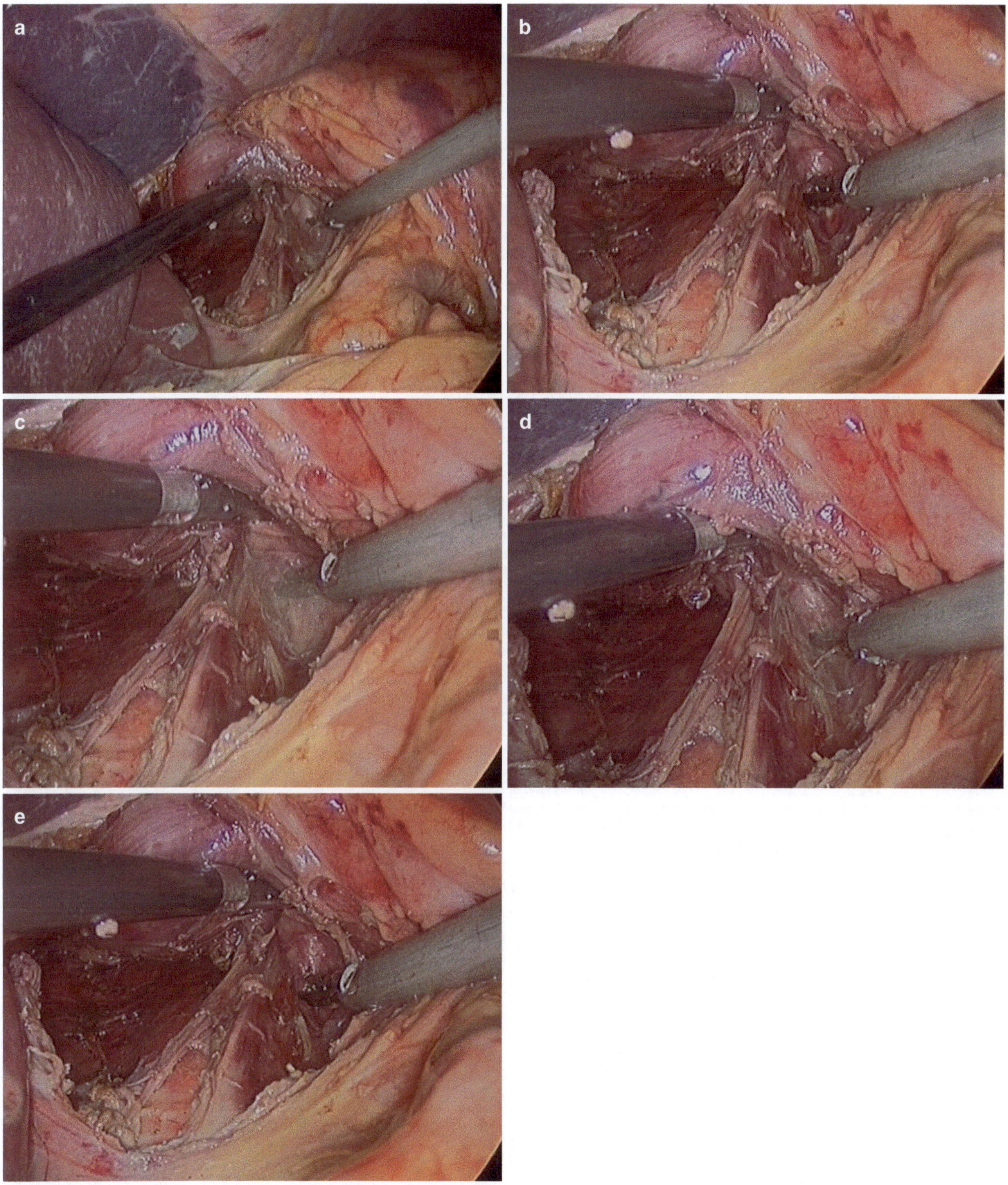

Photo 5.15 (a-e)

15. A posterior window is created and extended to the left till the left dome of diaphragm is seen. The window is enlarged by sweeping the left hand toward the diaphragm and the right hand pushing the esophagus upward. This movement helps to open the avascular plane which exists between the dome of diaphragm and the fundus (Photo 5.15a–e).

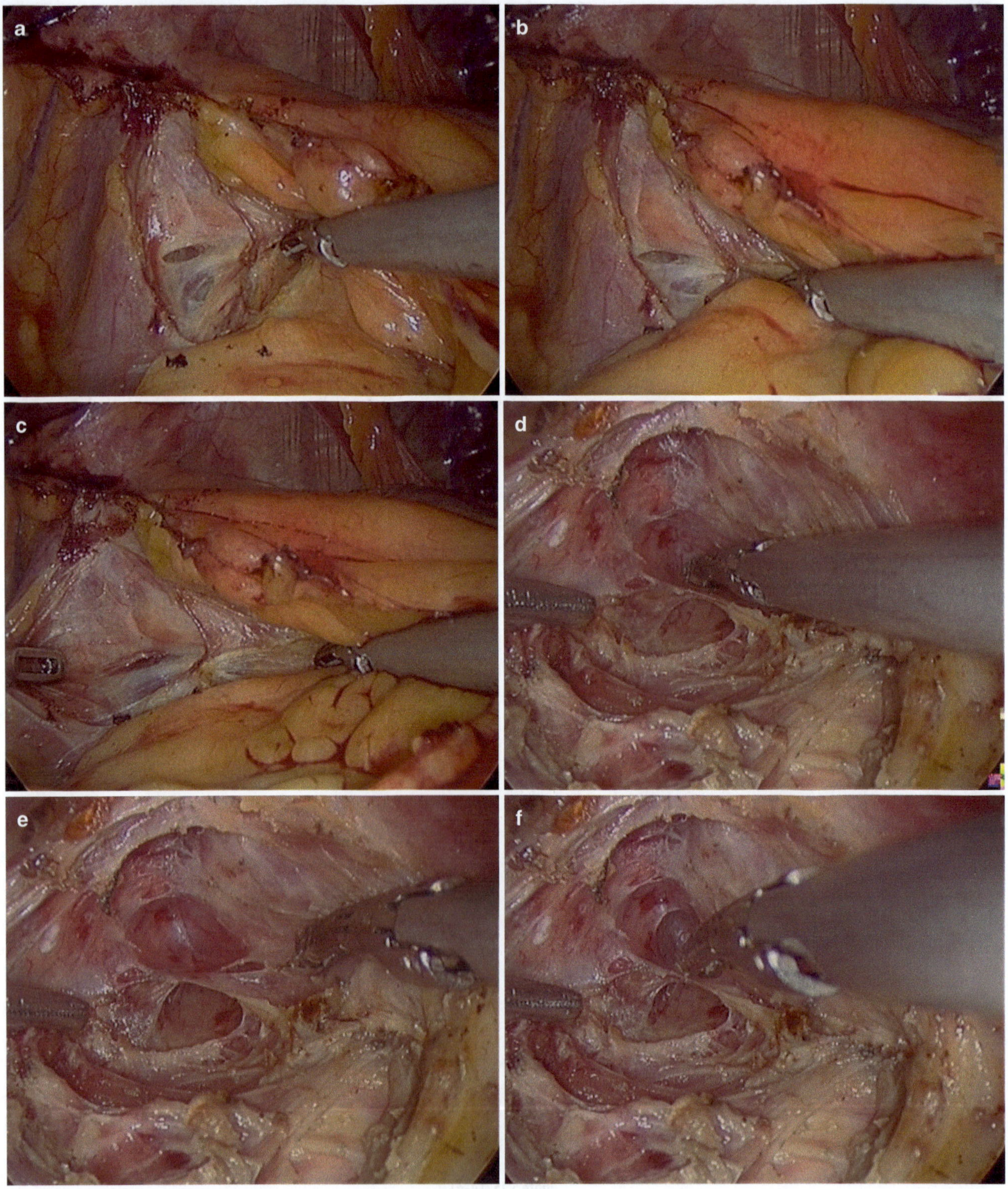

Photo 5.16 (a–f)

16. Opening of the posterior space allows the esophagus to be retracted to the left side. This opens the plane on the right side of the esophagus. The dissection is then continued on the right side. The left-hand grasper pushes the right pleura while the right-hand instrument pushes the esophagus toward the left (Photo 5.16a–f).

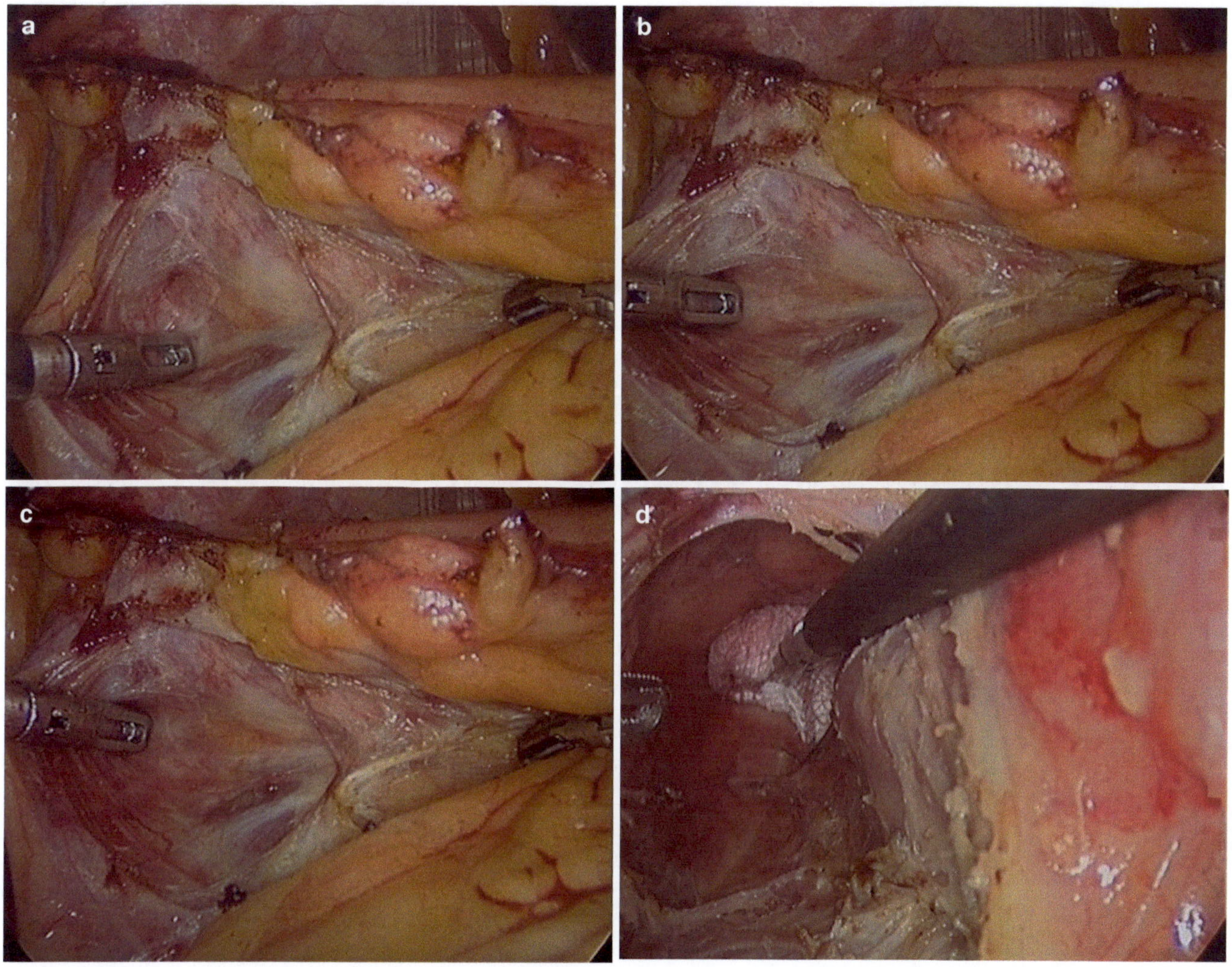

Photo 5.17 (a–g)

17. This dissection is to be done gently till the right pleural reflection is identified. The right pleura is pushed with the right hand grasper. This dissection should be done bluntly, since the pleura is vulnerable to injury at this level. The CO_2 insufflation helps to open this plane further. Alternatively a gauze piece may be used for dissection (Photo 5.17a–g).

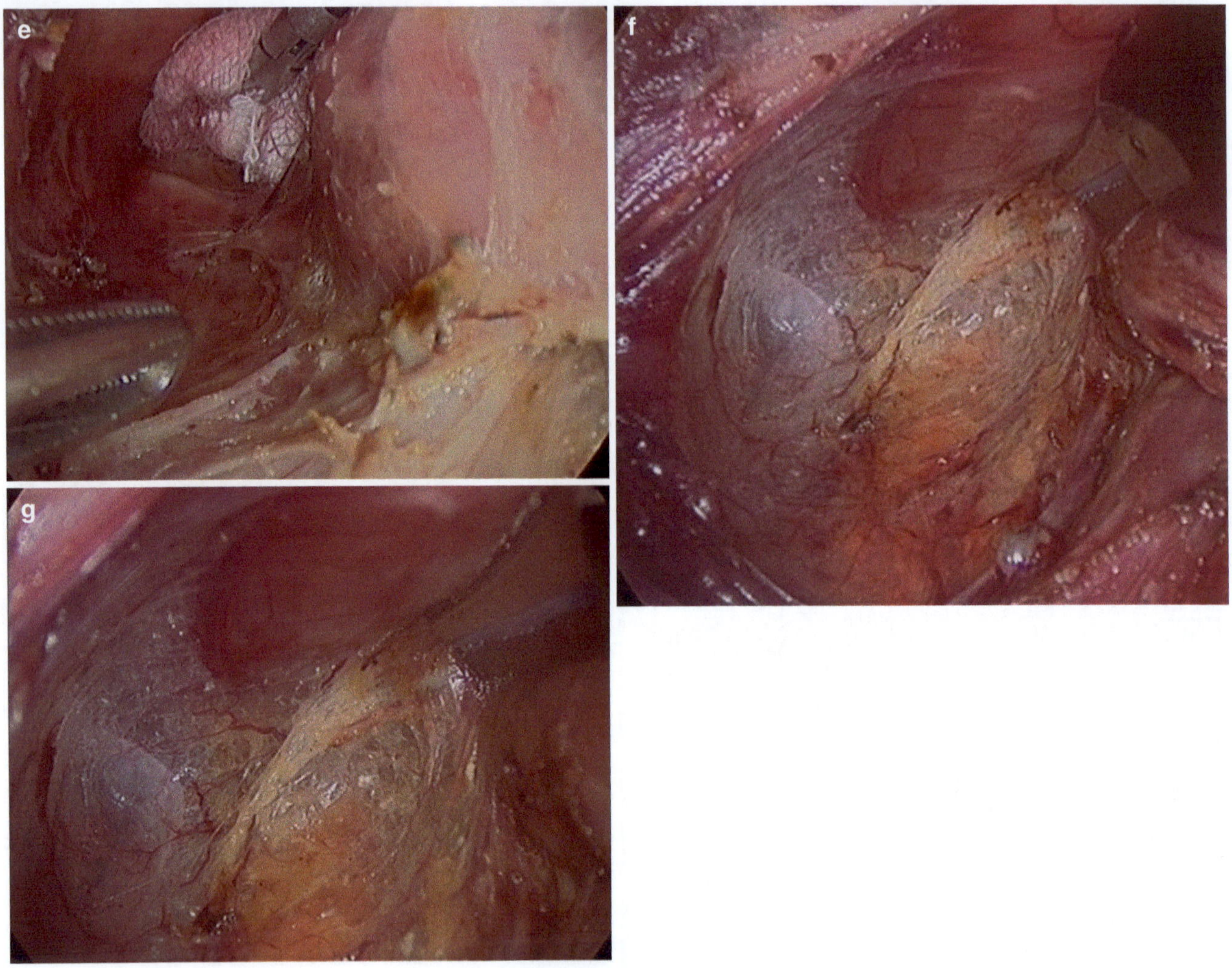

Photo 5.17 (Continued)

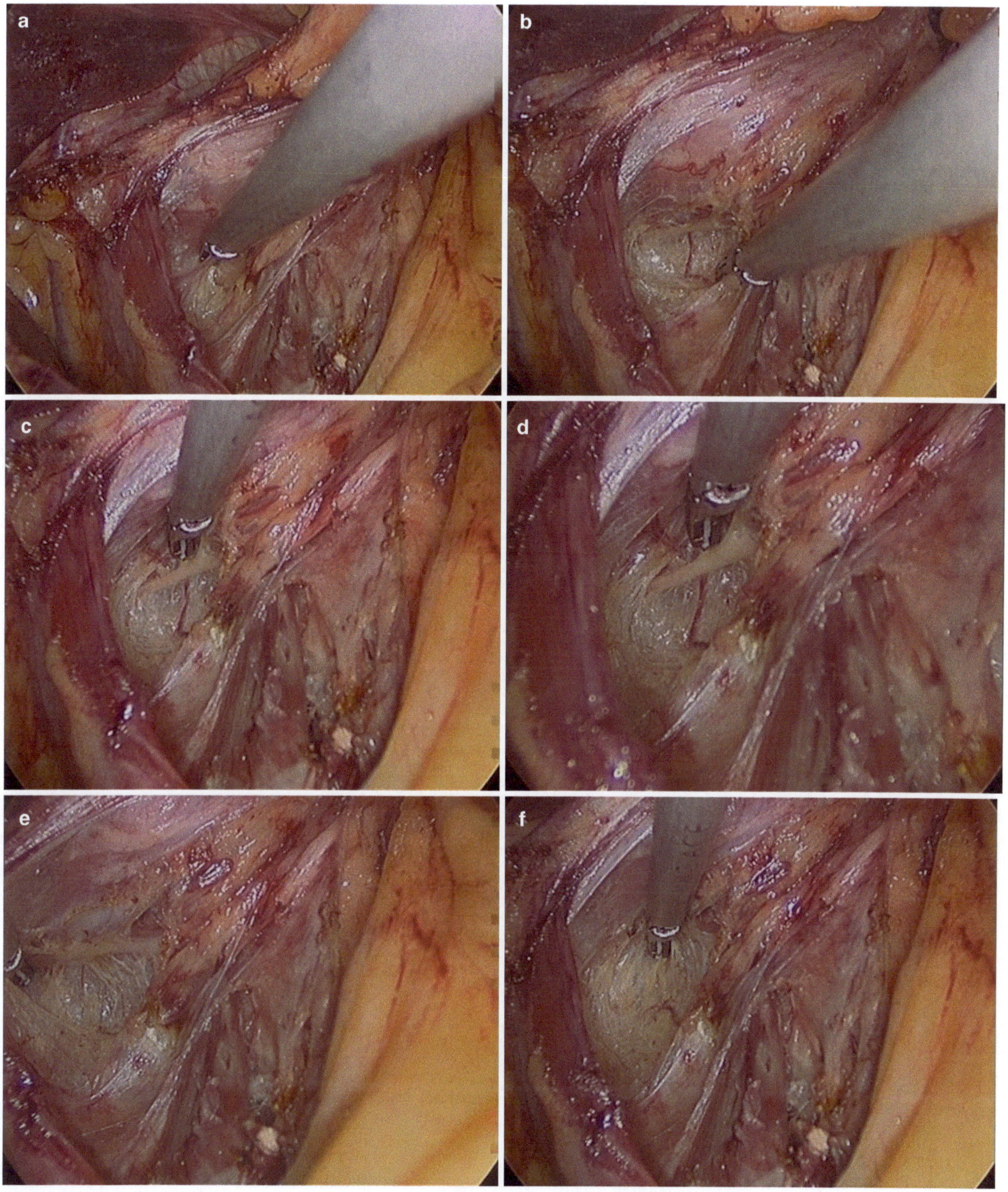

Photo 5.18 (a–r)

18. The dissection is continued posteriorly between the esophagus and the aorta (Photo 5.18a–r).

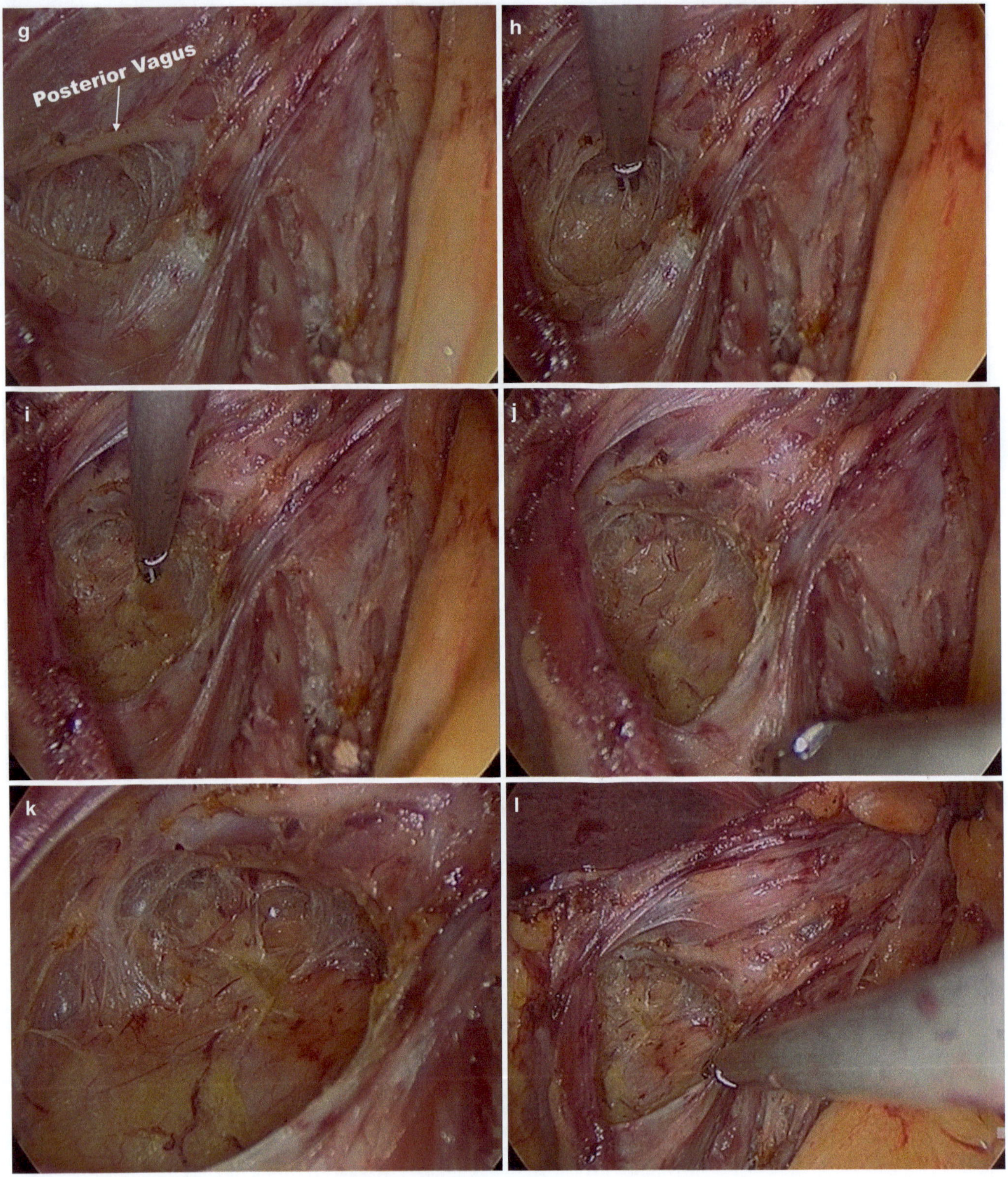

Photo 5.18 (Continued)

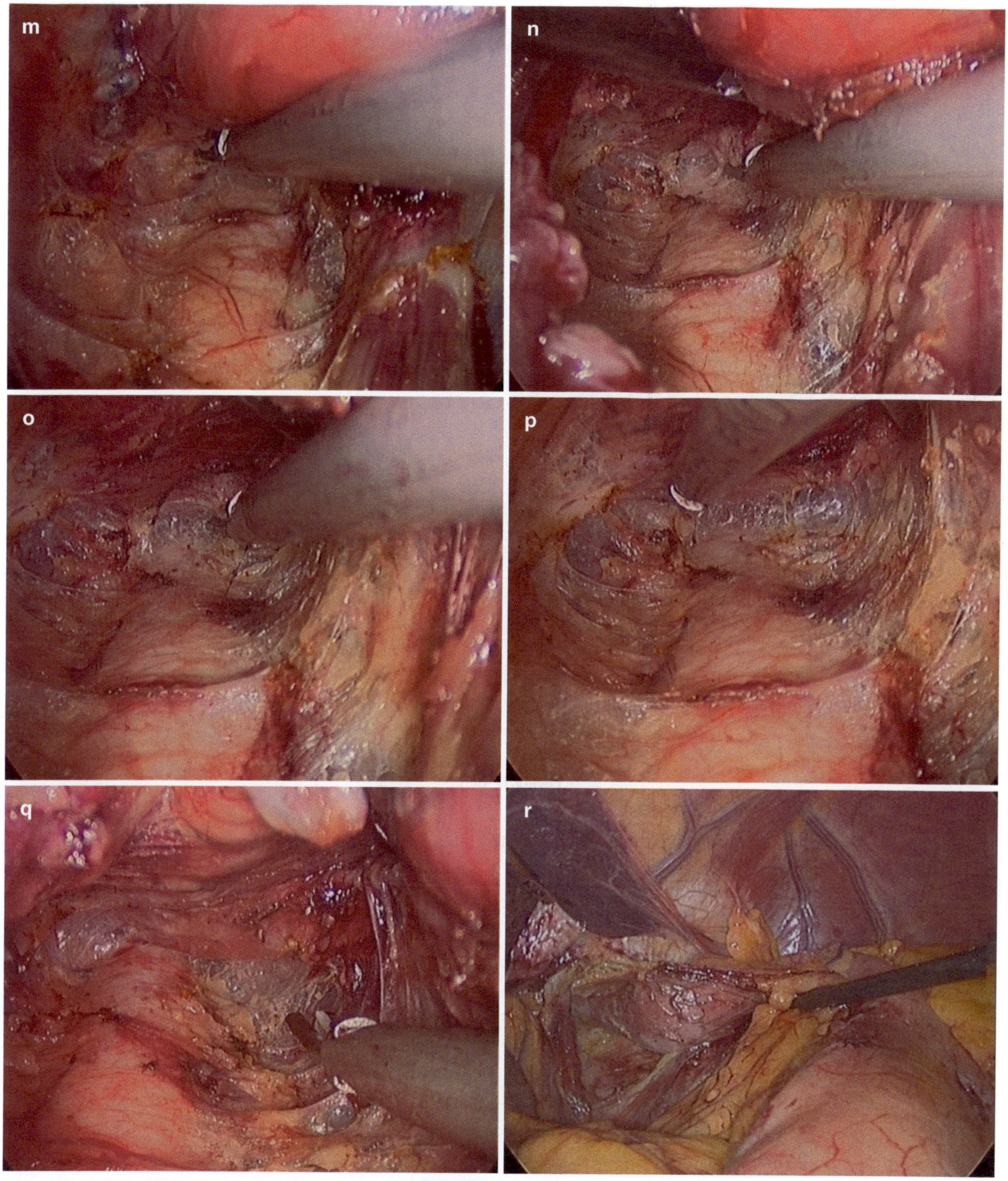

Photo 5.18 (Continued)

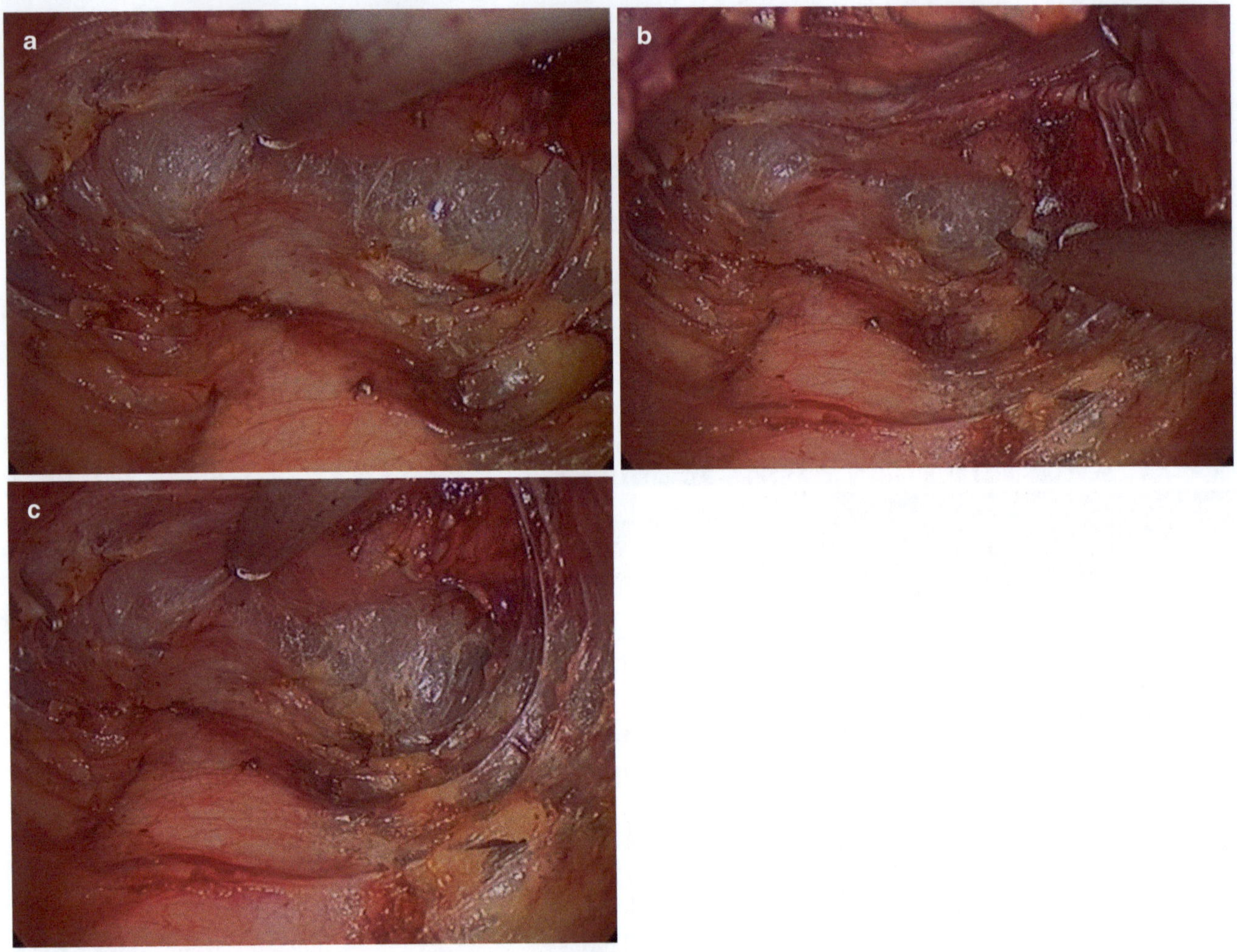

Photo 5.19 (a–c)

19. The entire fibro-fatty tissue over the aorta is lifted along with esophagus (Photo 5.19a–c).

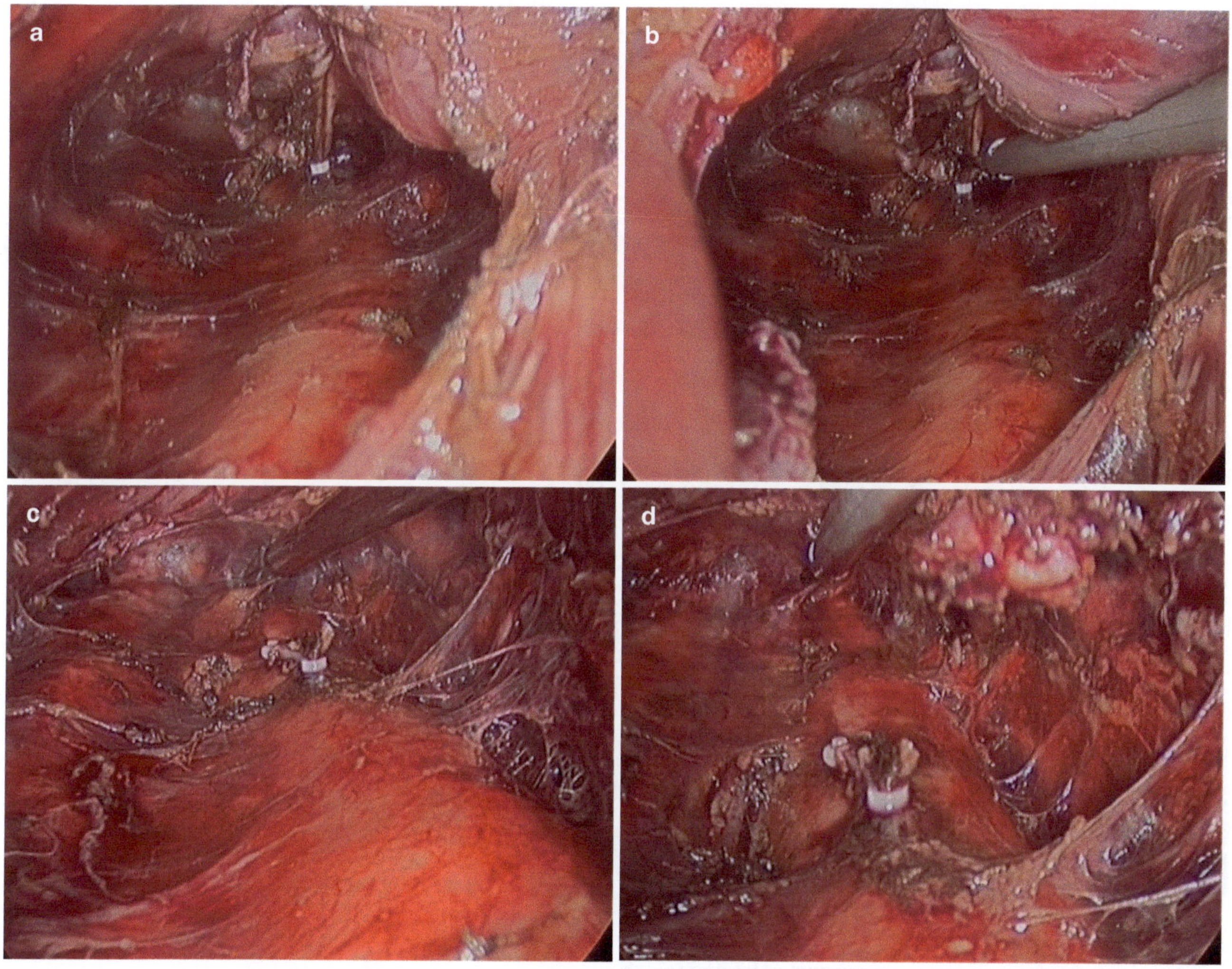

Photo 5.20 (a–d)

20. Few direct branches from the aorta can be clipped and cut (Photo 5.20a–d).

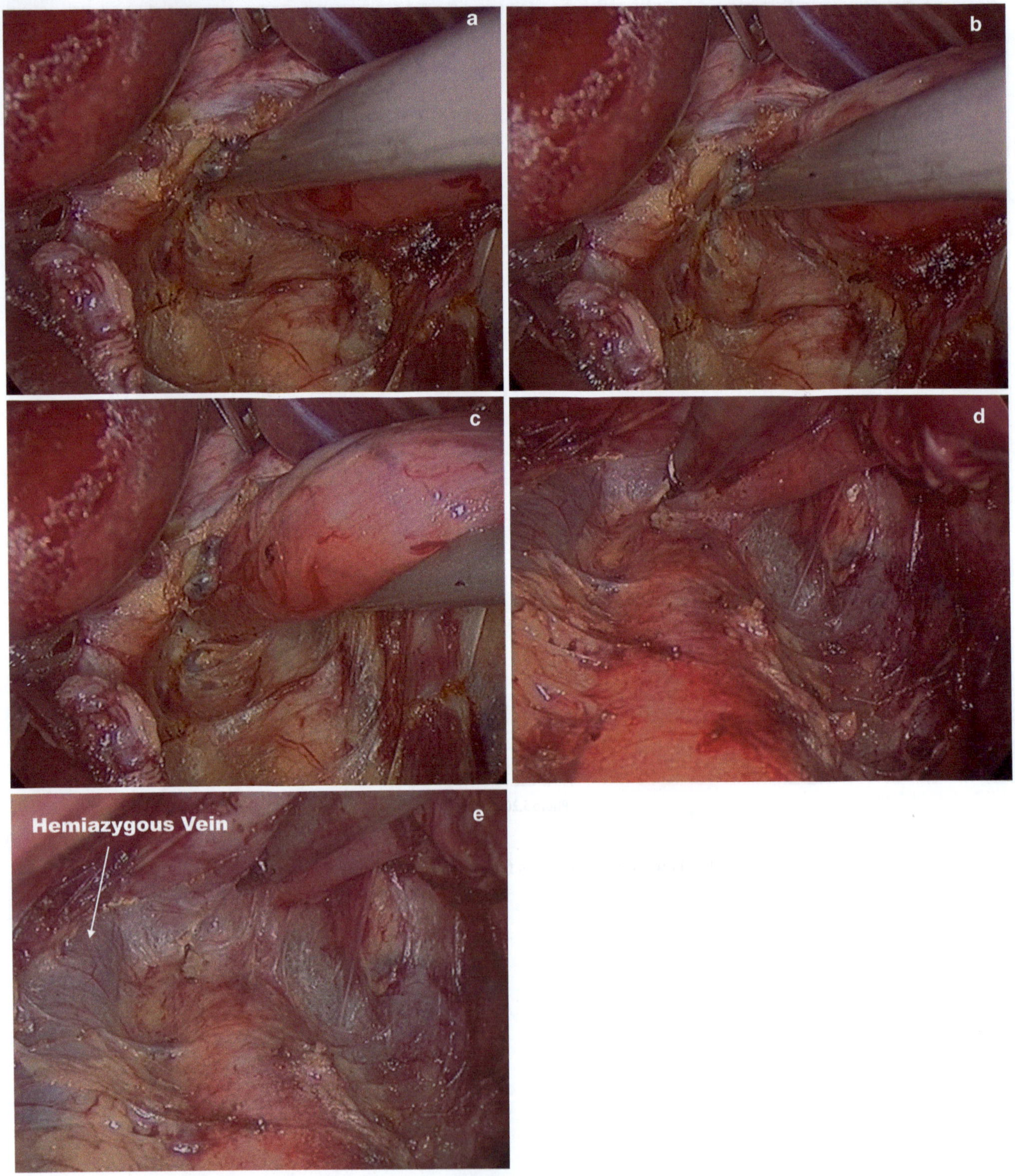

Photo 5.21 (a–e)

21. The direction of the dissection should be from the aorta towards the esophagus, sweeping all the tissues towards the esophagus (Photo 5.21a–e).

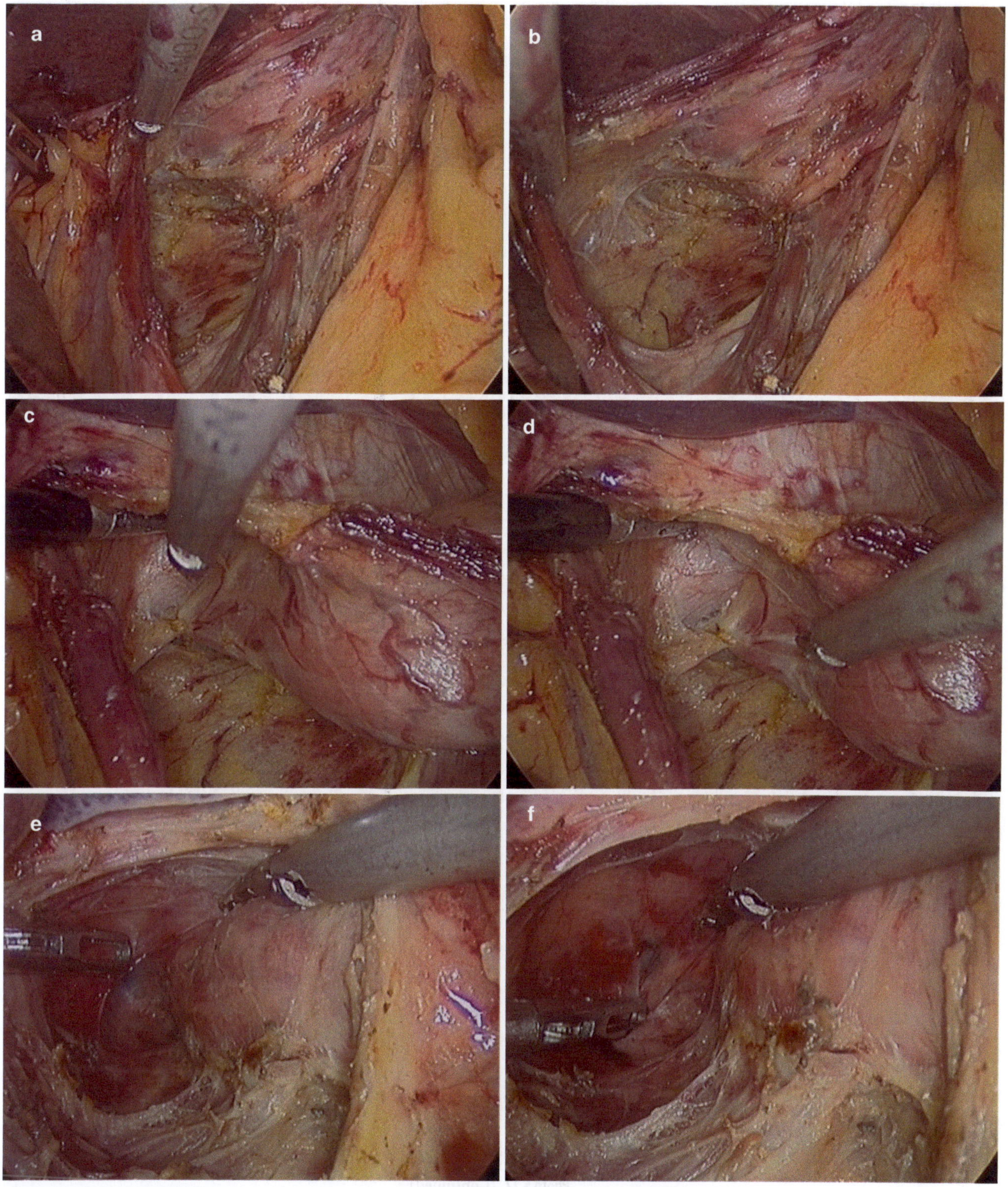

Photo 5.22 (a–o)

22. Once the esophagus is freely mobilized posteriorly, the same dissection is continued on the right side of esophagus reflecting off the pleura. There is no specific upper limit of the dissection but one should continue the dissection as far cranially as one can go. Anatomically, the right main bronchus is the limiting factor and the left-hand grasper can some times feel the cartilages of the right main bronchus. As the esophagus gets separated from the right side, the caudal traction can be enhanced further by the assistant (Photo. 5.22a–o).

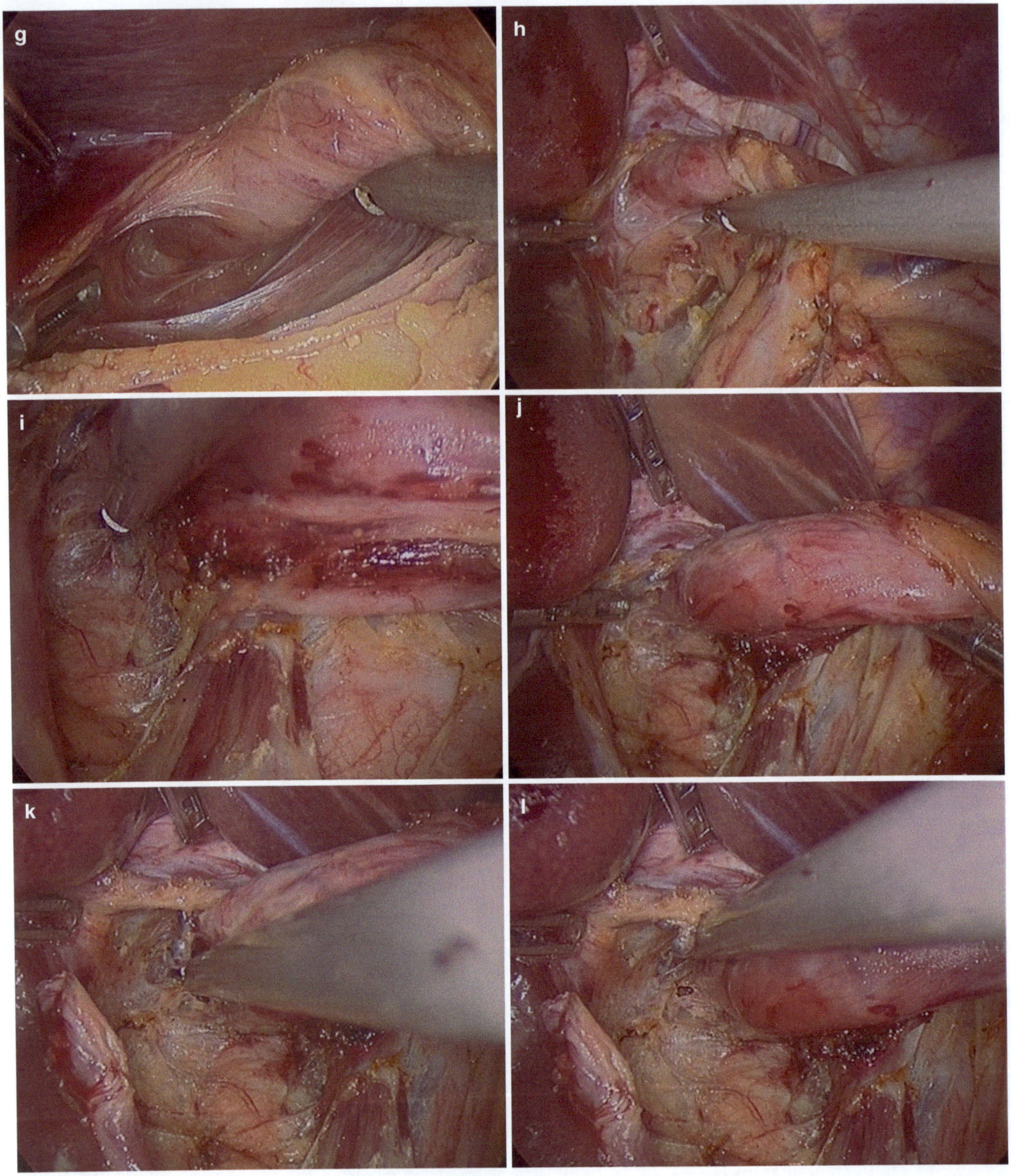

Photo 5.22 (Continued)

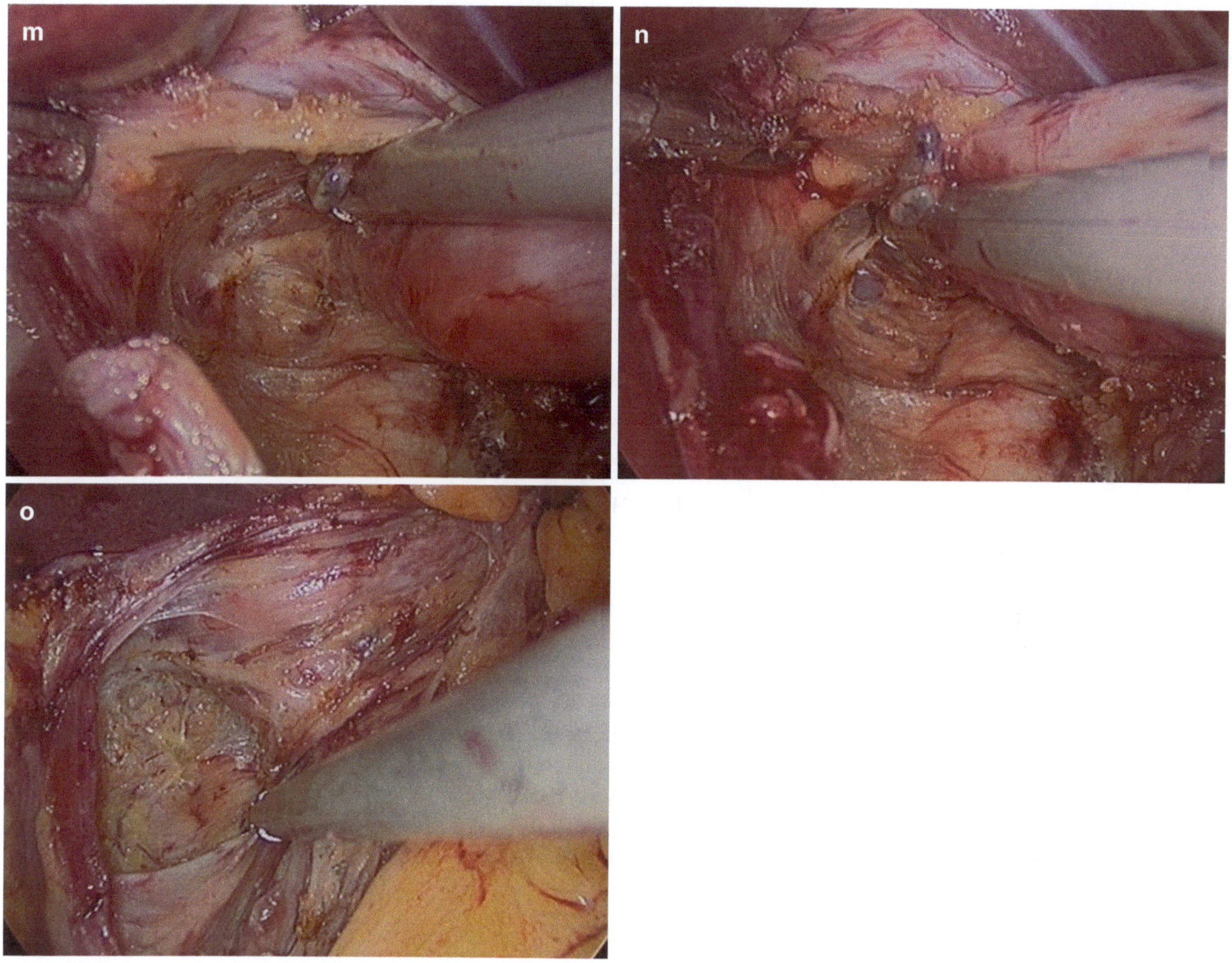

Photo 5.22 (Continued)

23. The caudal tributary of the Azygous vein can be seen on the right side of the aorta at this stage. The thoracic duct can be seen to the right of aorta (Photo 5.23a, b).

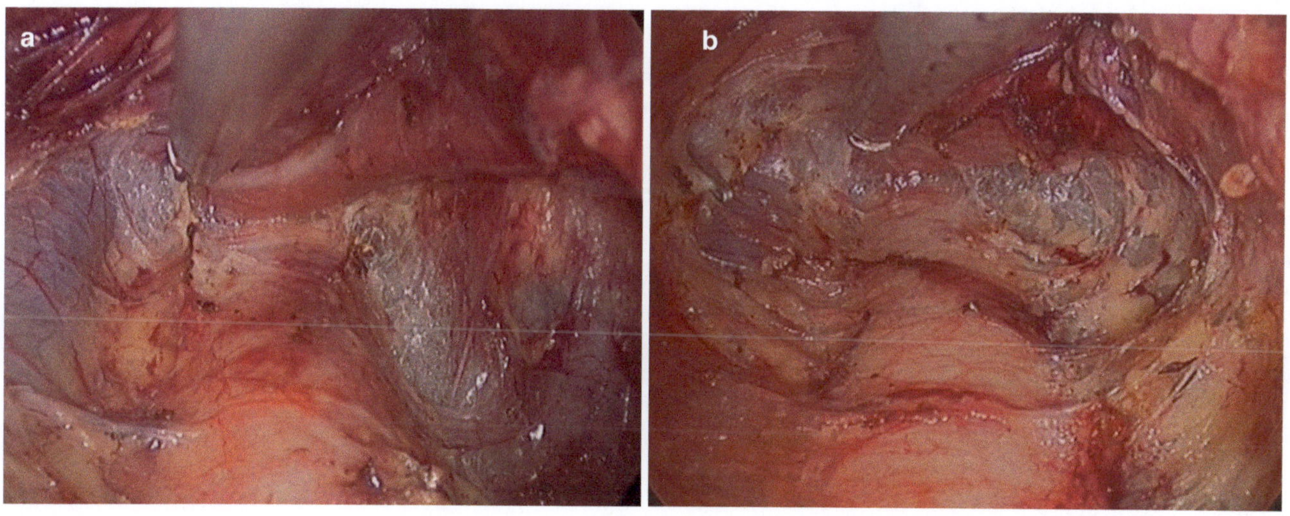

Photo 5.23 (a, b)

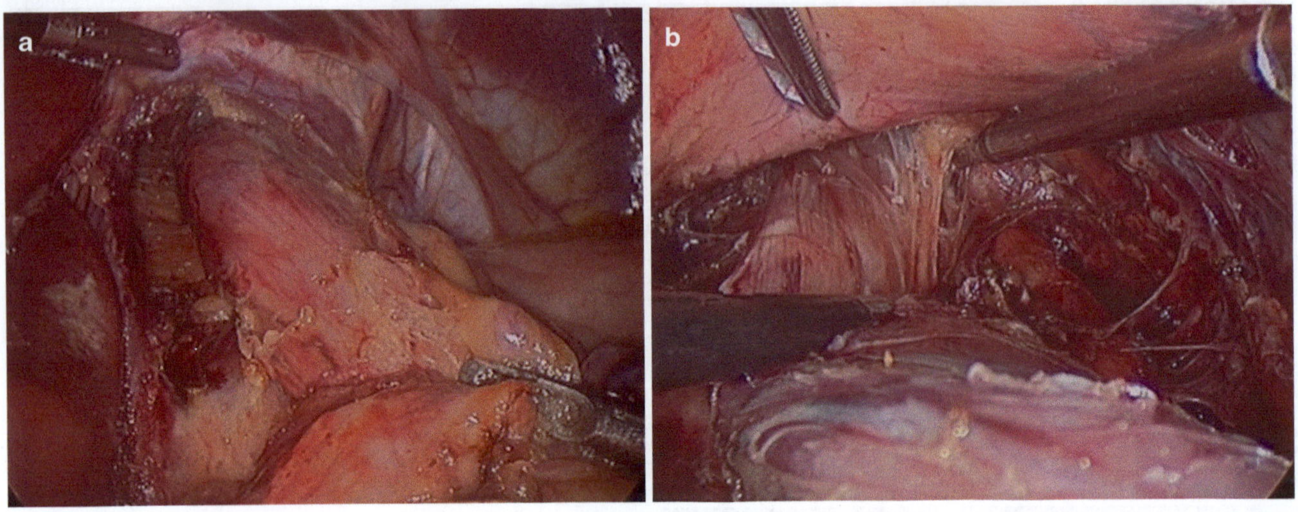

Photo 5.24 (a, b)

24. The esophagus is then pulled caudally and posteriorly. This is achieved by the left-sided assistant pushing the fundus downward and posteriorly. The grasper retracting the liver is now put at the upper end of the hiatus (Photo 5.24a–b).

25. The anterior dissection between the heart and esophagus is commenced. The dissection is done using the same principle of traction and countertraction. The traction is applied by the left-hand grasper pushing the hiatus anteriorly and the countertraction is achieved by the right hand pushing caudally and posteriorly. A few paraesophageal nodes can be easily removed along with the esophagus. The pericardium should not be retracted with the instrument, as it may lead to arrhythmias. The plane between the pericardium and the esophagus is devoid of any vessels, and hence this dissection is bloodless (Photo 5.25a–n).

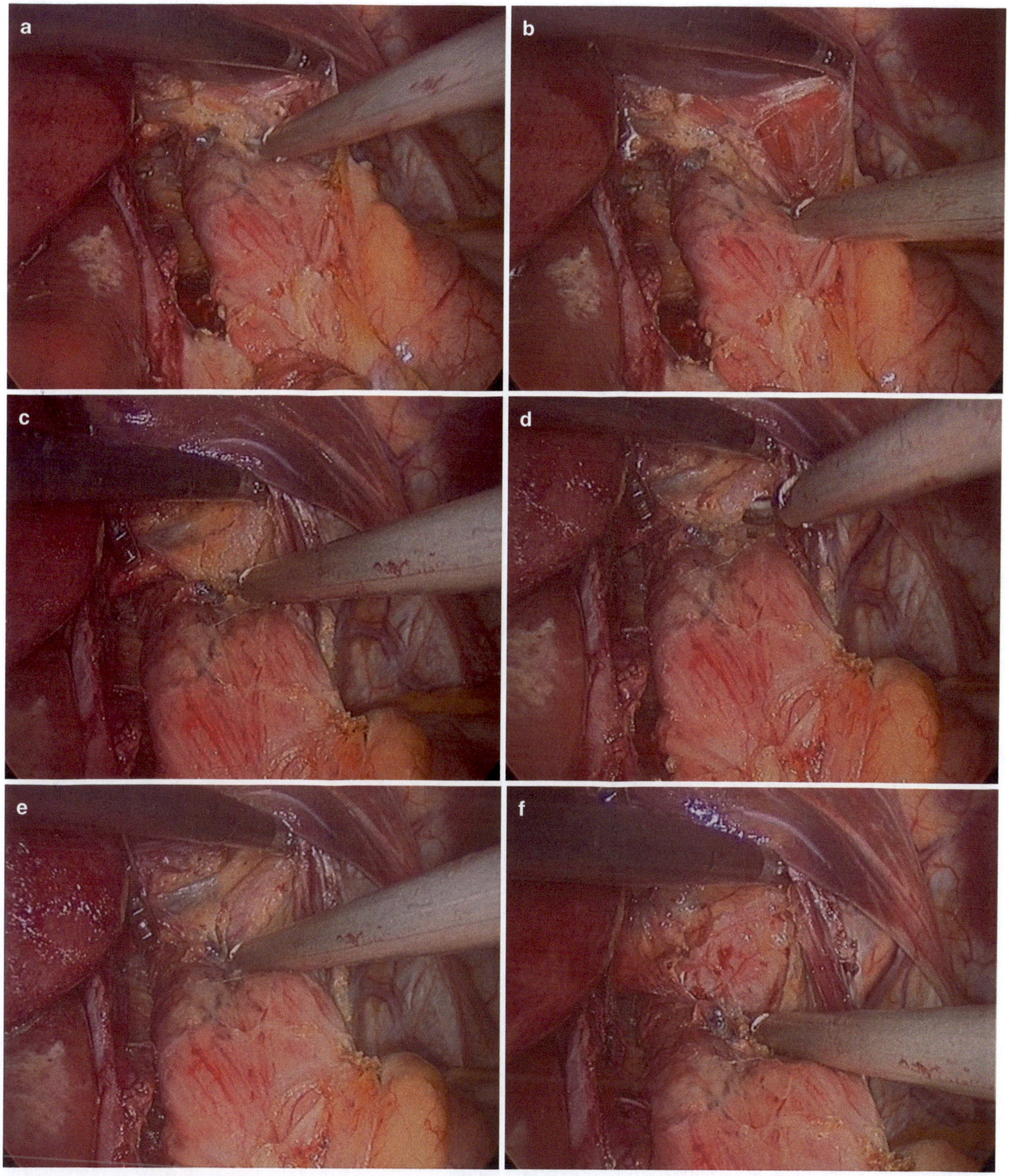

Photo 5.25 (a–n)

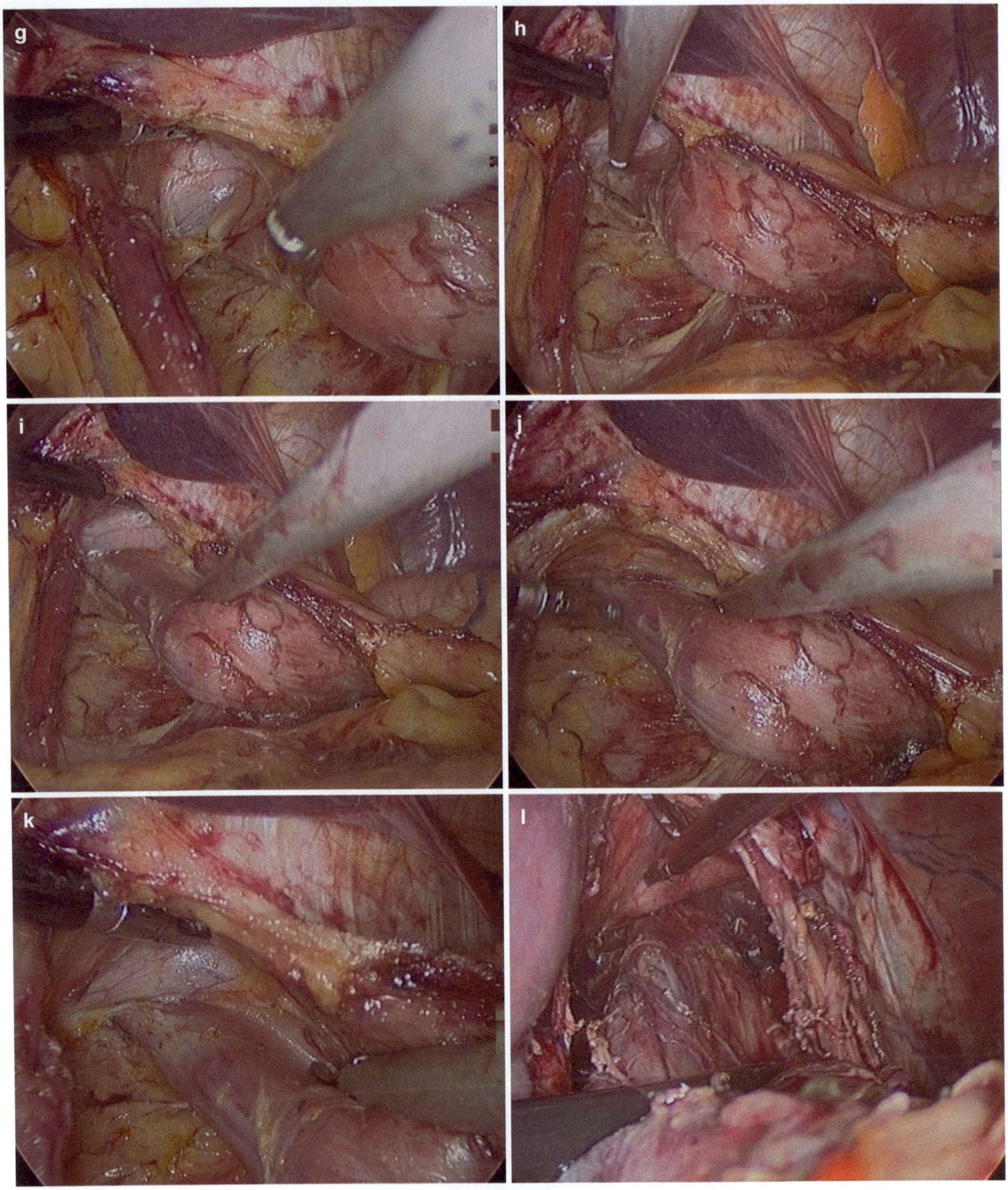

Photo 5.25 (Continued)

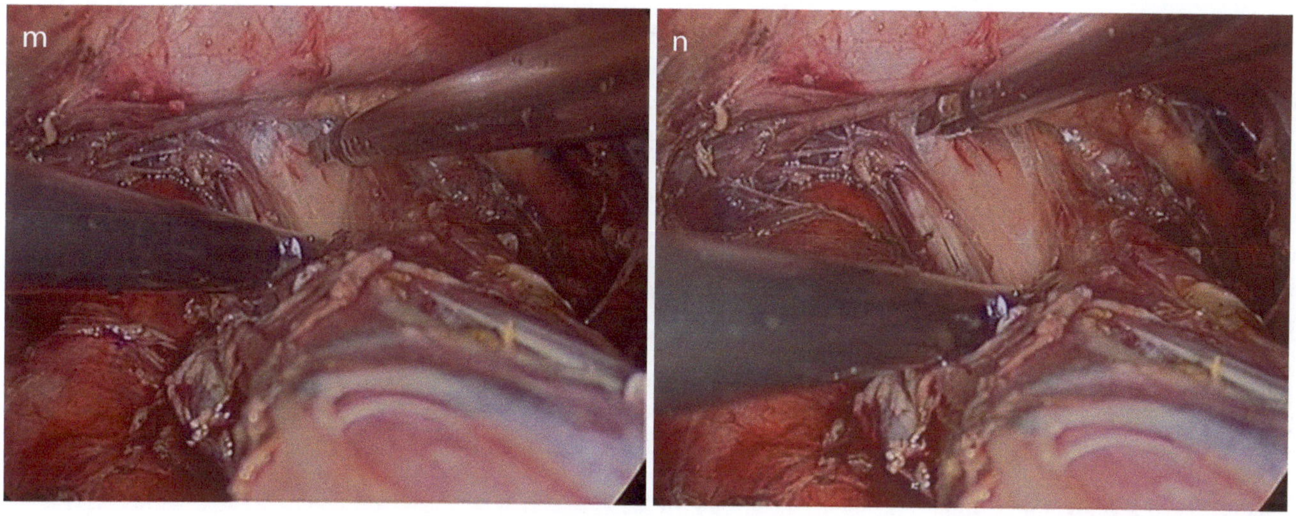

Photo 5.25 (Continued)

26. Dissection of the left side of the esophagus is started by cutting the peritoneum over the left crus. The left pleura is very close and may be damaged at this level. The right-hand grasper pushes the pleura while the left-hand grasper pulls the esophagus to the right side. This maneuver helps to open the space on the left side of the esophagus (Photo 5.26a–g).

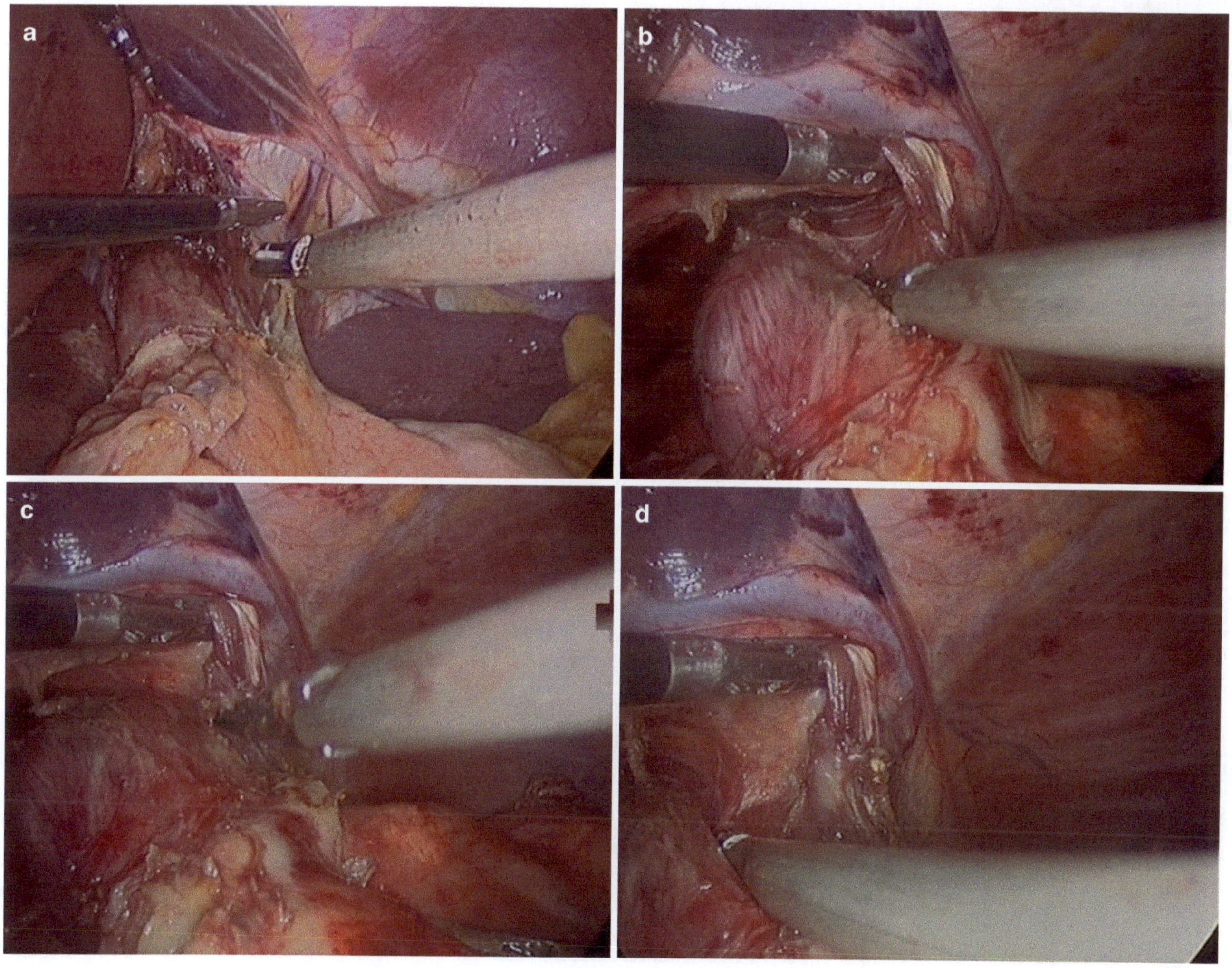

Photo 5.26 (a–g)

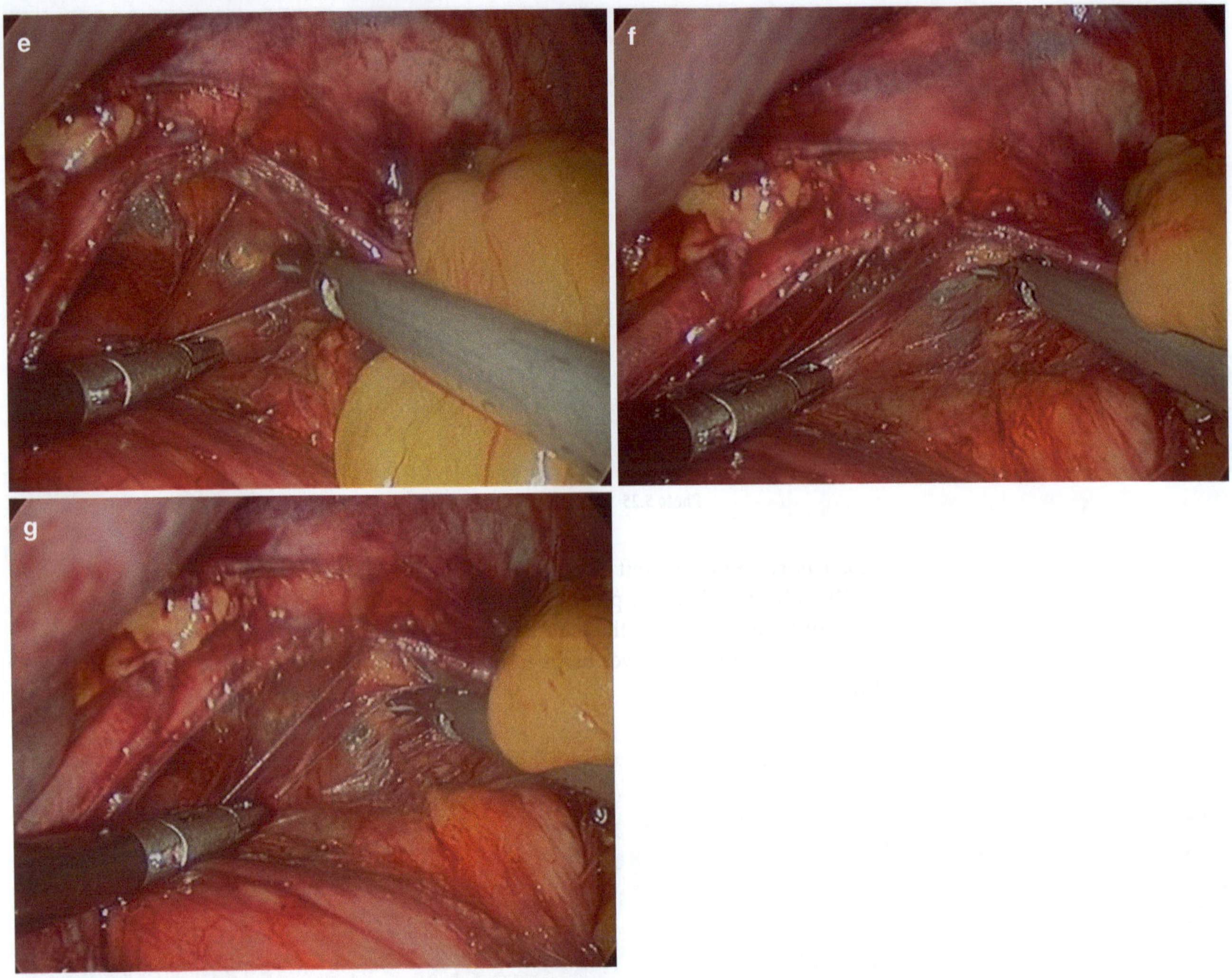

Photo 5.26 (Continued)

27. The left pleura is identified and reflected away from the esophagus (Photo 5.27a–j).

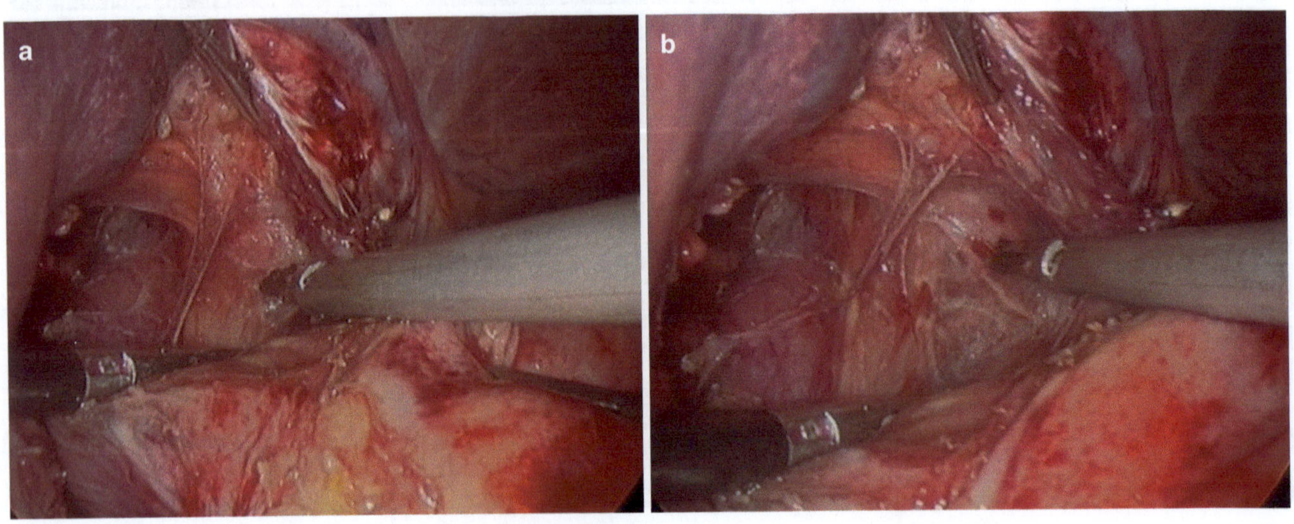

Photo 5.27 (a–j)

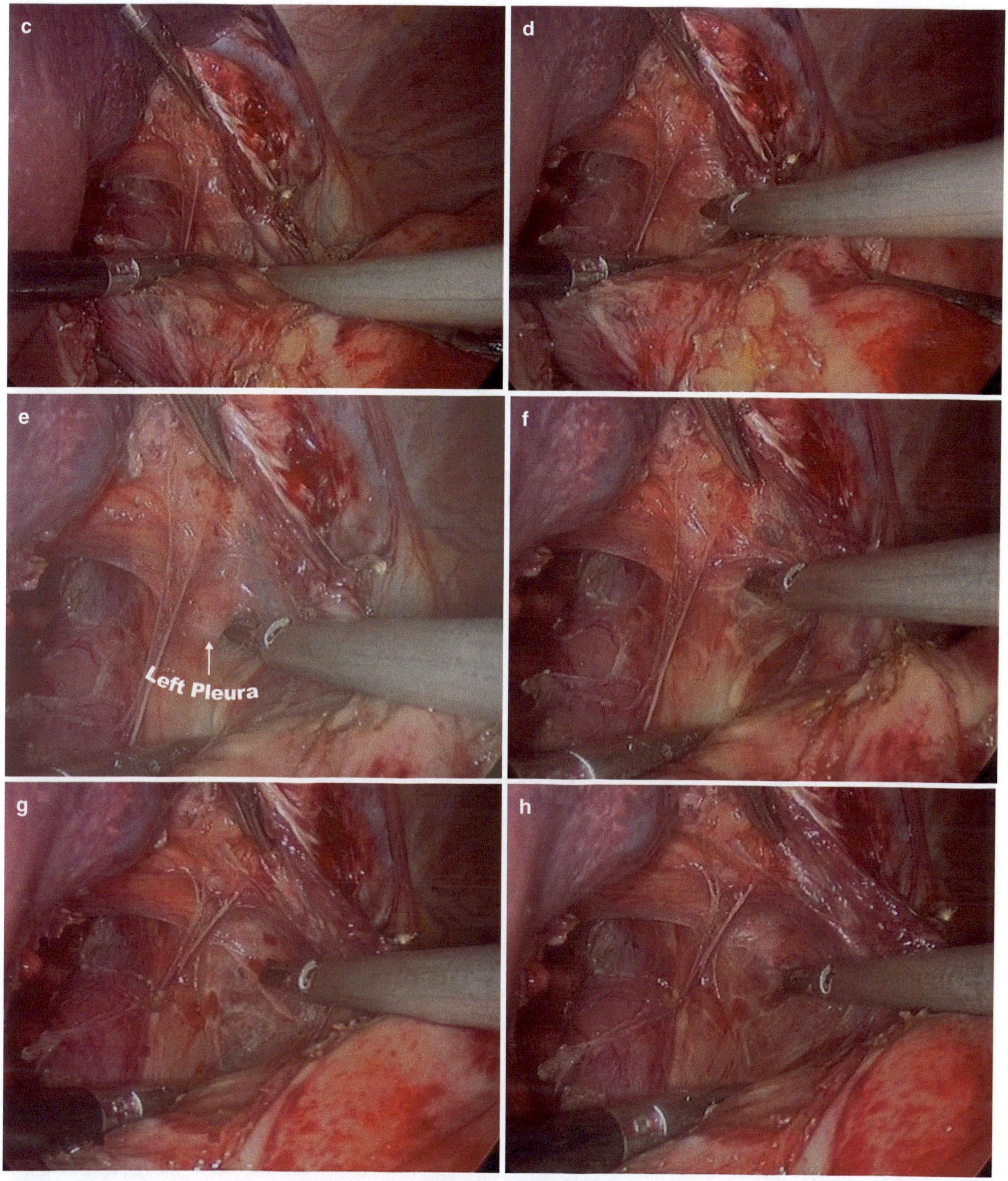

Photo 5.27 (Continued)

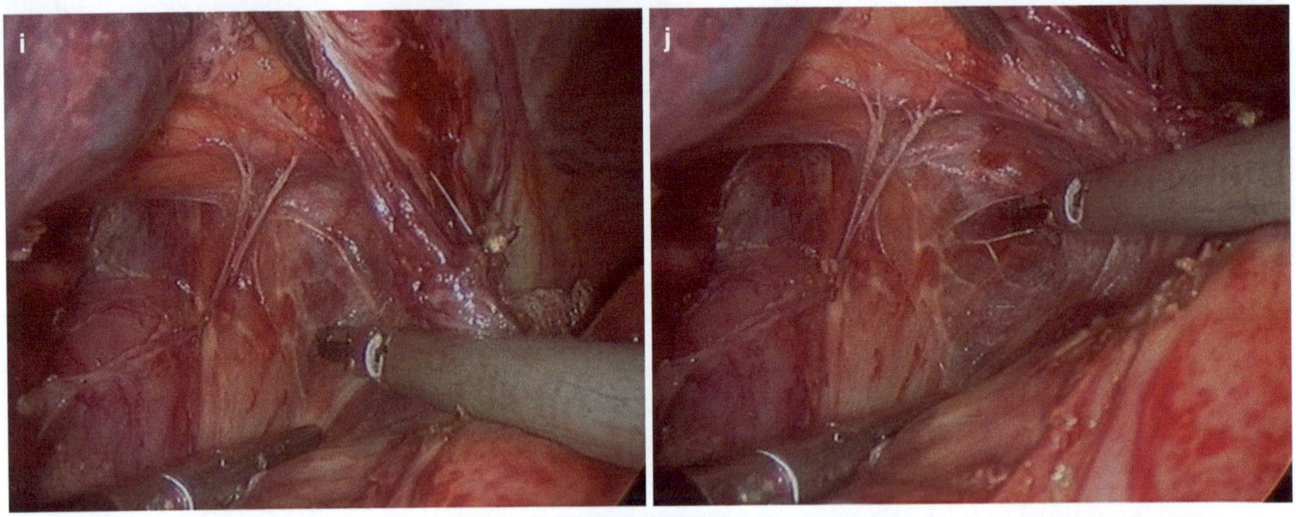

Photo 5.27 (Continued)

28. The dissection is then continued in the plane between the pericardium and the esophagus, proceeding toward the left side. The anterior vagus is identified. Dissection is then continued parallel to the left margin of the esophagus, taking care not to damage the left pleura (Photo 5.28a–g).

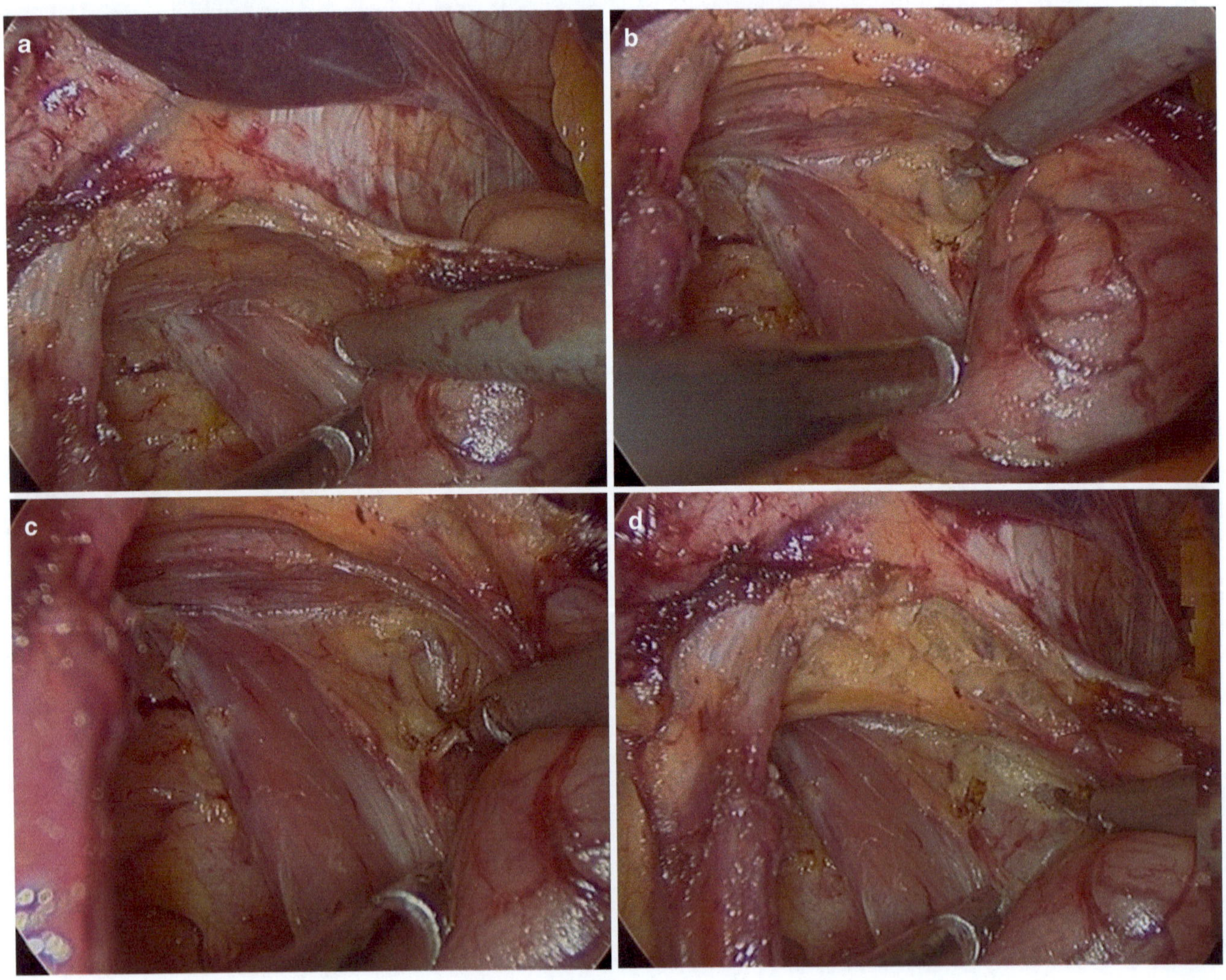

Photo 5.28 (a–g)

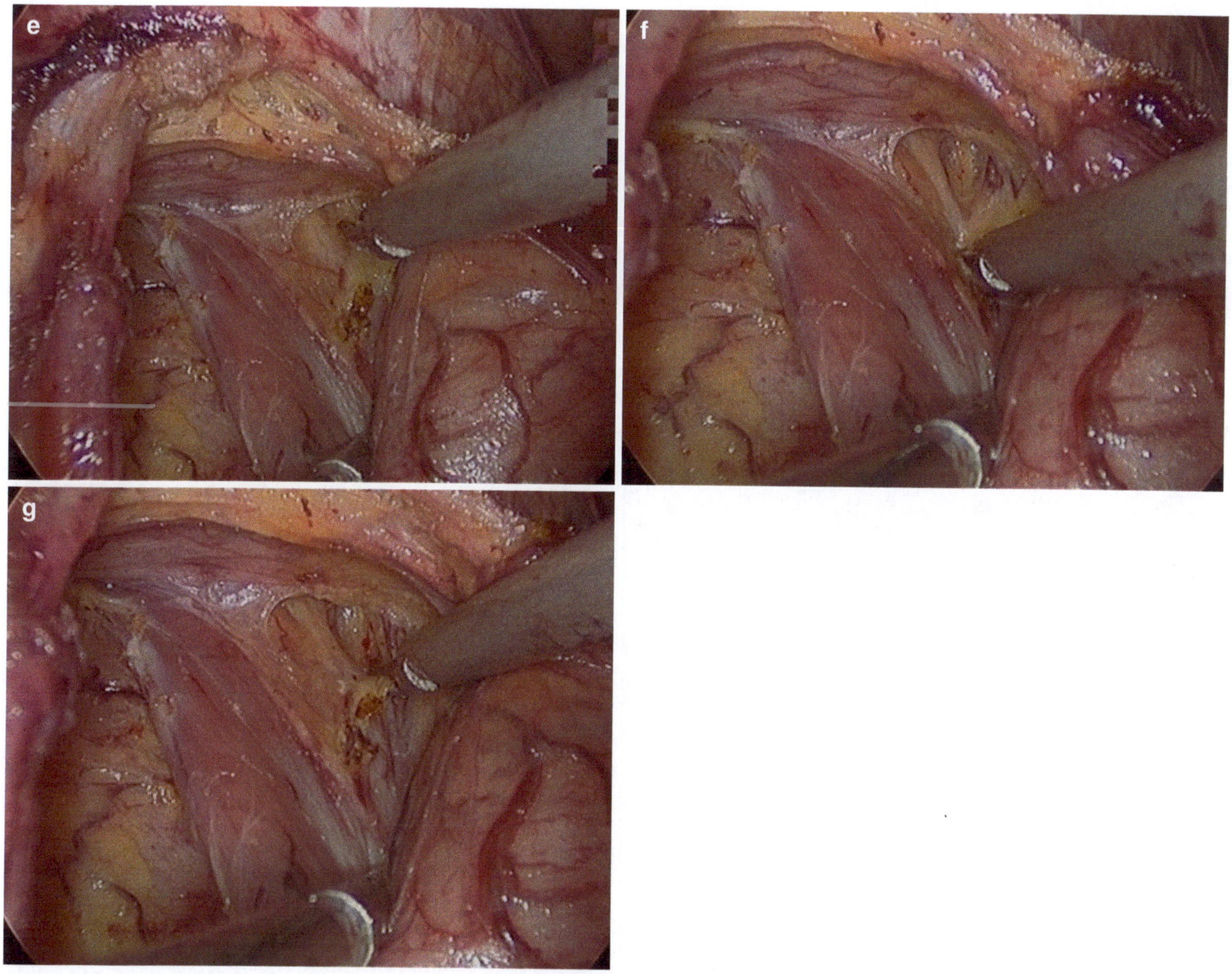

Photo 5.28 (Continued)

29. The anterior vagus is identified and dissection is done outside the vagus nerve. The vagus nerve is cut at the highest level of left-lateral mobilization. On cutting the vagus, release phenomenon can be experienced by the surgeon. Anatomically, this preserves the branches of the vagus to the trachea and left main bronchus. The esophagus is further mobilized. The plane of dissection now lies between the vagus and the esophagus (Photo 5.29a–h).

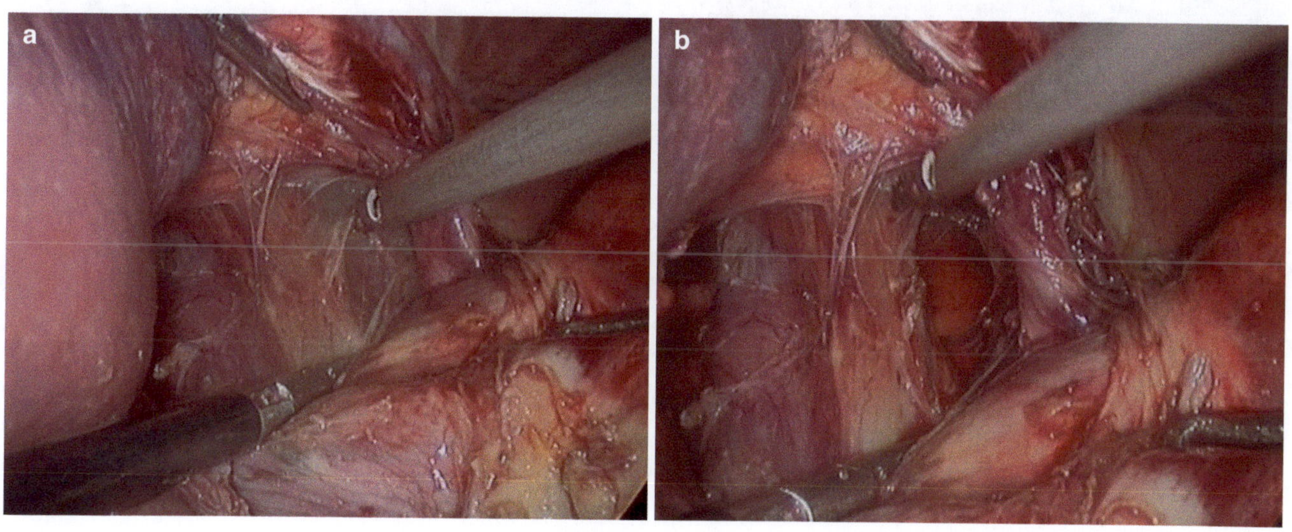

Photo 5.29 (a–h)

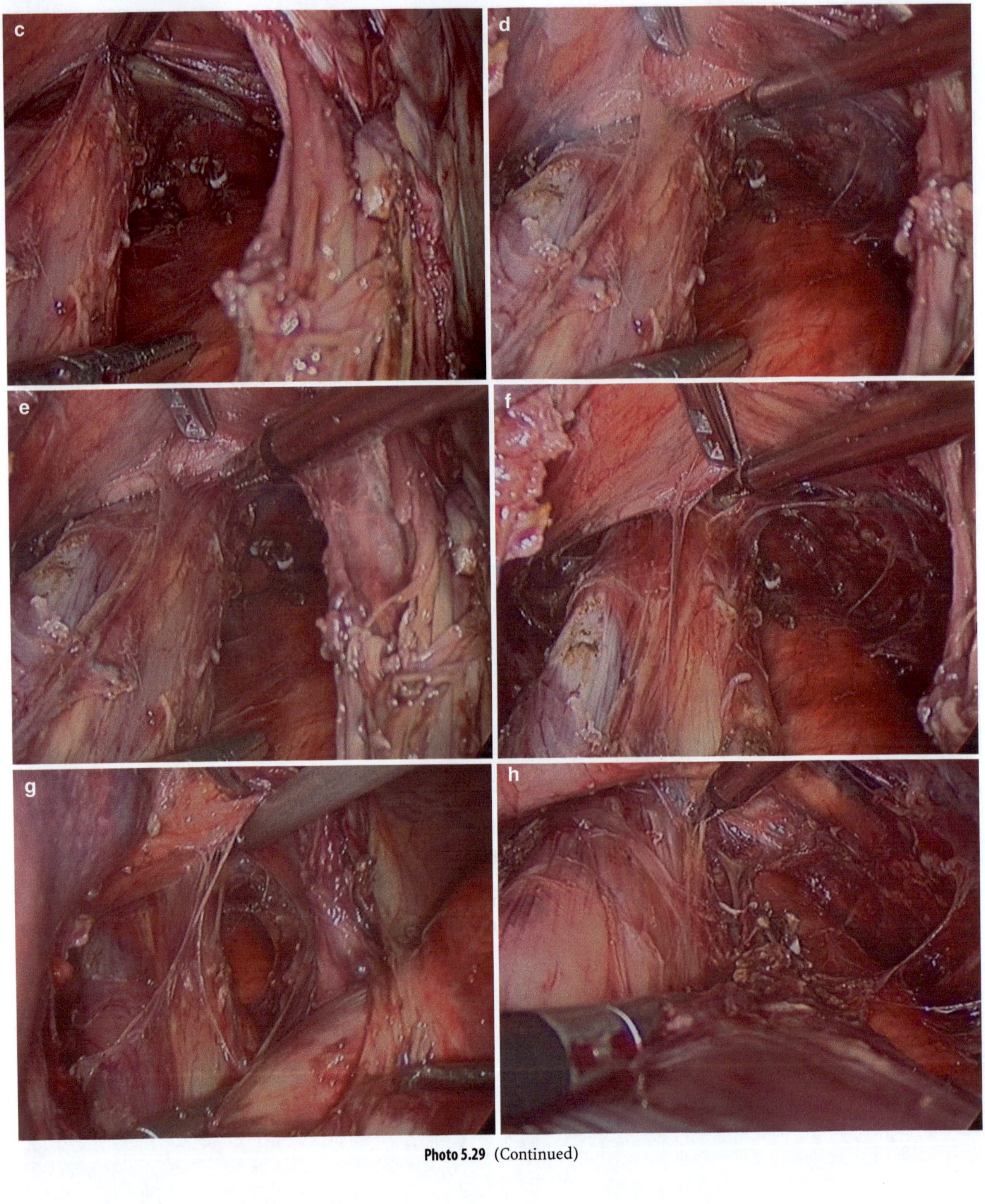

Photo 5.29 (Continued)

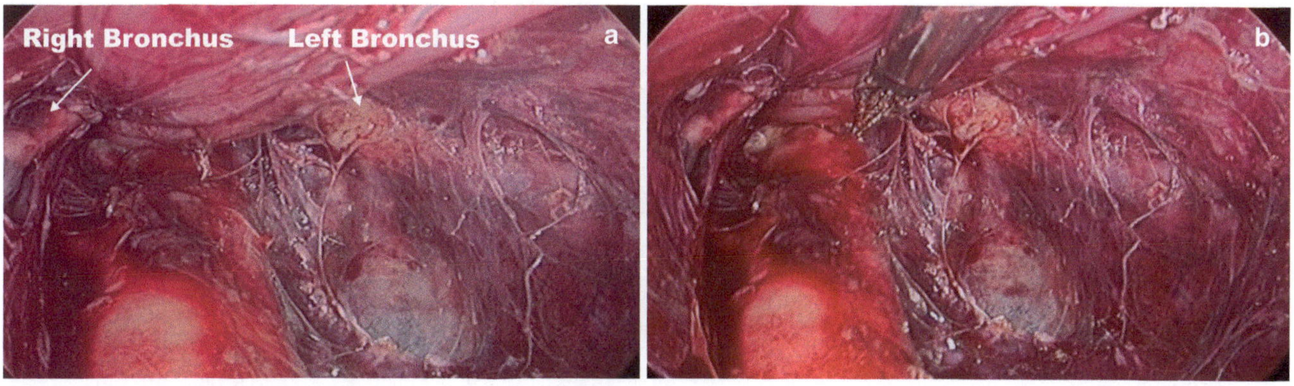

Photo 5.30 (a, b)

30. The dissection proceeds cranially till the identification of the left main bronchus (Photo 5.30a, b).

31. The sign of complete dissection all around is the visualization of descending aorta from the left side of esophagus (Photo 5.31a–d).

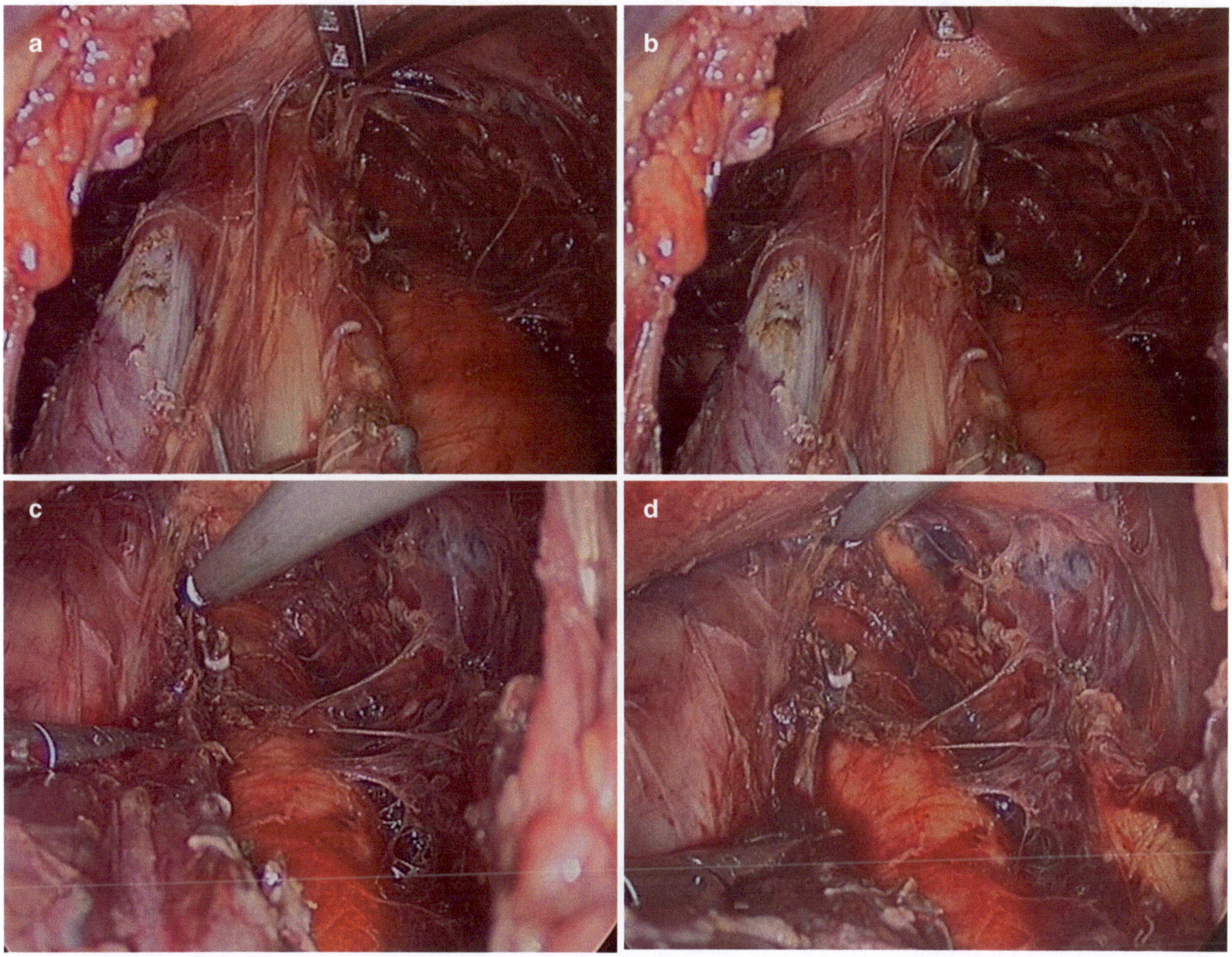

Photo 5.31 (a–d)

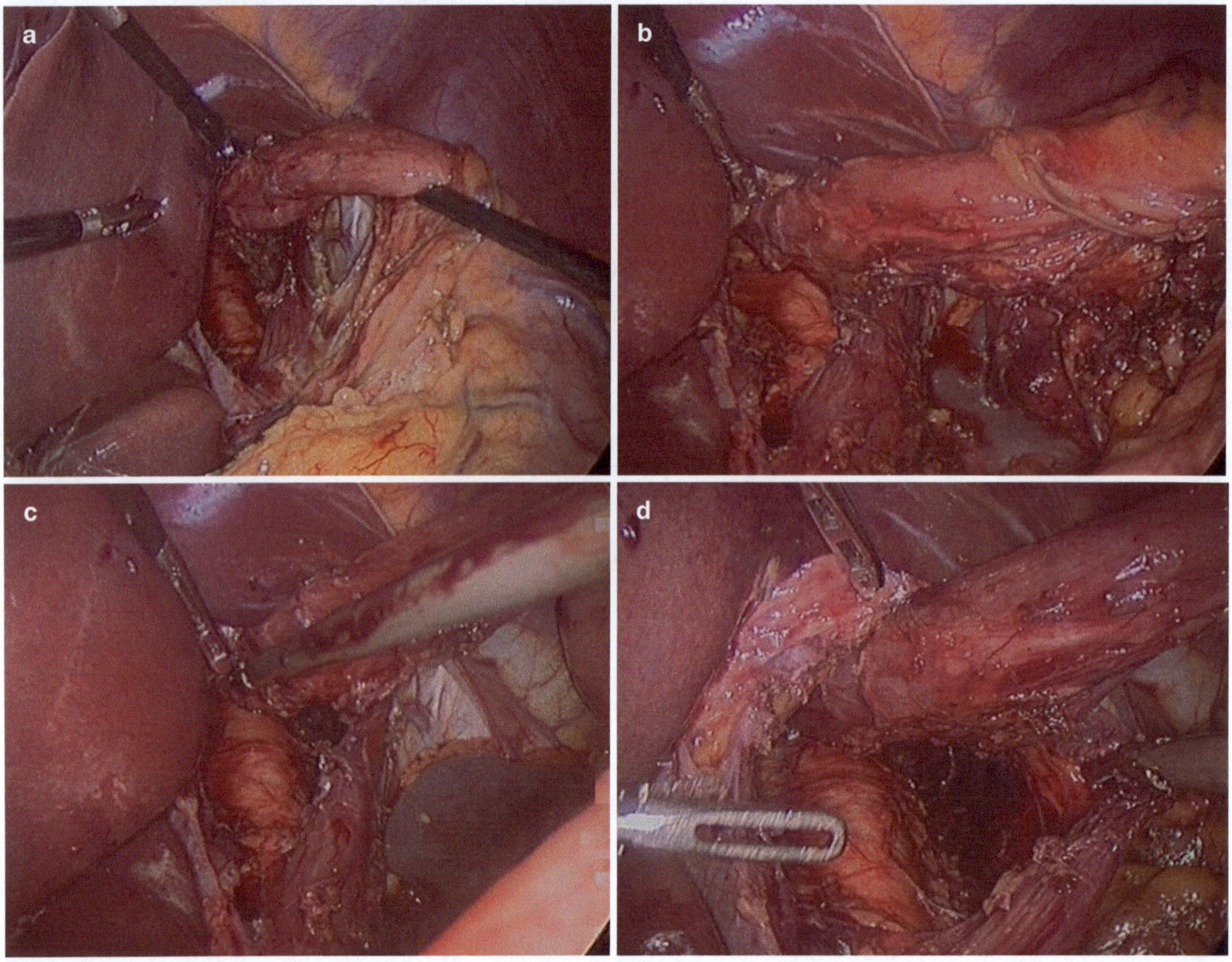

Photo 5.32 (a–d)

32. Completely mobilized esophagus can now be pulled downward and laterally, with the complete visualization of the aorta (Photo 5.32a–d).

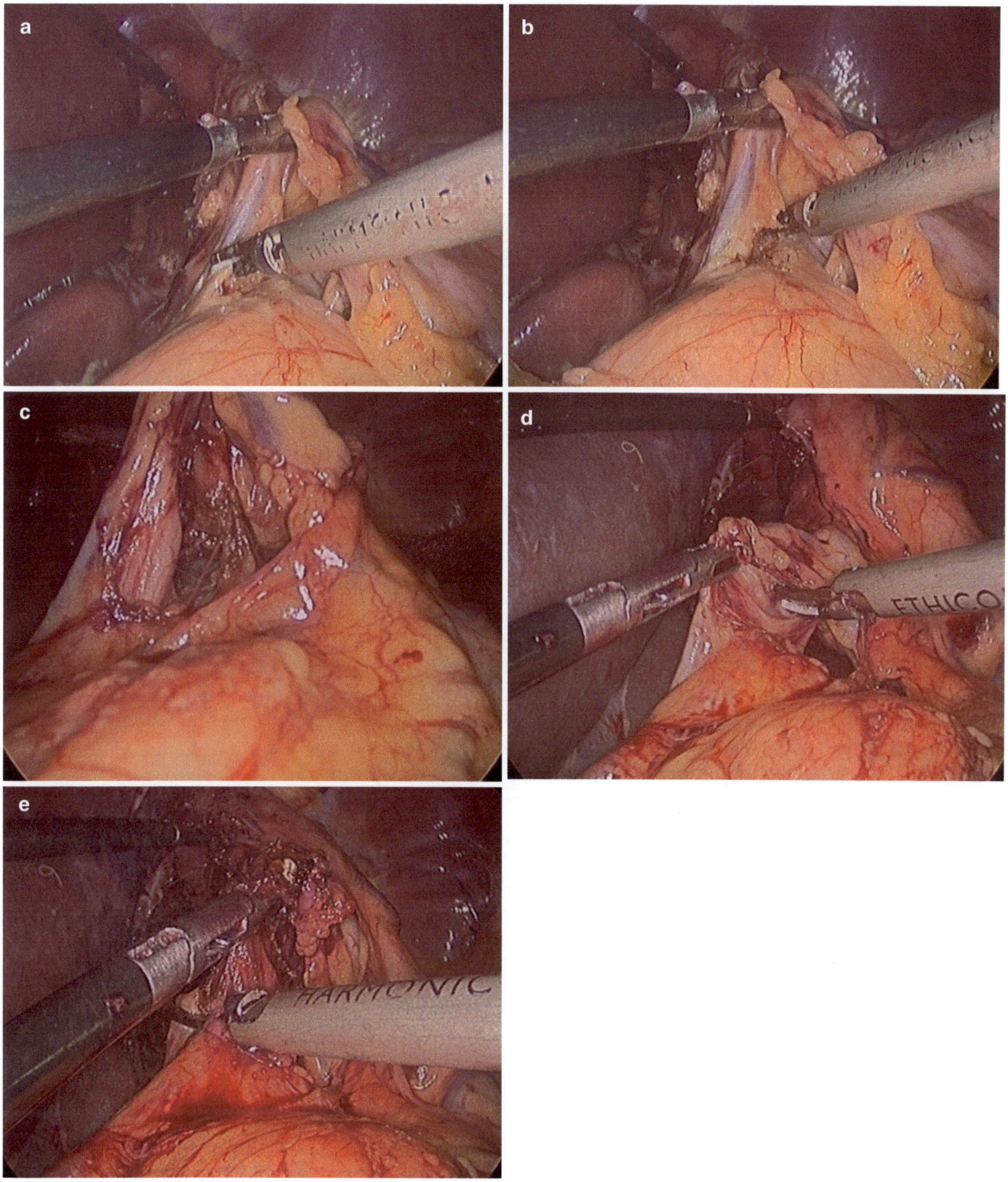

Photo 5.33 (a–e)

33. Commencement of the Celiac dissection (Photo 5.33a–e).

Stomach mobilization, mobilization of the esophagus in the neck, specimen retrieval, and creation of the stomach tube, esophago-gastric anastomosis in the neck and the postoperative management are the same as described for thoracoscopic esophagectomy (See Chap. 4).

6

Thoracoscopic Esophageal Resection for Cancer in Prone Decubitus Position: Operative Technique

Miguel A. Cuesta, Joris J. G. Scheepers, Wolter Oosterhuis, Surya S.A.Y. Biere, Donald L. van der Peet, and Bob H.M. Heijnen

Minimally invasive approach for esophageal resection for cancer is increasingly used in many centers because it can resect the esophageal cancer along the same planes as in the conventional way, and perform the same type of one- or two-field lymphadenectomy (obtaining the same number of lymph nodes (LN)), but avoiding a thoracotomy and/or laparotomy. Consequences of this are less postoperative pain and possibly less respiratory complications.

Initial reports used the right lateral thoracoscopic approach with total lung block in order to visualize and dissect the esophagus [1–3]. The goal of this minimally invasive procedure was to resect the esophageal cancer, according to established oncological principles, with all postoperative advantages of the minimally invasive surgery.

However, the reports of the initial pioneers were followed by others who were critical about the procedure and others who were especially disappointed [4, 5] because the outcome (conversions to open approach in 10–17%, morbidity, especially respiratory, between 17 and 42% and mortality between 3 and 12%) were not better than the conventional approach.

They conclude that this approach was feasible but these initial results did not show a real benefit.

As a consequence of this, Cuschieri et al., attempted to change the thoracoscopic approach from a lateral to a prone position, without total collapse of the lung, in order to diminish the postoperative respiratory complications [6].

Prone decubitus position for conventional lung resection was initially described by Overholt in 1949 [7].

The advantages of this approach, in comparison with the standard lateral decubitus position were: (a) the attainable range of thoracic cage and diaphragmatic excursion is greater than in the side position; (b) the amplitude of mediastinal swing or displacement is less; (c) exposure of the posterior aspect of the hilum and esophageal area is facilitated; (d) the weight of the lung itself allows it to fall forward; and (e) in the event of hemorrhage the blood flows away from its source, thus permitting its control with greater ease.

The approach was not commonly used again until the introduction of the esophageal approach by prone decubitus right thoracoscopy.

Indication

All patients with esophageal squamous cancer or adenocarcinoma of the esophagus, with exception of the gastro-esophageal junction cancers Siewert type I, were considered for thoracoscopic-prone position (and laparoscopy plus cervical approach) resection.

Exclusion and Conversion

Patients operated on previously by right thoracotomy were excluded for this approach.

Extensive adhesions in the thoracic cavity, precluding an adequate partial collapse of the right lung were quickly converted to conventional right thoracotomy.

Operative Technique

1. After induction of general anesthesia, standard intratracheal single lumen intubation follows.

Patient is then positioned in prone decubitus position on a standard apparatus in order to support on the head, thorax and pelvis. Abdomen is maintained free for breathing excursions. Position of the arms is very important in order to get abduction of the scapula. The arms are positioned on a support device in flexion of the shoulders and elbows (Fig. 6.1a, b).

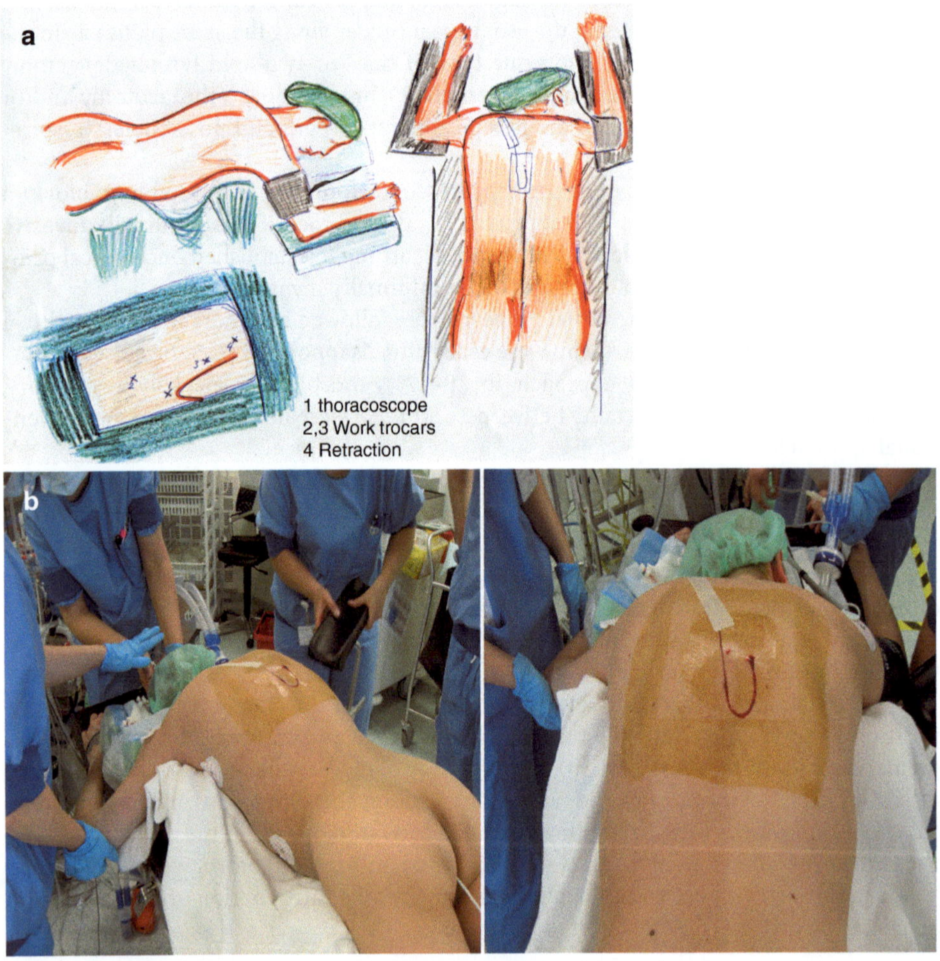

Fig. 6.1 (a–d) Placement of patient in the prone position. Operating room set-up during operation. Surgeon (and the first assistant) stand at the right side of the patient, looking at the monitor in front of them. Position of trocars along the medial border of the scapula

Fig. 6.1 (Continued)

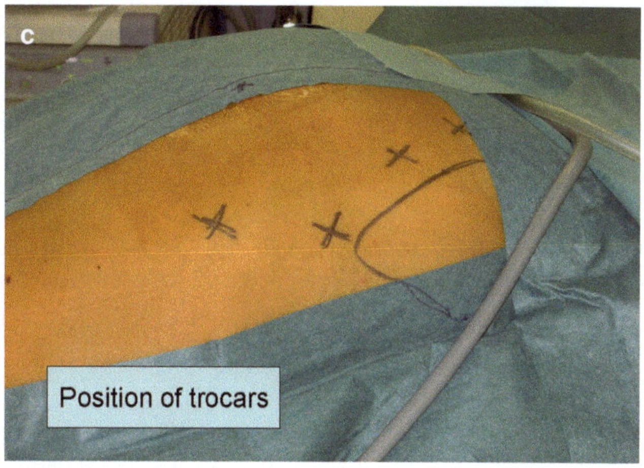

In this way the area between the spine and the inner edge of the scapula is broadened.

2. Surgeon stands on the right side of patient with the first assistant on his/her right side looking to the monitor in front of them. Scrub nurse stands on the left side of the surgeon (Fig. 6.1d).

3. Four trocars are placed along the inner edge of the right scapula (Fig. 6.1c). The first at the level of the lowest point of the scapula, a 10 mm, (can be 5 mm) for the thoracoscope. The second, at the level of 4th intercostal space, 5 mm; the third, at the level of 8th intercostal space, 12 mm and the last, at the level of 2th intercostal space as work trocar for assistant (suction, lung retraction etc). The first trocar is introduced open in the thoracic cavity after control by finger palpation that the space is free of adhesions. After introduction of the first trocar a positive insufflation of 5–8 mmHg is initiated in order to retract enough the right lung for an adequate visualization of the posterior mediastinum. A thoracoscope of 30° is used.

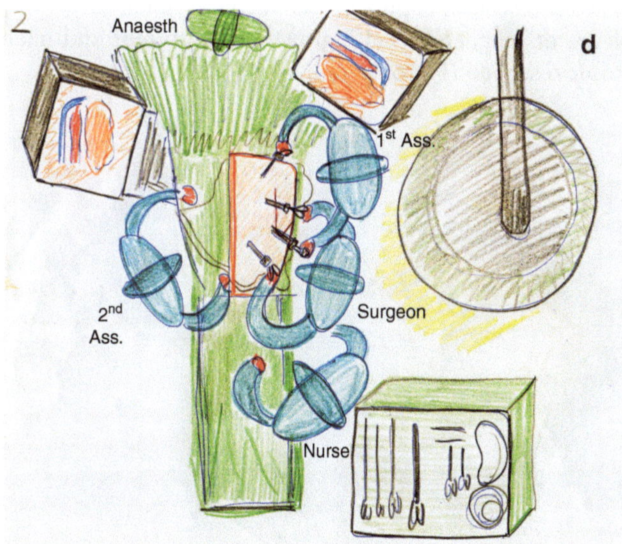

Fig. 6.1 (Continued)

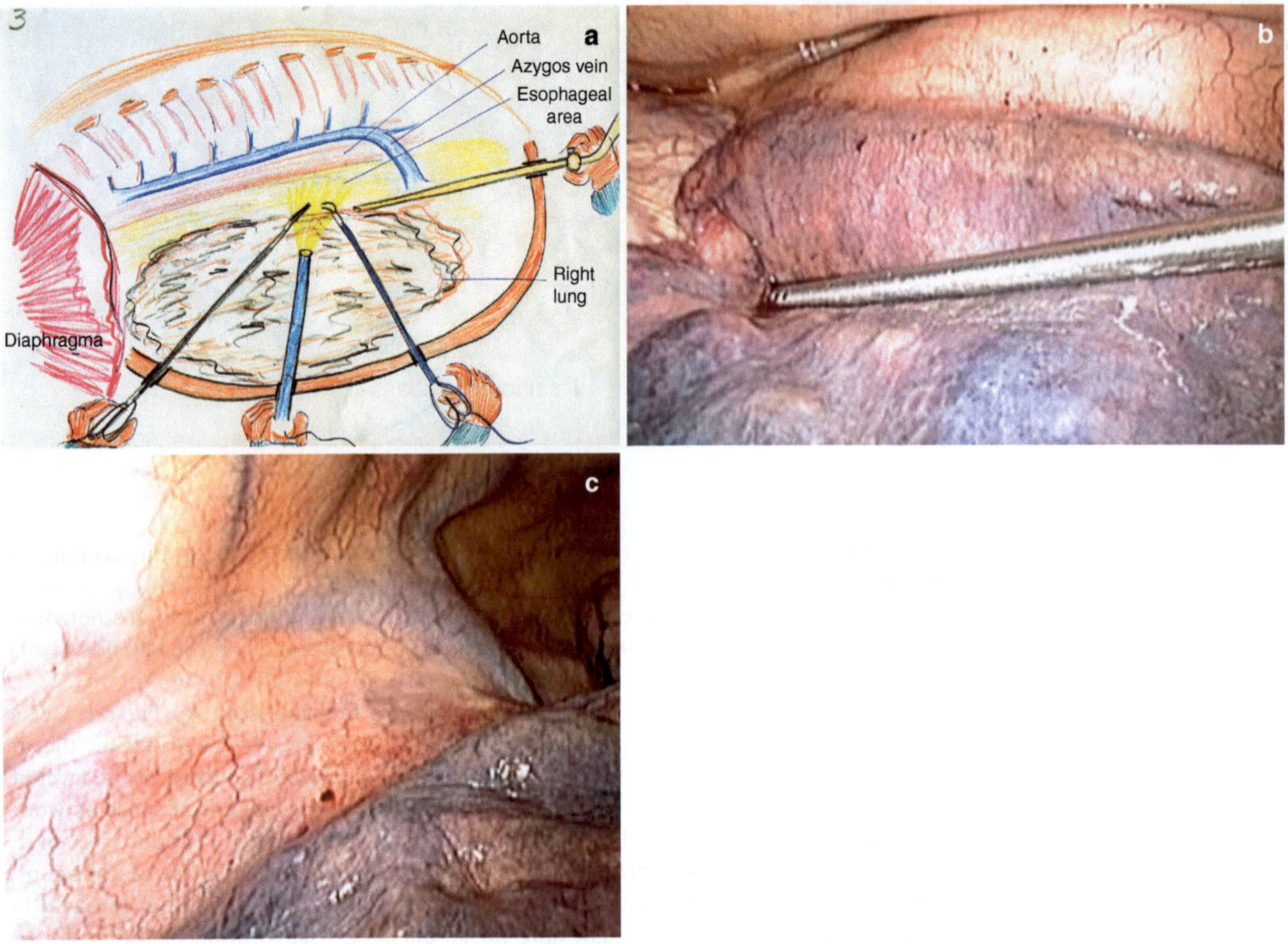

Fig. 6.2 General inspection of the thoracic cavity, distal part and aspects of esophageal area, at the level of the carina and azygos vein (**a**–**c**). The right lung falls due to the insufflation of the cavity (pressure between 5 and 8 mm) and the position of the patient. (**d**–**h**)

4. Inspection is performed of the thoracic cavity and the esophageal area in order to assess if resection is possible As in conventional surgery, presence of metastases, in the pleura or lung, and local ingrowth of the tumor and fixation will preclude a thoracoscopic resection (Fig. 6.2a–c).

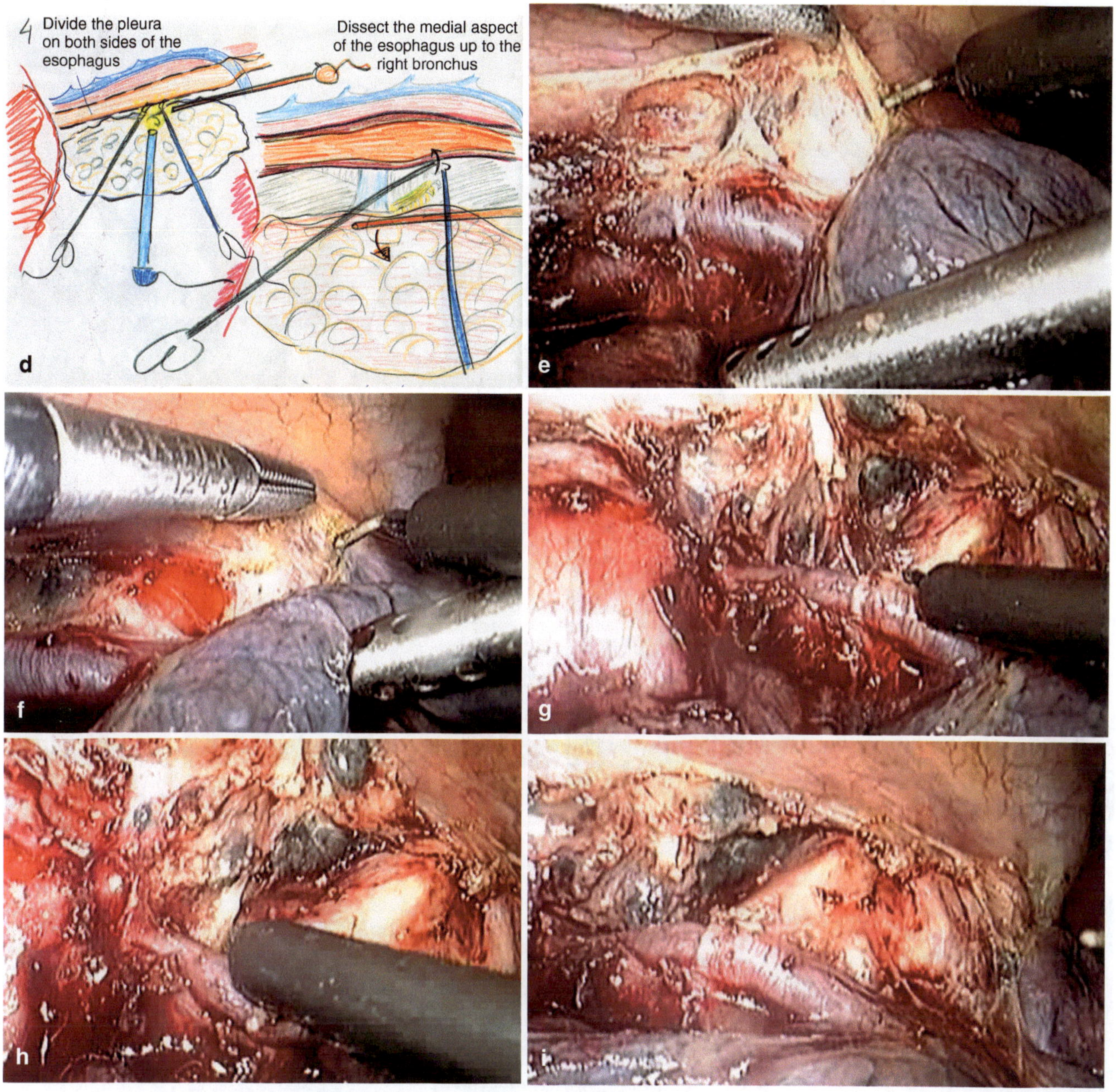

Fig. 6.2 (Continued)

Dissection starts anteriorly by cutting the pulmonary ligament, and the anterior pleura along the lung, from the pericard sac to the hilum of the right lung (right pulmonary vein and right bronchus) up to the azygos vein (Fig. 6.2d–i).

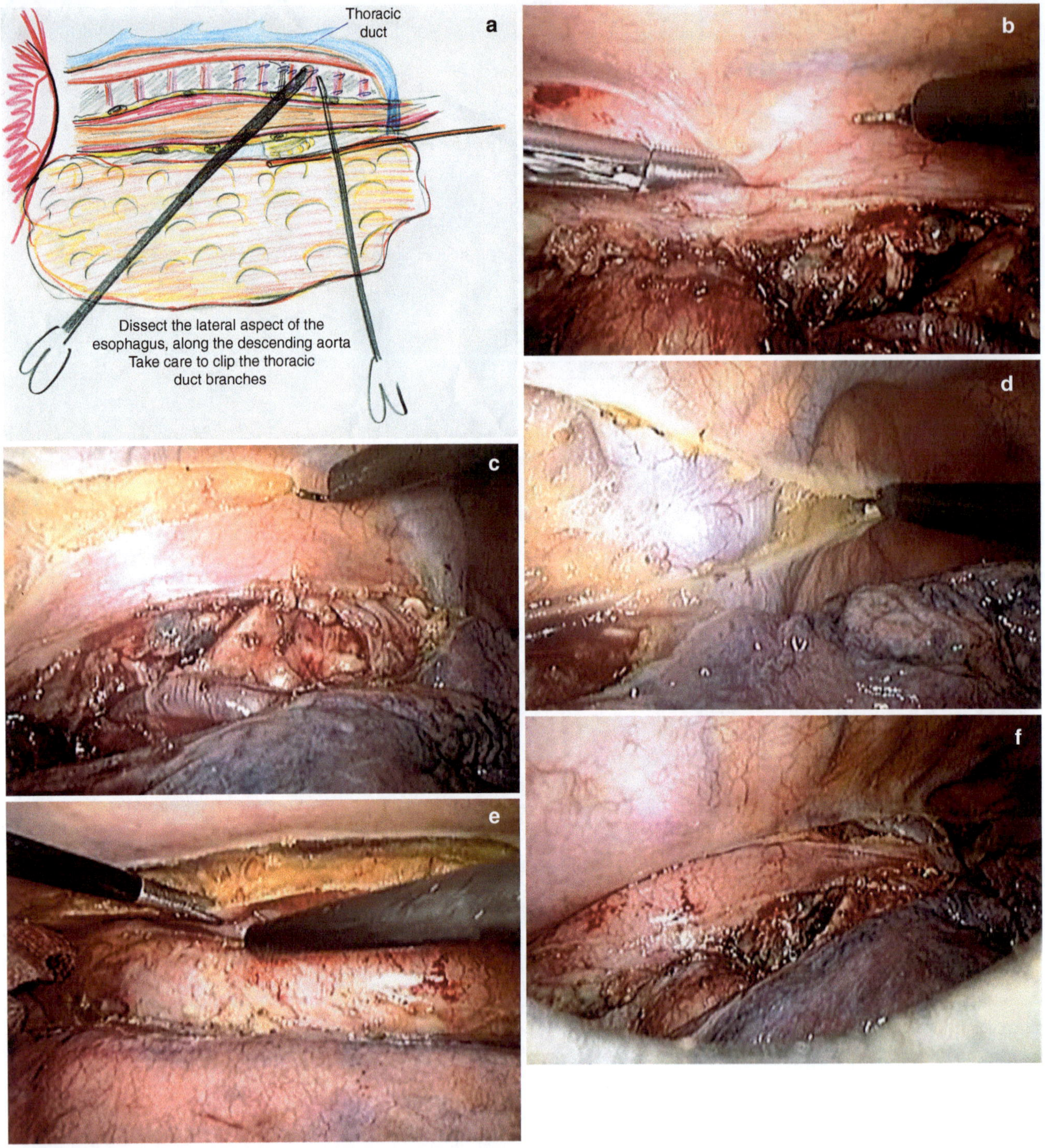

Fig. 6.3 The mediastinal pleura is open at the posterior aspect of the esophagus along the medial aspect of the azygos vein. Dissection takes place along the aorta plane, taking care to localize the thoracic duct, dividing all its branches at the level of the carina between clips (**a**–**h**). The posterior aspect of the dissection is reached (pericard sac, pulmonal veins and contralateral pleura), after dividing several esophageal vessels (**i**)

5. Posteriorly the mediastinal pleura is cut longitudinally at the posterior edge of the esophagus, anterior of the azygos vein from the costo-phrenic angle to the arch of the azygos vein (Fig. 6.3a–f). In this way a broad piece of pleura is resected with the specimen.

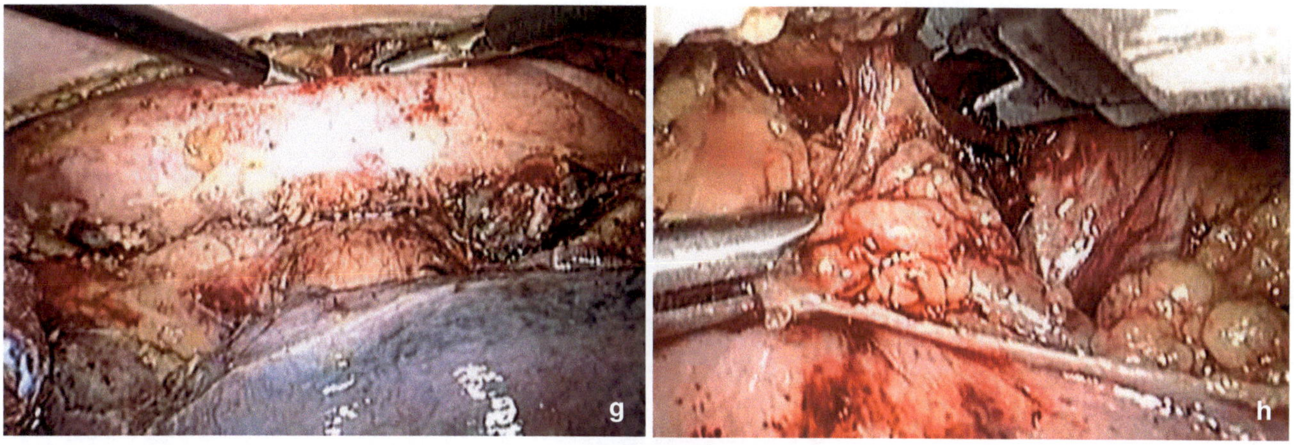

Fig. 6.3 (Continued)

6. Along the plane of the descending aorta, the esophagus with periesophageal lymphnodes and fat is dissected free, taking care with the control of the thoracic duct, and crossing branches from right to left at the carina level. Vascular branches from the aorta to the esophagus at this level have to be clipped in order to avoid lymph leakage (Fig. 6.3g–h). The rest of branches are divided by means of a Ligasure device®. In this way the posterior plane of the pericard, right atrium and contralateral pleura is reached (Fig. 6.3i).

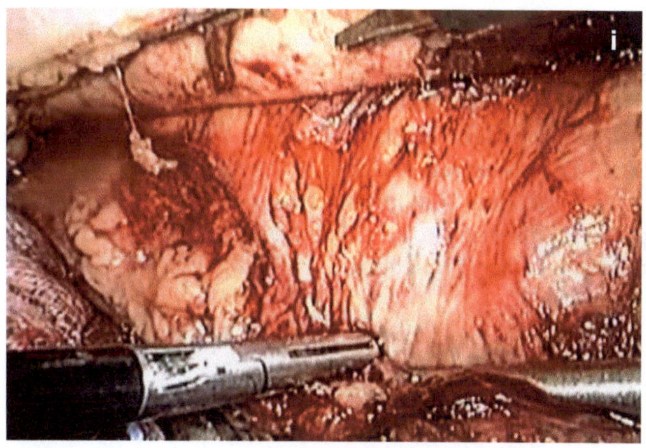

Fig. 6.3 (Continued)

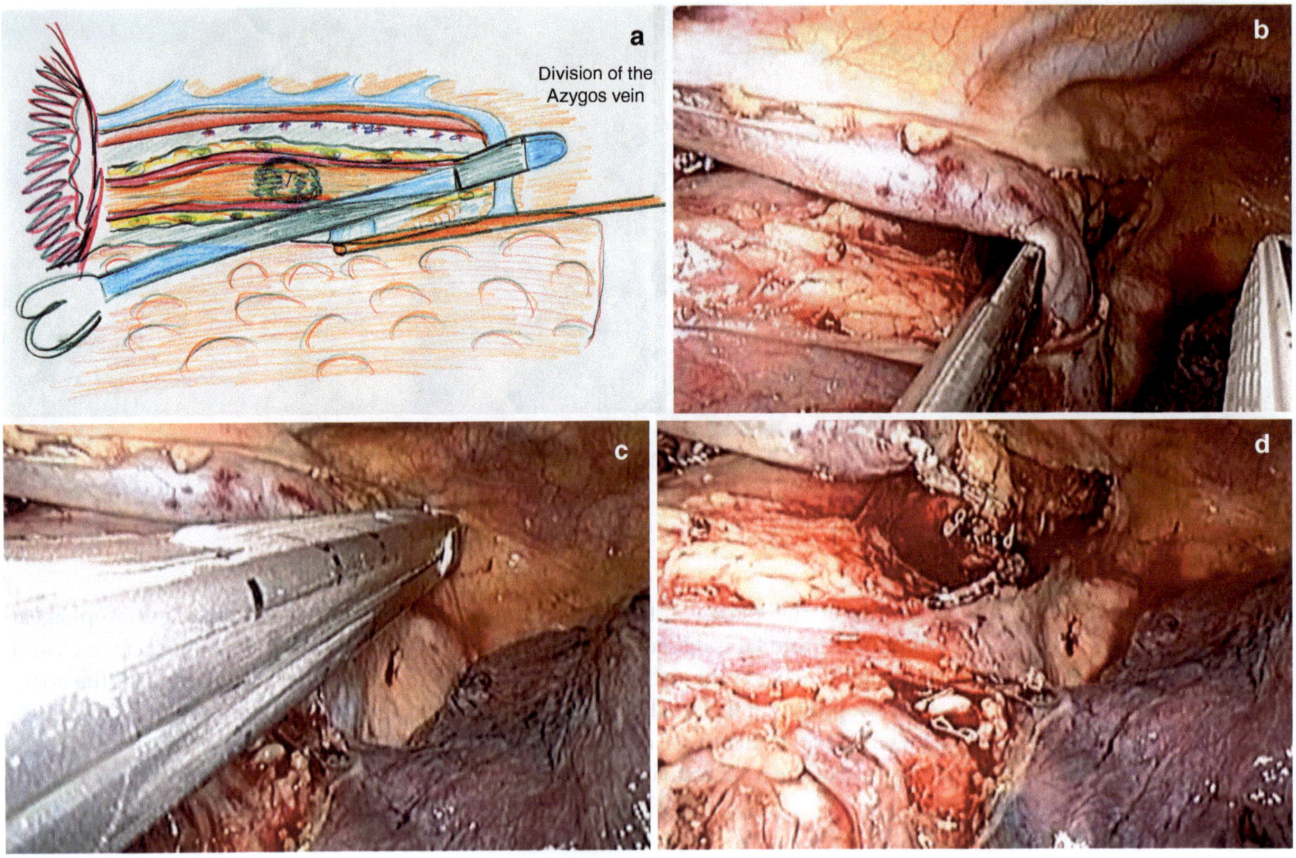

Fig. 6.4 (a–d) The azygos vein is dissected free and divided by means of vascular (white) endostapler

7. Furthermore the azygos vein is dissected free and cut by means of a vascular endostapler (Fig. 6.4a–d).

8. Dissection proceeds with extensive lymphadenectomy of the right bronchus, carina and left bronchus resection (Fig. 6.5a–f). Lymphadenectomy is not picking one but "en bloc," The LN remain attached to the specimen.

9. Dissection continues between esophagus and trachea (pars membranacea) in proximal direction, to stop 3 cm from the apex of the thoracic cavity, leaving a small cuff of pleura intact (Fig. 6.5g, h).

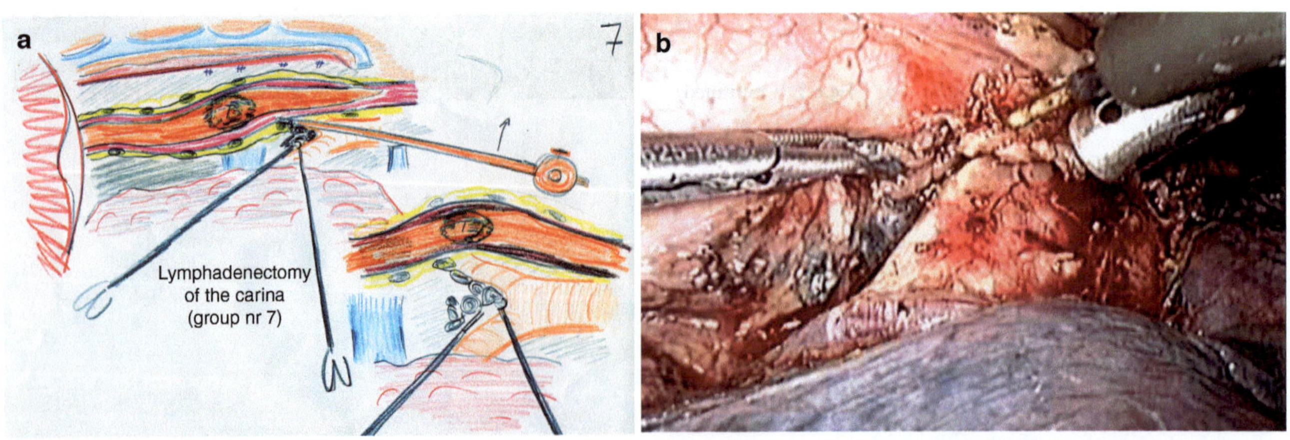

Fig. 6.5 (a–h) Lymphadenectomy of the carina is now performed, starting at the right bronchus, the carina and thereafter the left bronchus. The hook is used for this dissection. It is important to complete the dissection of the left bronchus not only behind the esophagus but also from the other side (posterior). In this way the lymphadenectomy of the carina is completed and the lymph nodes remain attached to the esophagus. The trachea is freed from the esophagus. In proximal tumors dissection must be very precise and careful in order to preserve the pars membranacea of the trachea

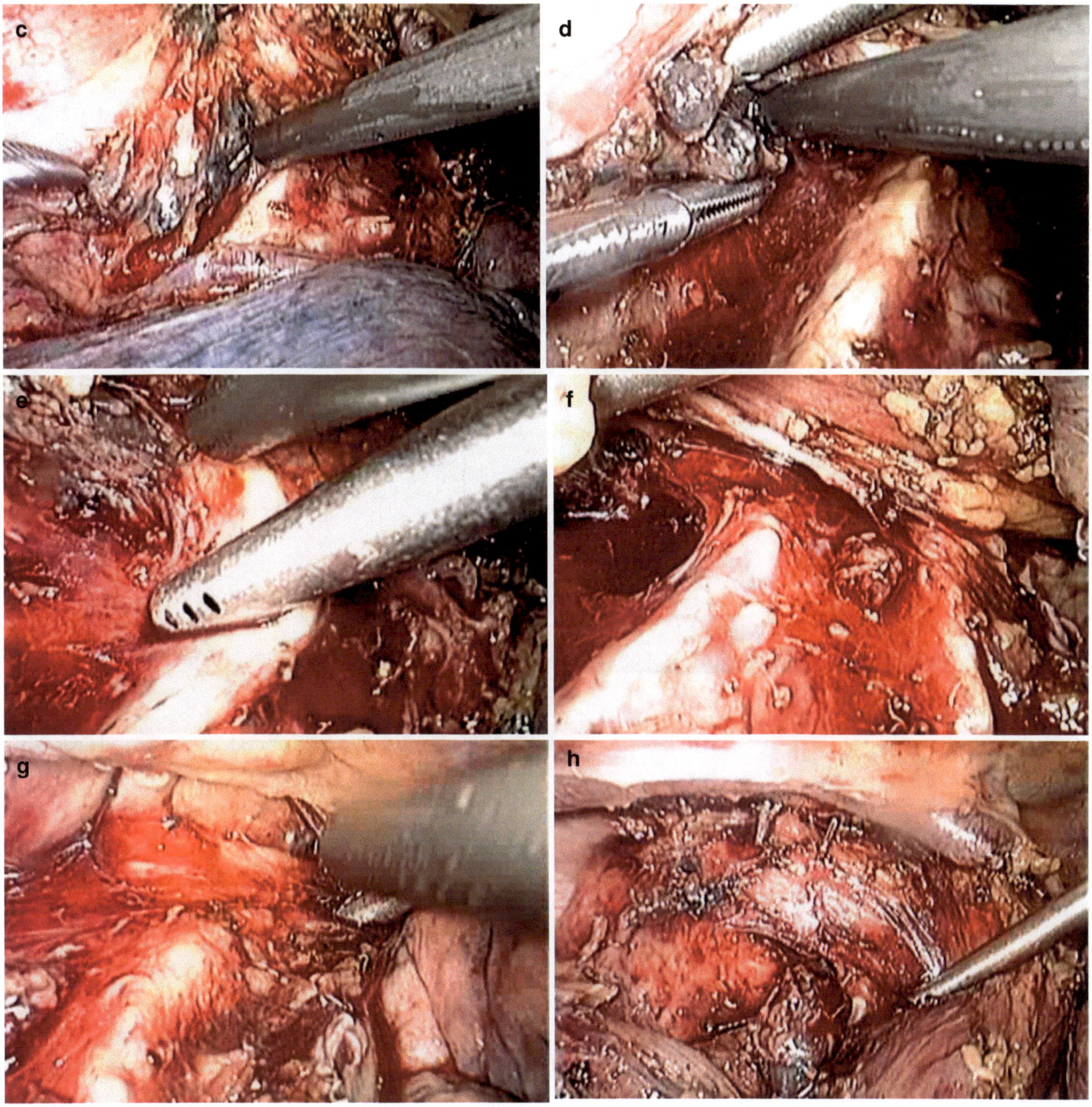

Fig. 6.5 (Continued)

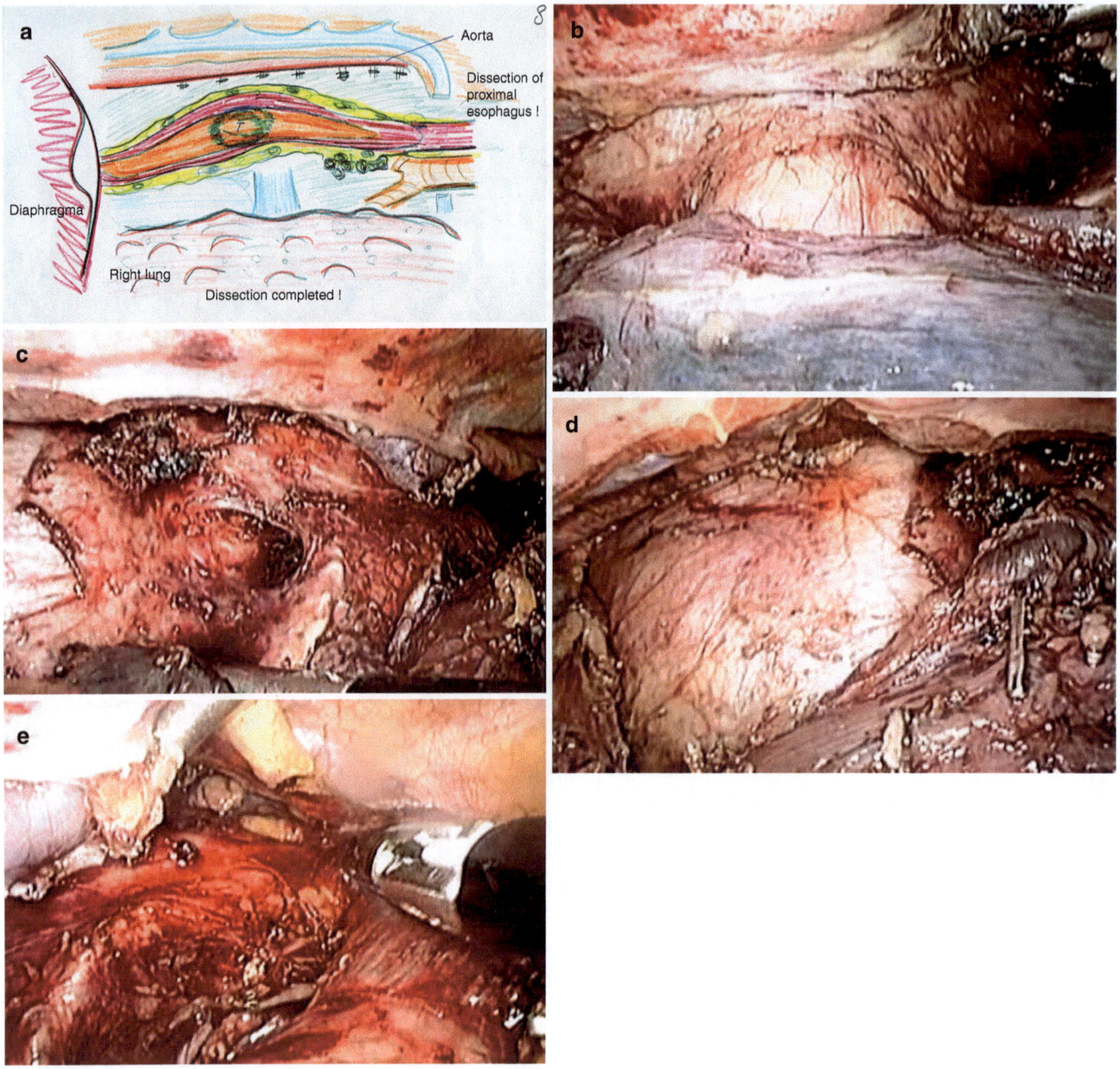

Fig. 6.6 (**a**) General inspection once the dissection is completed. (**b**) Right pulmonary vein; (**c**) carina; (**d**) pericard sac, left atrium and (**e**) trachea

10. After hemostasia control, a thoracic drain is left in the posterior mediastinum and the thoracoscopic phase is considered finalized after general inspection for hemostasia (Fig. 6.6a–e).

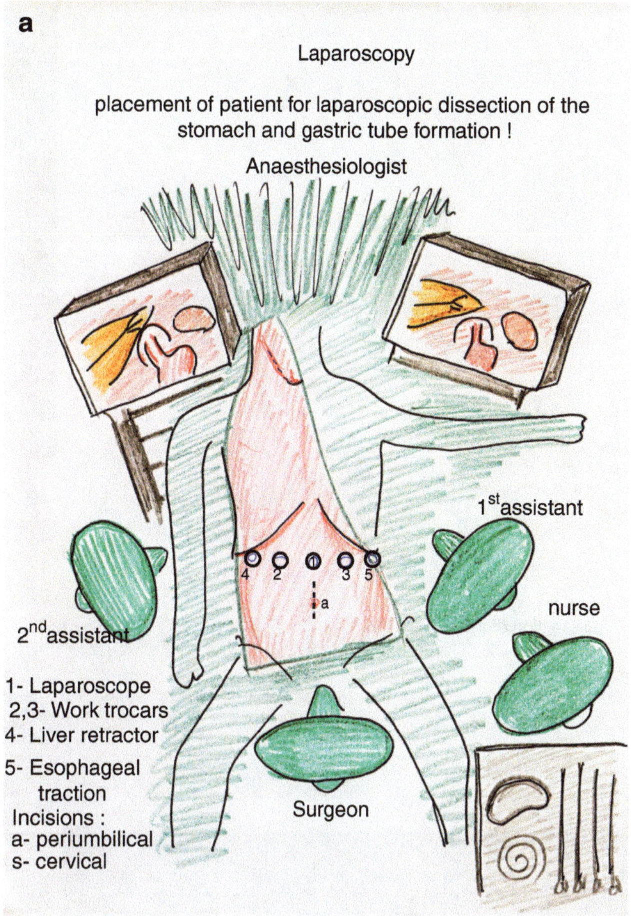

Fig. 6.7 Operating room set-up for laparoscopic dissection of the stomach (**a**), gastric dissection a long the greater curvature (**b-d**), performing an extensive lymphadenectomy of the celiac trunk (**e–f**)

11. Patient is placed for the laparoscopic and cervical phase of the operation (Fig. 6.7a). Stomach is mobilized completely with preservation of the gastro-epiploic vessels and an extensive lymphadenectomy of the celiac trunk is performed (Fig. 6.7b–f). Last part of the laparoscopic approach is the dissection of the hiatal area in which the hiatus is enlarged anteriorly and carefully a communication is made with the thoracic dissected area. Take care that all the specimen, esophagus, and stomach are completely free! At the end of the laparoscopic phase a second team will approach the esophagus at

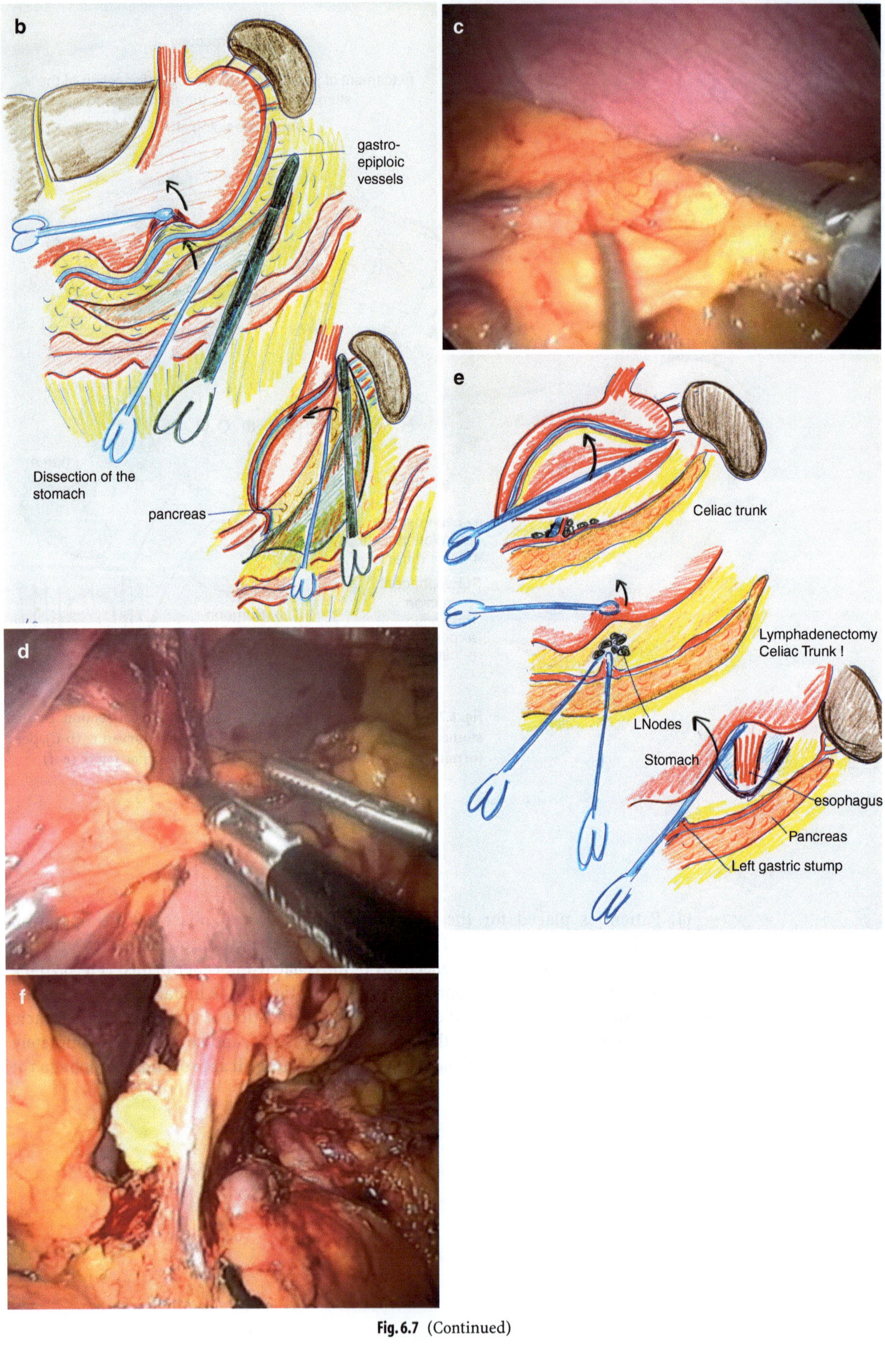

Fig. 6.7 (Continued)

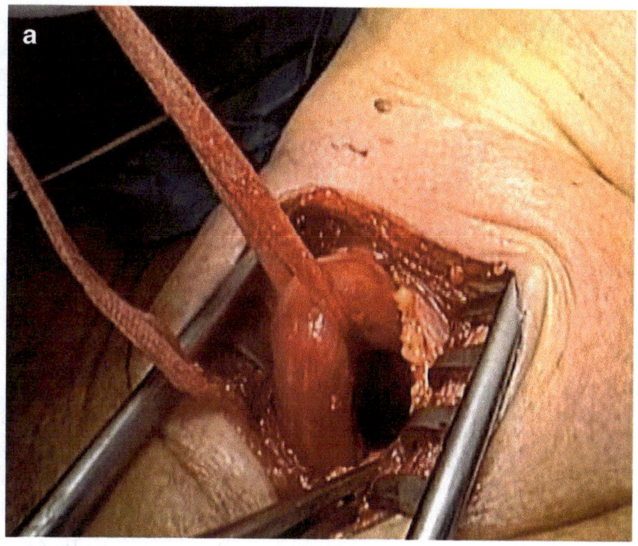

Fig. 6.8 Through a cervical incision the esophagus is dissected free (**a**). The specimen is retrieved through a hand assisted device transumbilical positioned (**b**–**e**). A gastric tube is created by means of GIA stapler (**f**–**g**) and pulled up (attached to a nasogastric tube) into the cervical wound (h) and anastomosed to the proximal esophagus. Aspect of the scars at 10 days postoperative (**i**, **j**)

the cervical area (Fig. 6.8a) and after division of the esophagus (and attached a NG tube to the distal part of the divided esophagus) the specimen is retrieved by the abdominal surgeon through a transumbilical incision of 7 cm, protected by a hand assisted device

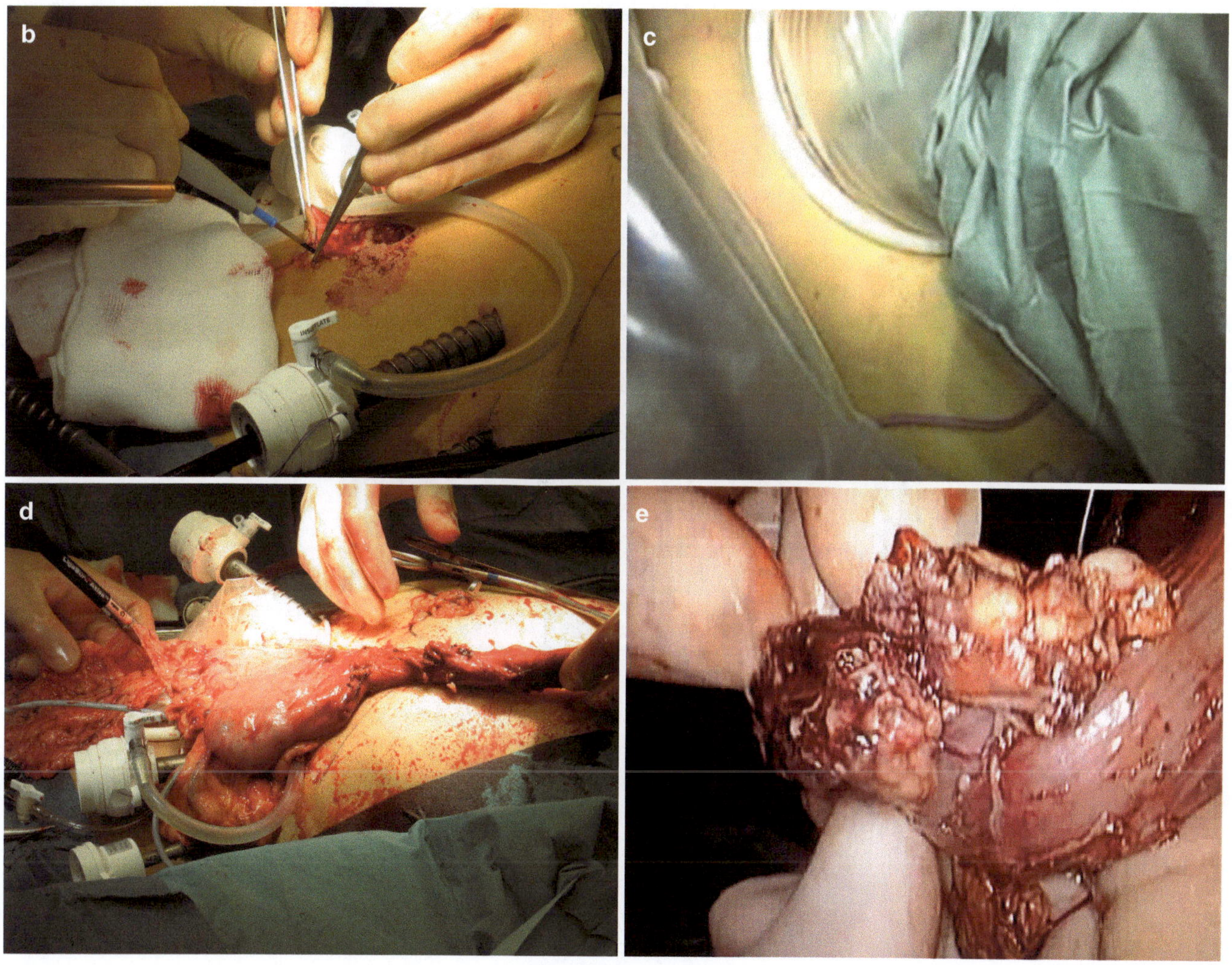

Fig. 6.8 (Continued)

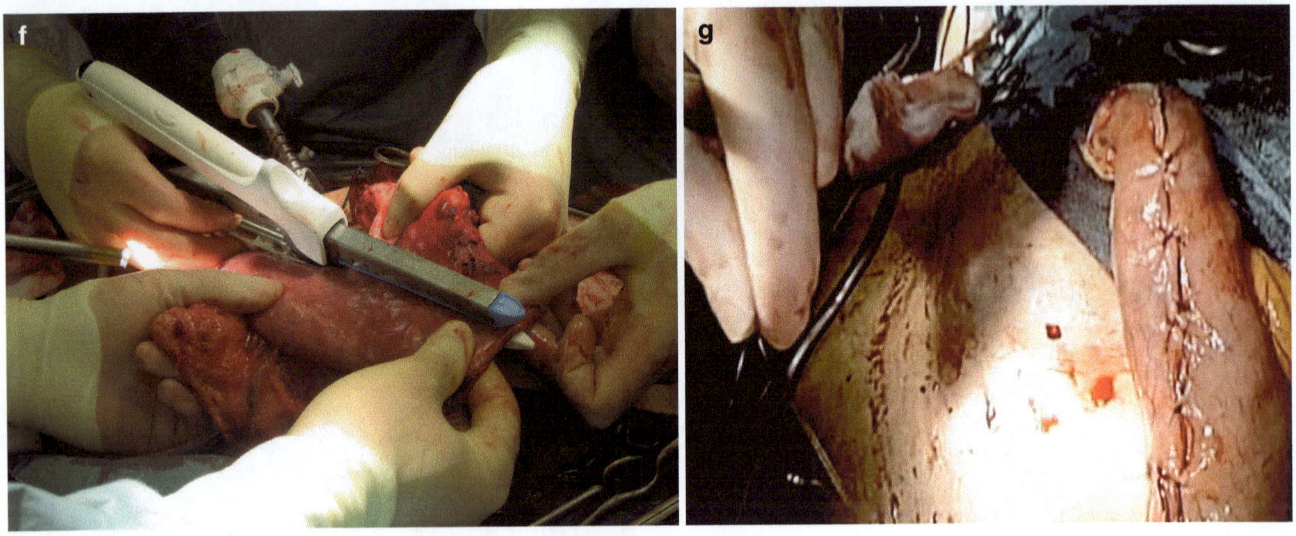

Fig. 6.8 (Continued)

(Fig. 6.8b–e). A 4 cm wide gastric tube is created extracorporeally by means of a 10 cm linear stapler device (Fig. 6.8f–g). No pyloromyotomy or pyloroplasty or Kocher maneuver are performed. After closure of the abdominal wound, insufflation is restarted and under laparoscopic control, the gastric tube, fixed to the NG tube is transhiatal placed into the cervical region (Fig. 6.8h). Final situation is depicted in Fig. 6.8i–j.

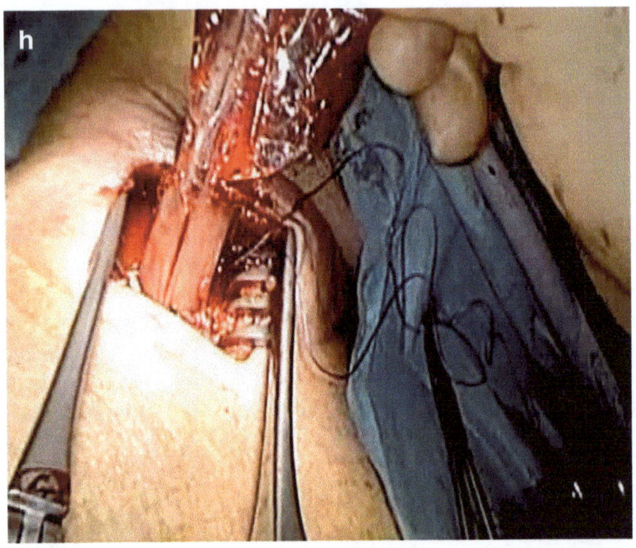

Fig. 6.8 (Continued)

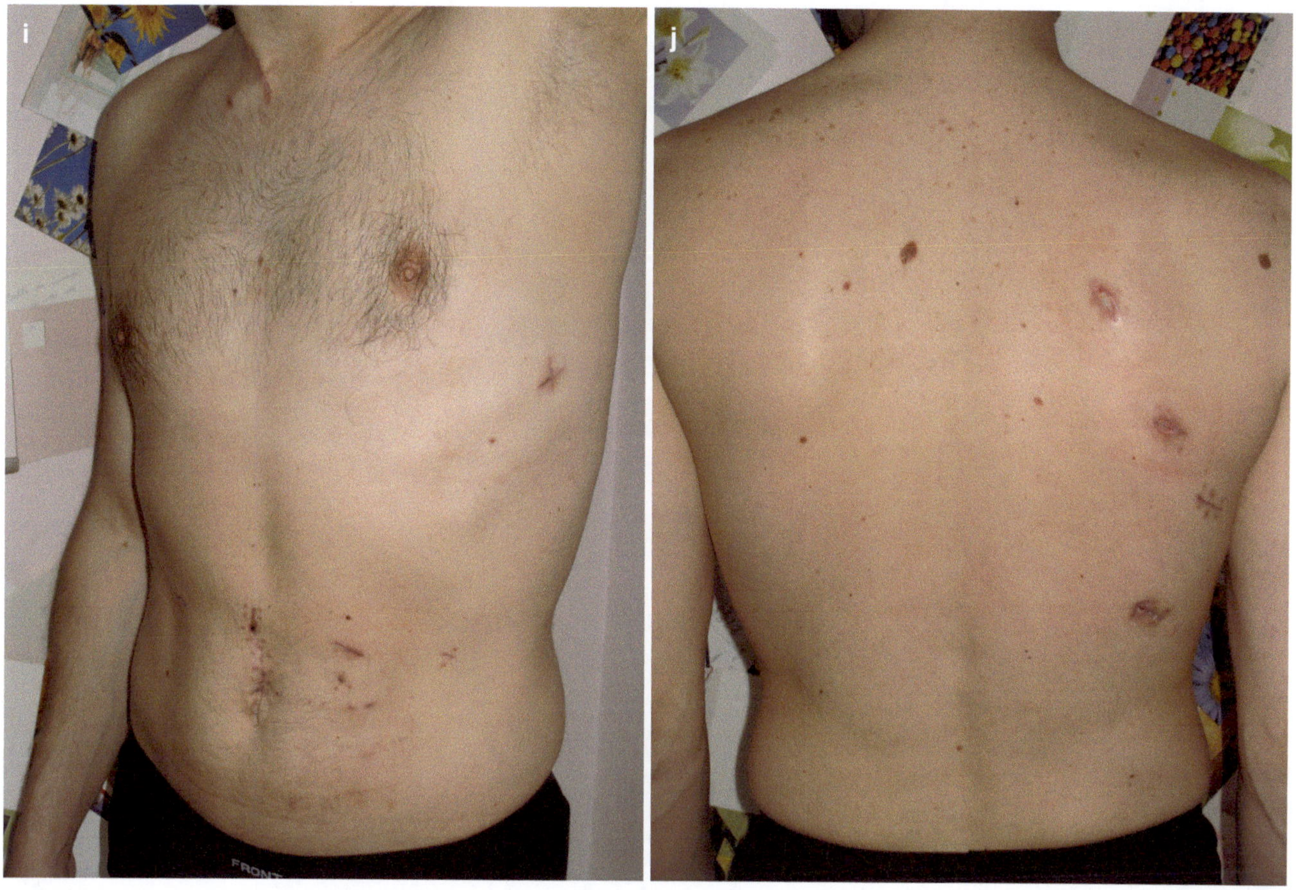

Fig. 6.8 (Continued)

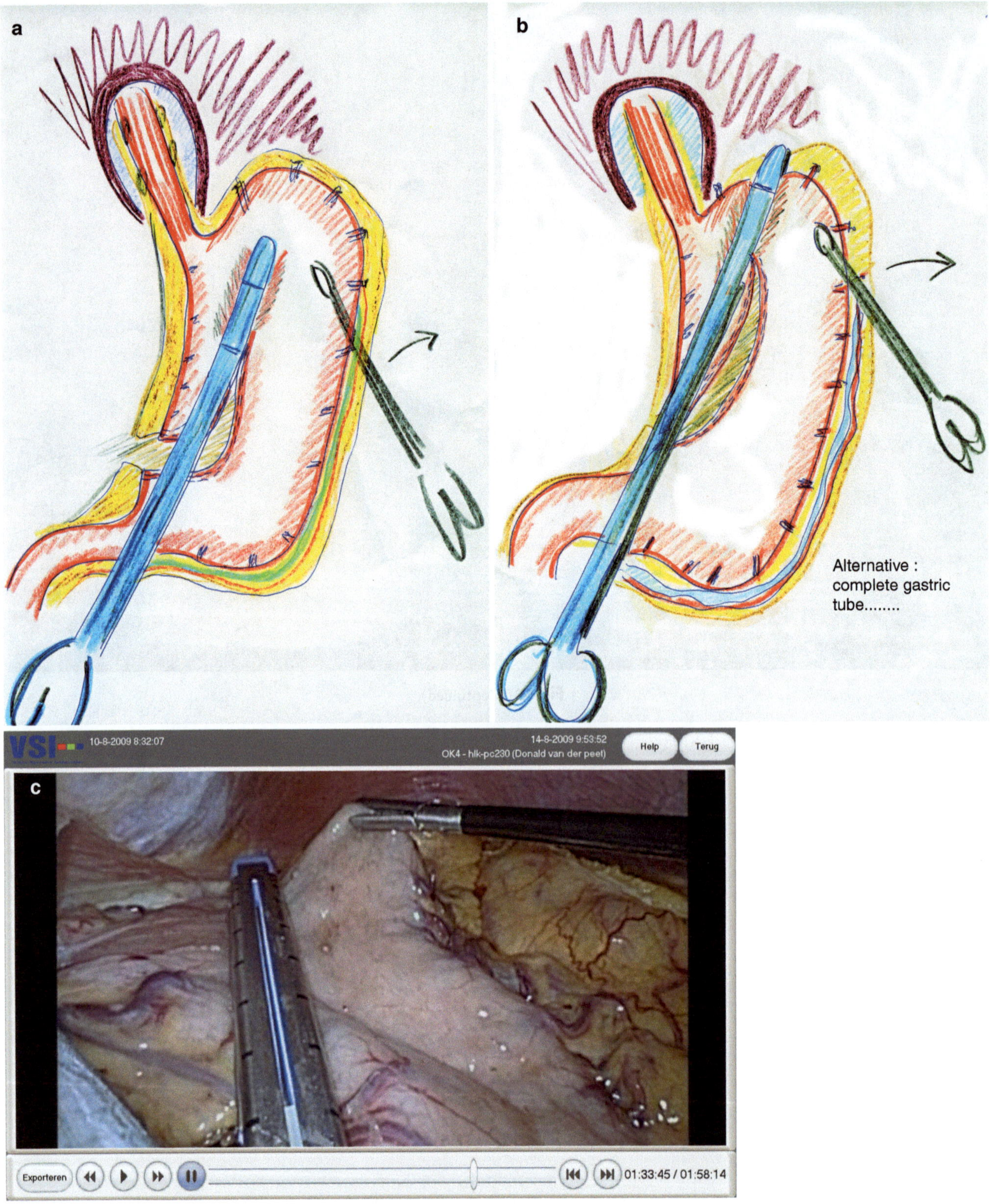

Fig. 6.9 Alternative for the extracorporeal created gastric tube is the total laparoscopic creation of the gastric tube by means of division of the stomach by means of the endostapler (**a–c**). The gastric tube is attached to the fundus and retrieved through the cervical wound (**d–f**)

12. Other option will be to create the gastric tube totally intraabdominal. Once the gastric mobilization has been accomplished, the stomach is divided by means of a 6 cm endostapler in order to create a gastric tube 4 cm wide along the greater curvature (Fig. 6.9a–c). Once this is done the gastric tube is left attached to the gastric fundus by two strong

Fig. 6.9 (Continued)

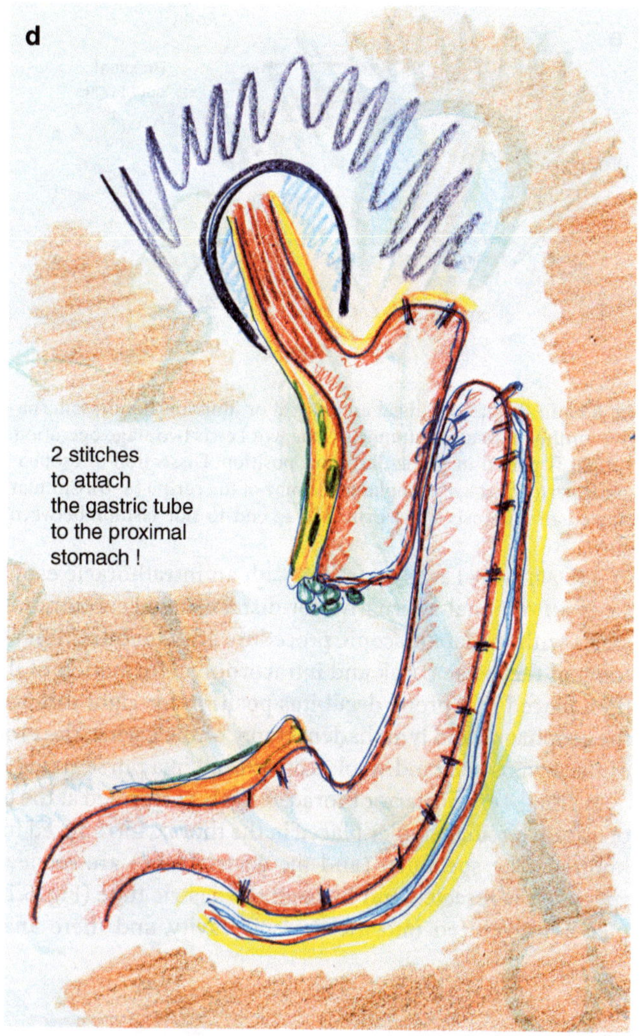

stitches or by a small bridge of fundus (Fig. 6.9d). Through the neck the specimen and the gastric tube can be retrieved and both exteriorized in the neck. After resection, an esophago-gastric tube anastomosis is performed (Fig. 6.9e–f).

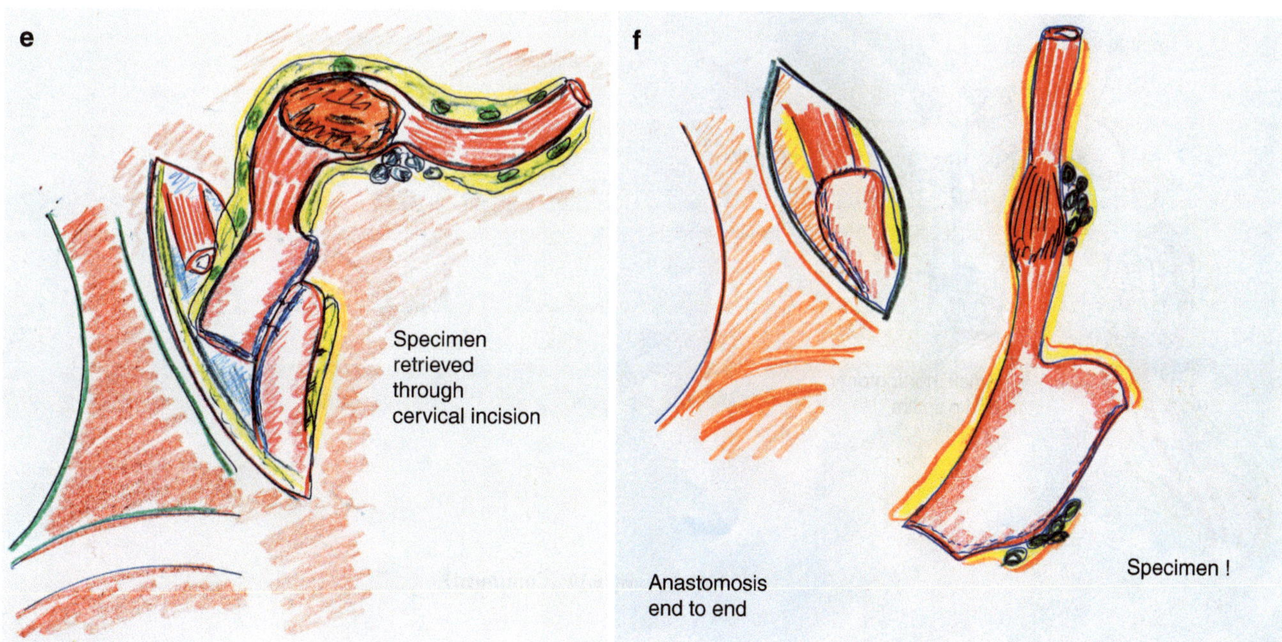

Fig. 6.9 (Continued)

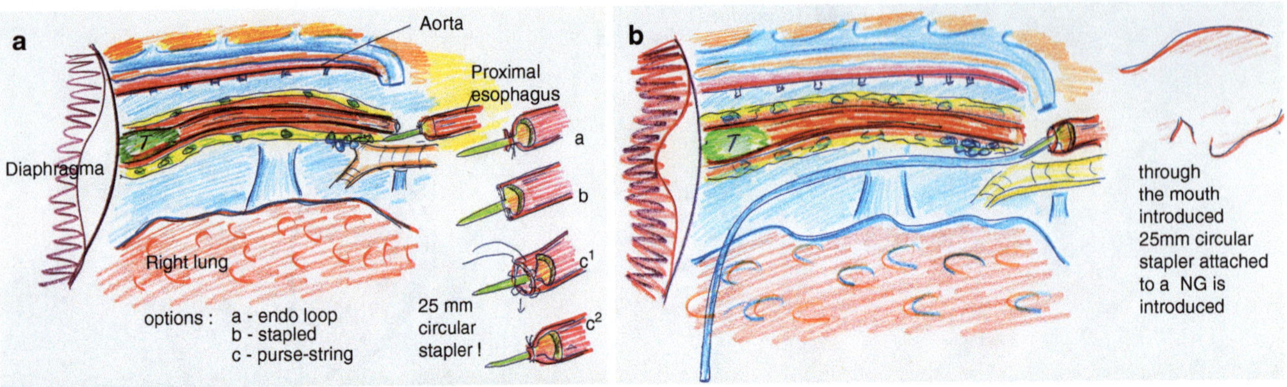

Fig. 6.10 In the case of distal esophageal or junction tumors, alternative for the cervical anastomosis is the Ivor Lewis two stage operation. Patient is placed in prone decubitus position. Dissection of esophagus is performed with lymphadenectomy of the carina (**a–b**). Circular stapled anastomosis is performed in an end-to side fashion between the proximal esophagus and the gastric tube through a protected 4 cm posterior thoracotomy (**c–d**) after retrieval of the specimen. There are different ways to perform the anastomosis (endo-loop, stapled esophagus or purse string), our choice is the purse string method (**e–h**)

13. An Ivor–Lewis approach with an intrathoracic esophago-gastric tube anastomosis is an optional alternative for distal esophageal tumors (see video 4). The operation starts with the laparoscopic procedure with mobilization of the stomach, lymphadenectomy of the celiac trunk and intracorporeal formation of the gastric tube. The patient is then placed in a prone decubitus position for right thoracoscopy. After mobilization of the esophagus and lymphadenectomy of the carina, the esophagus is divided at the level of the azygos vein and stapled or sutured in a purse string fashion (Fig. 6.10a, b).

A small 4 cm posterior thoracotomy is performed at the 6th intercostal space, the anvil of 25 mm circular stapler placed in the thorax, introduced in the proximal esophagus and knotted. The specimen (and the gastric tube) are retrieved through the incision, the specimen is resected and through the gastric tube (Fig. 6.10c,d) the 25 mm circular stapler is introduced into the thoracic cavity, and there anastomosed in an end to side

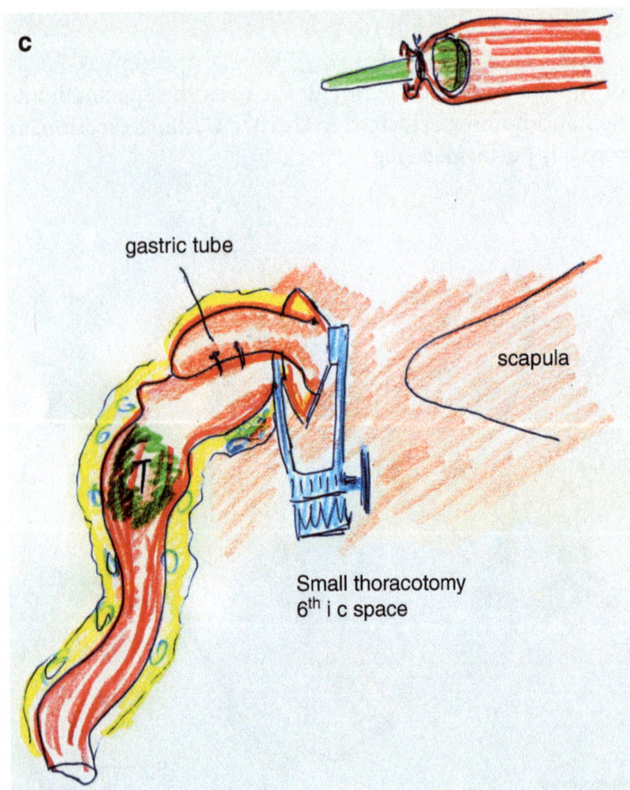

Fig. 6.10 (Continued)

Fig. 6.10 (Continued)

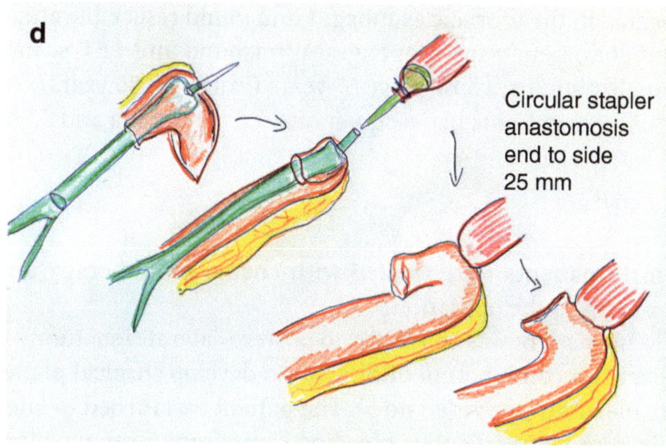

fashion (Fig. 6.10e). The rest of the loop will be excised by means of an endo-stapler (Fig. 6.10d). It is important to check-up the anastomosis by control of the donuts and methylene-blue in order to detect any leakage.

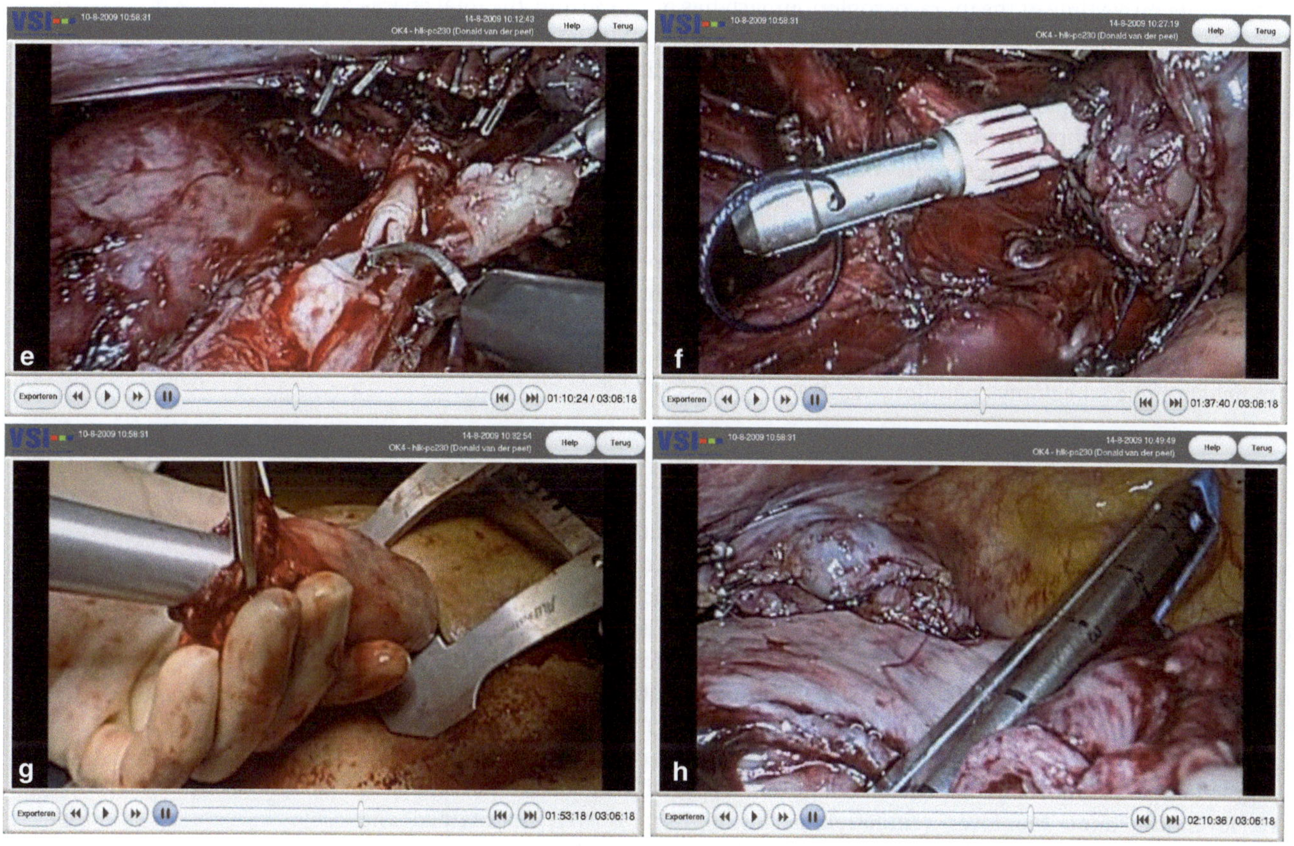

Fig. 6.10e (Continued)

Own Experience

In the period between March 2007 and July 2009, 40 patients have been approached by right thoracoscopic approach in the prone position because of esophageal cancer. Selection of patients has not been made on basis of the stage of the process. Tumors were located in the thoracic esophagus and found resectable and curable by CT-scan of thorax and abdomen, trans-esophageal ultrasound and PET-scan. There were 30 males and 10 female patients, average age 67 years (range 48–80 years).

Fifteen patients had a squamous cell carcinoma and 25 had adenocarcinoma.

Results

Thirty patients were treated with chemo-radiotherapy and seven with chemotherapy previous to the operation.

One patient was converted to postero-lateral right thoracotomy, after chemoradiation, because a combination of difficult to develop surgical plane along the aorta and moderate bleeding (see video no 5). The patient was turned to lateral position and conventionally approached. Venous bleeding came from a venous plexus at a location between the aorta and azygos vein. Pathological examination showed a complete response of the tumor without any active tumor rest.

In 25 patients abdomen was approached laparoscopically and in fifteen through a median laparotomy because of relative contraindications for laparoscopy such as extreme obesity, PET positive LN at the prepyloric small curvature and previous laparotomy. In one patient conversion to laparotomy was performed because the presence of extensive fibrosis in the celiac trunk after chemotherapy.

Mean operative time of the thoracoscopic approach has been 130 min, the total operative time of 290 min (range 240–460 min). Blood loss was 220ml (range 250–400).

Median ICU stay was 1 day (range 1–37 days) and a median hospital stay of 13 days (range 12–78 days). There is no mortality recorded.

Postoperative complications were seen in six patients: three anastomosis leak at the cervical wound; a fourth patient with an ischemia/necrosis of the proximal gastric tube, being explored by cervico-laparotomy, with resection of 5 cm of the top of the gastric tube, reanastomosed and protected with a Choo® stent and a limited chylothorax, treated conservatively in the other two patients. In the case of high output chylothorax, the leak can be approached and threated thoracoscopically (see video no 6).

Pathological examination showed an R0 resection in 36 patients with a complete response after chemoradiation in eight patients. Median number of LN resected, in this two field lymphadenectomy operation, was 21 (range 15–33).

Comment

If a comparison has to be made between the right prone and the right lateral thoracoscopic approaches for esophageal cancer, it seems that the prone position may cause less pulmonary complications than the lateral approach in which the right lung has to be blocked. Luketich et al., reports, in a series of 222 patients, an incidence of pulmonary complications in 7.6% of the patients after right lateral thoracoscopy with collapse of the lung [9]. Palanivelu et al., using the prone position in 130 patients, report only (1.5% in their series) [10]. Possible explaination for this difference may be the use of a single endotracheal tube with possible two-lung ventilation. The partial ventilation of the right lung, obtained during the prone decubitus thoracoscopy, will reduce the possibility of arteriovenous shunt. Moreover ventilation–perfusion ratio is well maintained and hypoxia and hypercarbia avoided. This may reduce the extent of pulmonary dysfunction and athelectasia postoperatively. Other important advantages of the prone position may be shorter anesthesia time, excellent exposure of the operative field and better ergonomy for the surgeon.

The early results in our series of 40 patients will confirm the outcome of the aforementioned series: pulmonary complications seems lower in the thoracoscopic prone position than in the lateral position and lower than in the open three-stage procedure, higher than 50% [11]. Obviously, complications of the anastomosis are related to the gastric conduit and will remain the same as in the open conventional approach.

References

1. Cuschieri A, Shimi S, Banting S. Endoscopic oesophagectomy through a right thoracoscopic approach. J R Coll Surg Edinb 1992;37:7–11
2. Dallemagne B, Weerts JM, Jehaes C. Thoracoscopic esophageal resection. In: Cuesta MA, Nagy AG, eds. Minimally Invasive Surgery in Gastrointestinal Cancer. Edinburgh: Churchill Livingstone, 1993, pp 59–68
3. Azagra JS, Ceuterick M, Goergen M, et al Thoracoscopy in oesophagectomy for oesophageal cancer. Br J Surg 1993;80:320–321
4. Gossot D, Fourquier P, Celerier M. Thoracoscopic esophagectomy: technique and initial results. Ann Thorac Surg 1993;56:667–670
5. McAnena OJ, Rogers J, Williams NS. Right thoracoscopically assisted oesophagectomy for cancer. Br J Surg 1994;81:236–238
6. Cuschieri A. Thoracoscopic subtotal oesophagectomy. Endosc Surg Allied Technol 1994;2;21–25
7. Muller JM, Erasmi H, Stelzner M, Zieren U, Pichlmaier H. Surgical therapy of oesophageal carcinoma. Review. Br J Surg 1990;77(8):845–857
8. Bizekis C, Kent MS, Luketich JD, et al Initial experience with minimally invasive Ivor Lewis esophagectomy. Ann Thor Surg 2006;82:402–406
9. Luketich JD, Alvelo-Rivera M, Buenaventura PO, et al Mnimally invasive esophagectomy. outcomes in 222 patients. Ann Surg 2003;238:486–494
10. Palanivelu Ch, Prakash A, Senthilkumar R, et al Minimally invasive esophagectomy: thoracoscopic mobilization of the esophagus and mediastinal lymphadenectomy in prone position-experience of 130 patients. J Am Coll Surg 2006;203:7–16
11. Hulscher JB, van Sandick JW, de Boer AG, Wijnhoven BP, Tijssen JG, Fockens P, et al Extended transthoracic resection compared with limited transhiatal resection for adenocarcinoma of the esophagus. New Engl J Med 2002;347:1662–1669

higher than 50% [11]. Obviously complications of the anastomosis are related to the gastric conduit and will remain the same as in the open conventional approach.

7

Laparoscopic Transhiatal Resection for Distal and Gastro-Esophageal Junction Cancer: Operative Technique

Miguel A. Cuesta, Donald L. van der Peet, Surya S.A.Y. Biere,
Joris J.G. Scheepers, Bob H. M. Heijnen

Introduction

Although different neoadjuvant therapies are being developed, surgical treatment remains the only curative therapy for esophageal cancer. For years, the procedure of choice for esophageal cancer was the Ivor-Lewis operation, later modified by McKeown [1]. In this modified procedure, the tumor is resected by means of a right-sided thoracotomy combined with a laparotomy using cervical esophago-gastric anastomosis. The advantage of this operation is the perfect exposure that allows complete esophageal dissection and possible en bloc resection. Disadvantages are the pulmonary complications related to the thoracotomy and collapse of the right lung. Pulmonary complications can be overcome by the transhiatal approach as described by Orringer, in which the esophagus is dissected free through the enlarged hiatus [2]. After the esophageal-proximal gastric resection, the created gastric tube is anastomosed with the cervical esophagus through a combined cervical–abdominal approach, thus avoiding a thoracotomy. Disadvantages of this approach are the partly blind resection of the esophagus and the tumor, and that it is limited to tumors of the distal esophagus and gastro-esophageal junction. Both procedures have high complication rates, varying from 40 to 80%, and the in-hospital mortality rate averages 7.5% to less than 5% in experienced centers [3].

The approach and extent of the resection that is necessary is still controversial. In a recent prospective randomized study by Hulscher et al [4], transthoracic esophageal resection with systematic abdominal and mediastinal lymph node dissection (two-field lymphadenectomy) was compared with the classic transhiatal approach. The transhiatal approach had lower morbidity than the extended lymphadenectomy. Even if a trend was observed with an advantage for the transthoracic approach in tumors located in the mid and distal esophagus, the median survival, disease-free, and quality-adjusted survival for the most common G–E junction cancers were not statistically significant.

In an attempt to lower the mortality and morbidity rates of conventional esophageal resection, advances produced in minimally invasive surgery have made possible a minimally invasive approach of the esophagus. Several minimally invasive approaches have been described, such as transhiatal, and right thoracoscopic procedures [5, 6]. A laparoscopically assisted transhiatal esophageal resection followed by a cervical anastomosis has been designed, in order to combine the advantages of the conventional transhiatal approach with a minimally invasive esophageal dissection, under direct vision of the camera, which allows the dissection in a correct surgical plane.

Indication

All patients with a squamous cell carcinoma or adenocarcinoma of the distal low third of the esophagus as well as type I G–E junction adenocarcinomas according to the Siewert classification were considered for laparoscopic transhiatal resection. Siewert I tumor was defined as an adenocarcinoma localized in the G–E junction with its center more than 1 cm above the gastro-esophageal junction.

Preoperative staging was performed by means of esophagoscopy and biopsies, endoscopic ultrasound, CT-scan of thorax and abdomen, neck ultrasound, and PET scan if considered necessary.

Exclusion and Conversion

Patients with previous upper abdominal surgery and those who needed a colon interposition may be excluded for this approach.

Operative Technique

The conventional operation technique described by Orringer and Sloan [2] is performed laparoscopically. (see video no 7)

1. The patient is positioned in the supine position with the legs in the French position and the neck extended with exposure of the right side of the neck. The operating surgeon stands between the legs of the patient looking at two monitors placed at shoulder level of the patient. Two assistants stand on both sides of the patient, with the nurse on the right side of the surgeon (Fig. 7.1a).

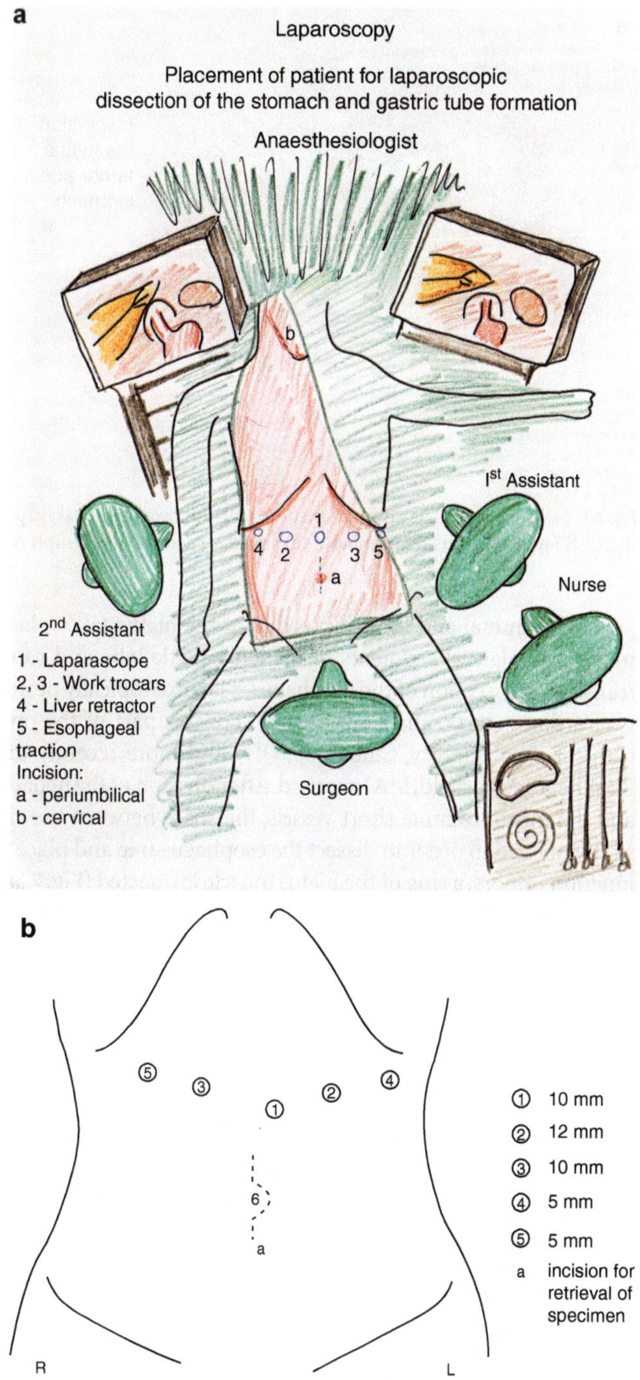

Fig. 7.1 The patient is placed for laparoscopic and cervical part of the procedure. The surgeon stands between the legs of the patient facing the monitor at the level of the patient's shoulders (**a**). Position of the trocars along both subcostal margins (**b**)

2. Pneumoperitoneum is created by a 10-mm incision 2/3–1/3 between the xiphoid and the umbilicus on the left side of the midline. Camera is introduced through this trocar, and four other trocars are placed in the upper abdomen (Fig. 7.1b).

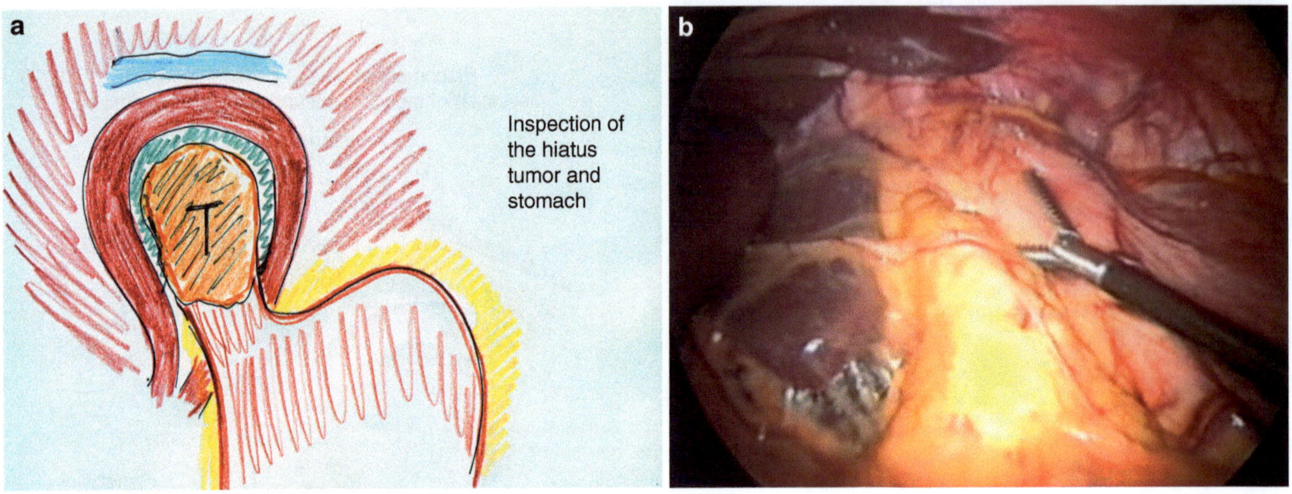

Fig. 7.2 (a, b) Complete abdominal inspection is followed by local inspection of the hiatal area. Especially attention is paid, if tumor is located in the G–E junction, to its relation with the hiatal structures and lymph nodes

3. Abdominal and local inspection at the hiatus takes place (Fig. 7.2a, b). After displacement of the lateral segments of the left hepatic lobe and caudal traction of the stomach, a transhiatal dissection of the esophagus is laparoscopically performed in the plane between the pericardium, aorta, and both pleurae. For this part of the operation, the Harmonic Scalpel (Ethicon Endosurgery, Cincinnati, OH) and more recently the Atlas Ligasure device (Tyco Healthcare, Mansfield, MA) are used. After division of the hepatogastric ligament (pars flacida) and the most proximal short vessels, the space between the right crus and the esophagus is gently opened in order to dissect the esophagus free and place a sling around it. In the case of junction tumors, a ring of the hiatus muscle is resected (Fig. 7.3a). The sling, placed around the esophagus, will permit traction of the esophagus in the caudal direction (Fig. 7.3b–d).

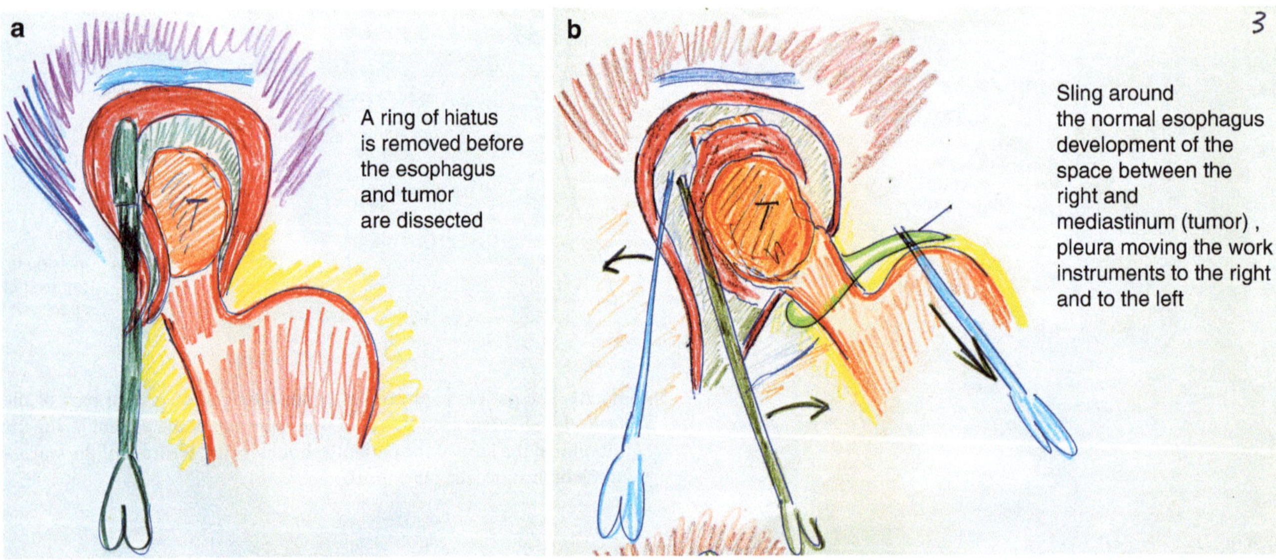

Fig. 7.3 (a–d) In the case of a G–E junction tumor, a ring of the hiatus is excised in continuity with the tumor. Very gentle dissection of the esophagus, makes it free and enables insertion of a sling around it for traction

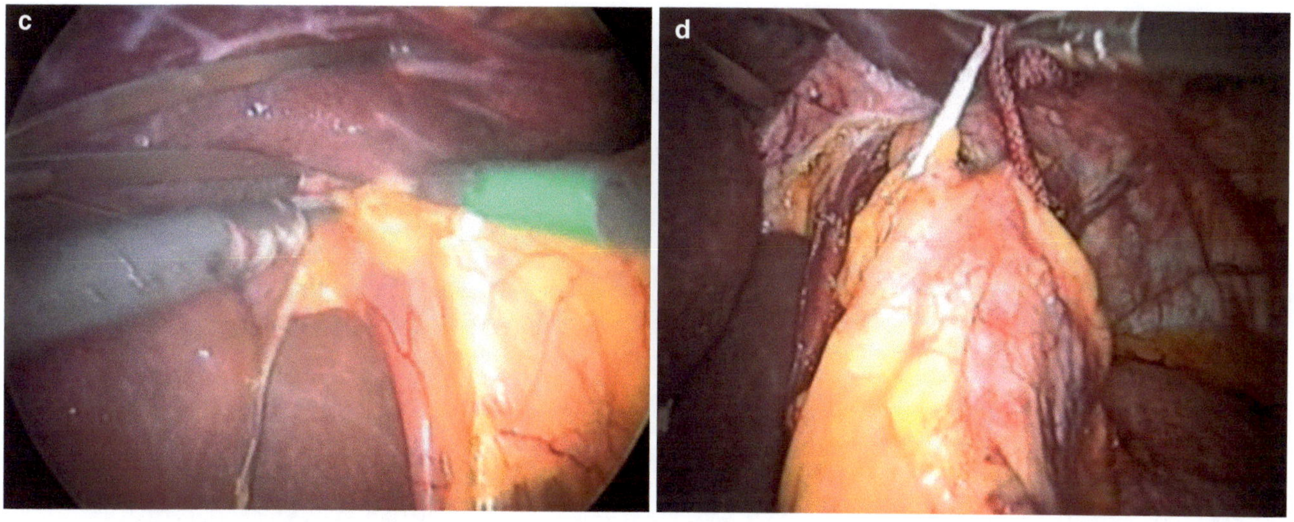

Fig. 7.3 (continued)

4. The hiatus is enlarged by dividing the anterior part with the division of the phrenic vein by means of the Ligasure device according to Pinotti [7] (Fig. 7.4a, b). Anteriorly, dissection is performed in an avascular plane in the anterior mediastinum with visualization of the pericardium and pulmonary vein (Fig. 7.5a, b). Dissection continues

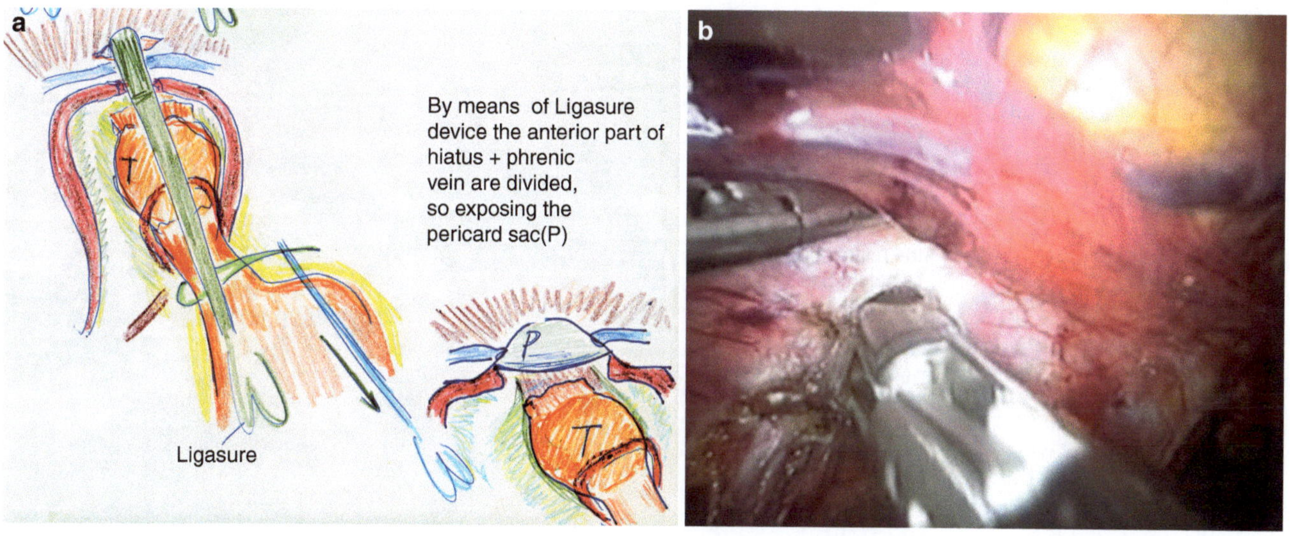

Fig. 7.4 (a, b) The hiatus is open anteriorly according to Pinotti; the phrenic vein being divided by means of Ligasure device

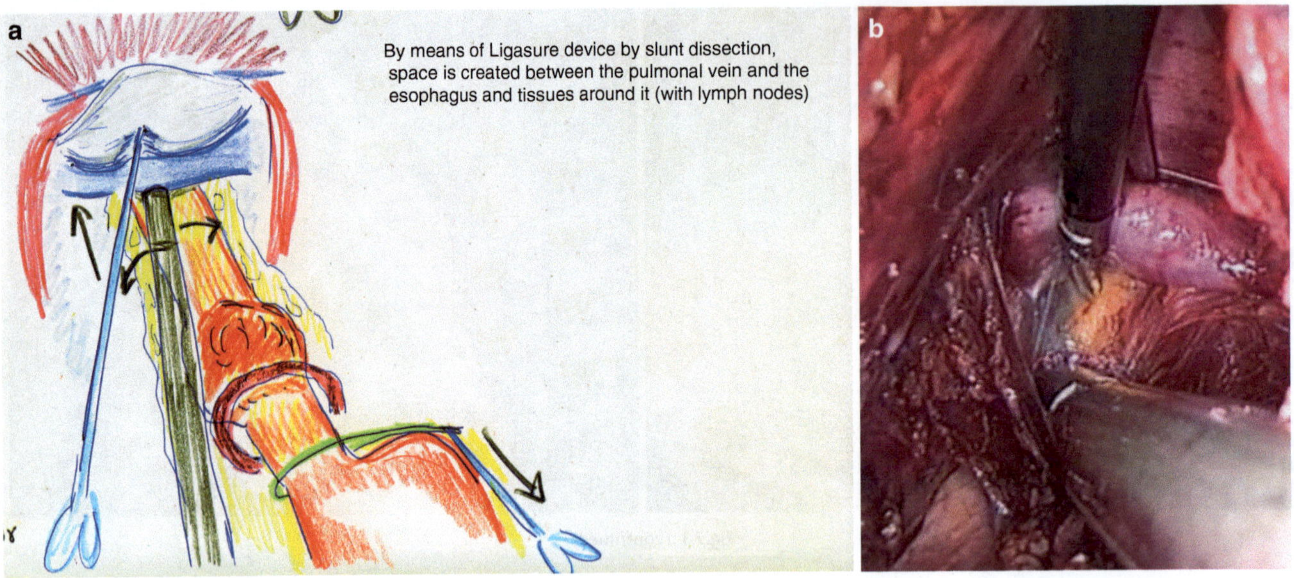

Fig. 7.5 (**a**, **b**) Gentle blunt dissection is anteriorly performed along the plane of the pericardial sac and inferior pulmonary vein

anteriorly up to the level of the carina, in which the lymph nodes can be visualized (Fig. 7.6a–d).

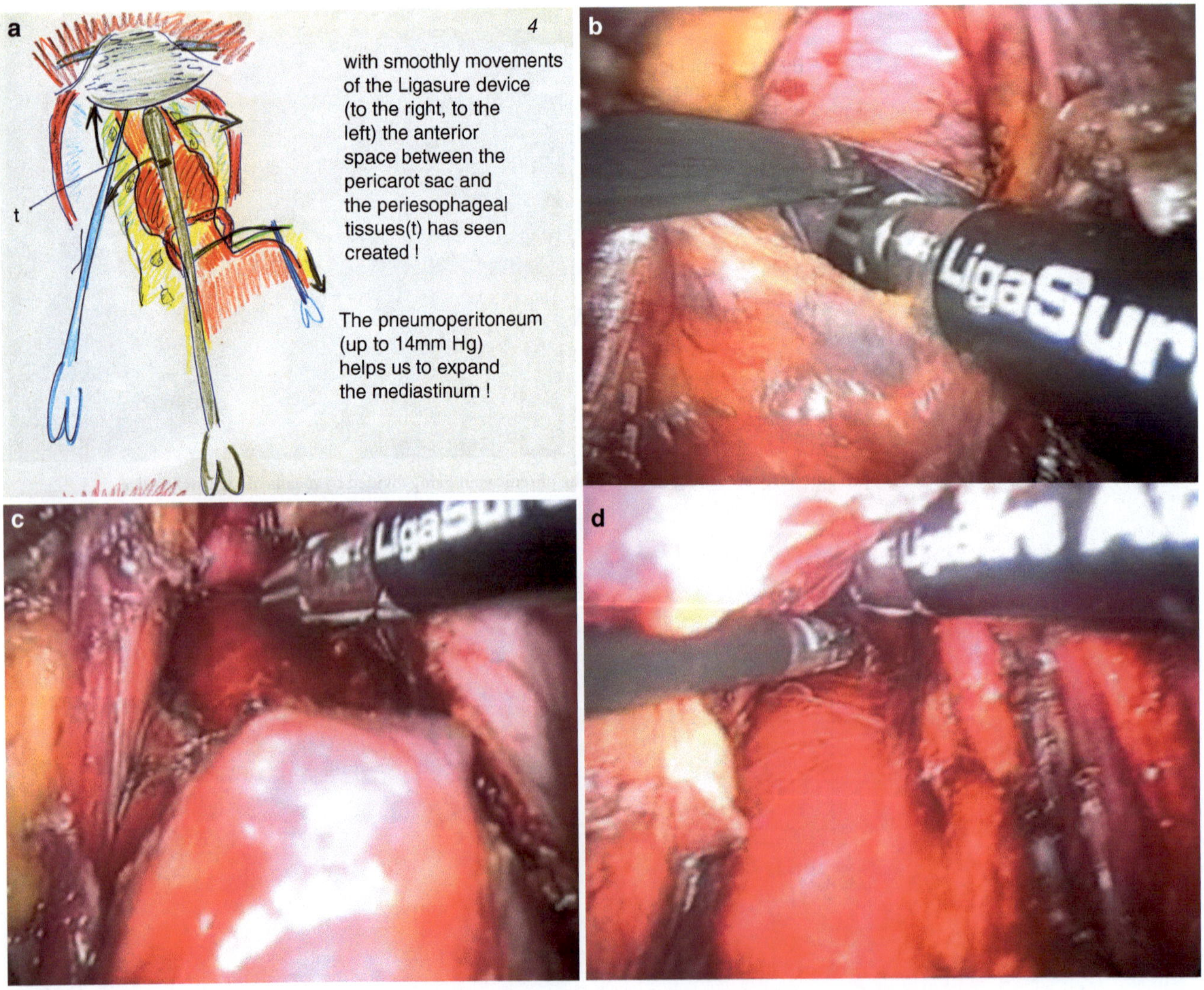

Fig. 7.6 (**a**–**d**) Dissection continues anteriorly above the pulmonary vein in direction to the carina

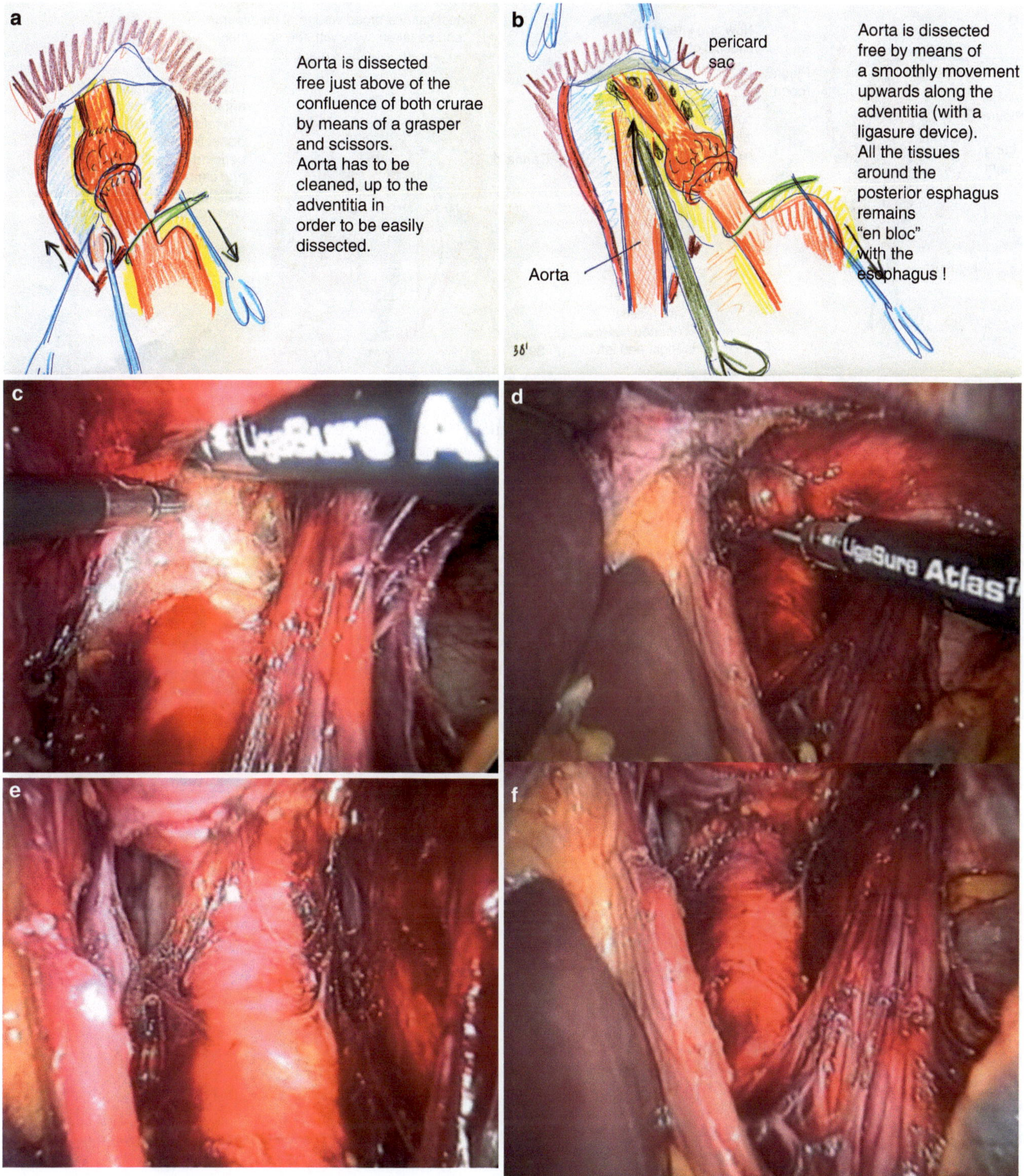

Fig. 7.7 Posteriorly the aorta is dissected free at the level of the hiatus and dissected bluntly in proximal direction (a–f)

5. On the right side of the esophagus, the aorta is approached at the level of the hiatus and in an avascular plane dissected free as high as possible in the posterior mediastinum (Fig. 7.7a–f).

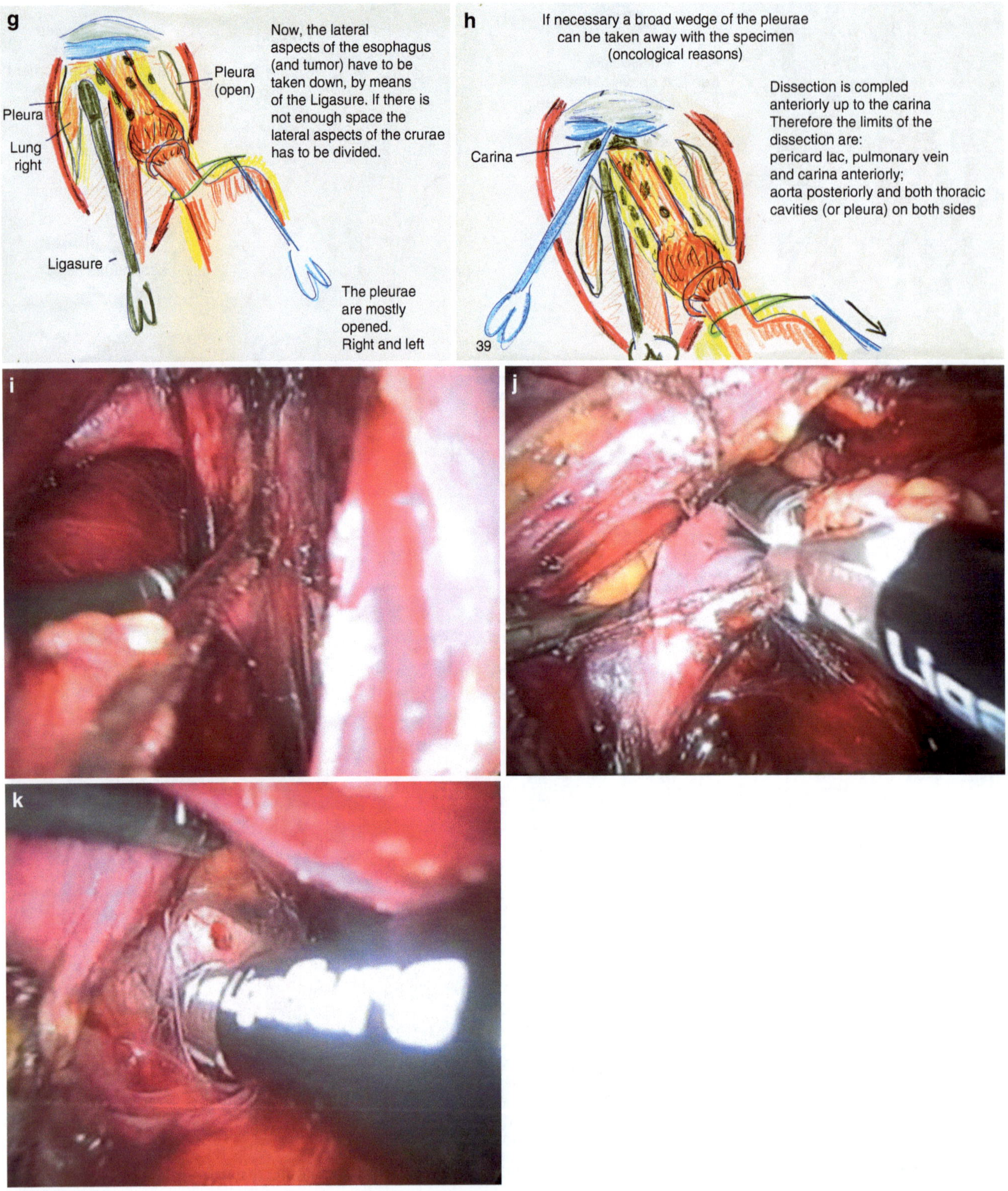

Fig. 7.7 Dissection proceeds at both lateral parts, taking down the lateral tissue (most of cases with a wedge of the pleura) by means of Ligasure device (g–j). (k) The carina is visualized (k)

6. Lateral dissection is performed on both sides at the level of the pleurae. The pleurae are always opened, on both sides in most cases, with resection of some part of it if necessary (Fig. 7.7g–j). Now it is possible visualize the carina completely (Fig. 7.7k). The anesthesiologist is warned of this situation because the mechanical ventilation must be adapted. Mechanical ventilation is corrected by means of increase of minute volume, use of positive end-expiratory pressure (PEEP), and decrease of the insufflation pressure to about 12 mmHg [8]. The esophagus is resected laparoscopically in this way, together with para-esophageal tissue and lymph nodes, to the level of the carina.

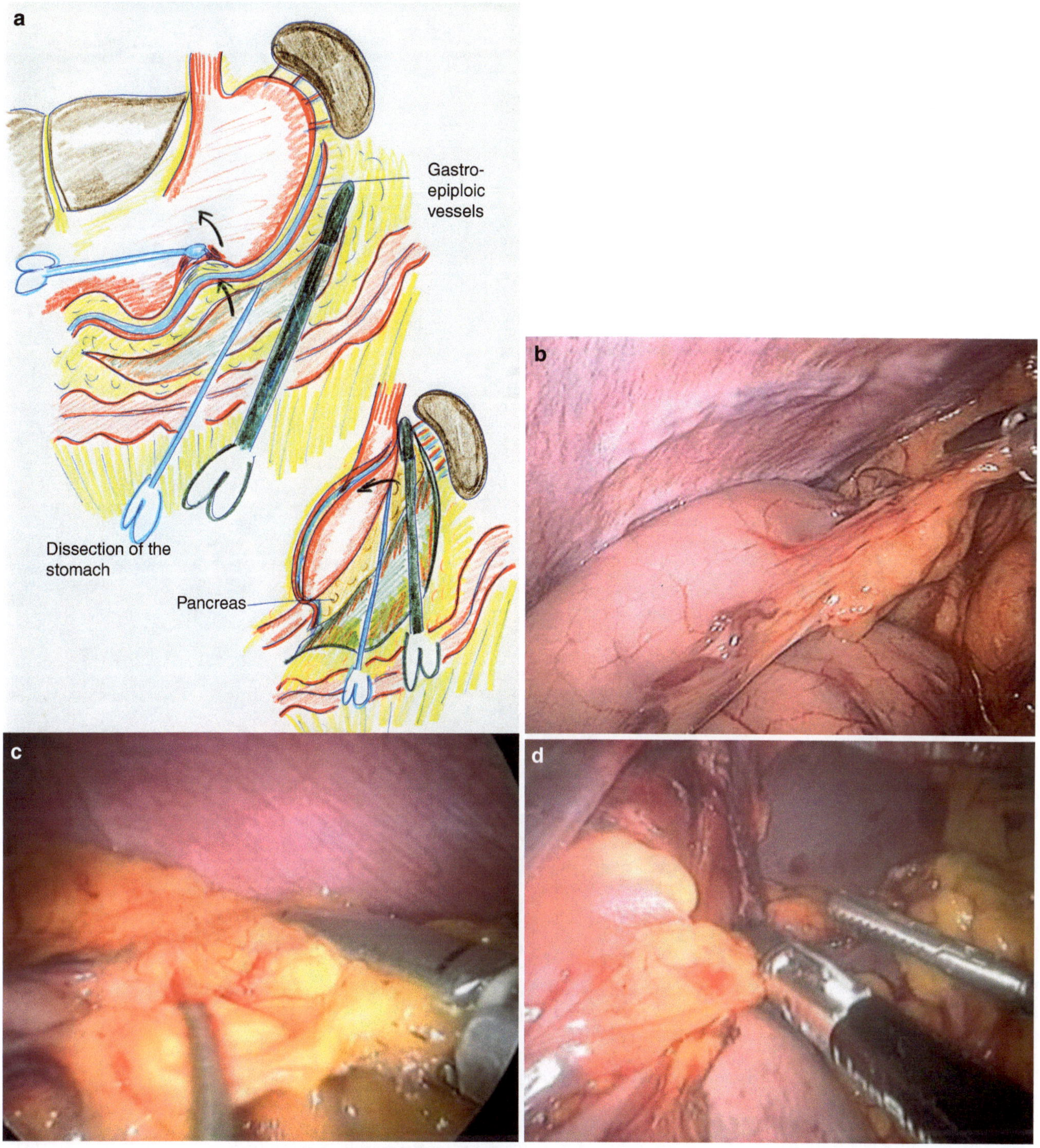

Fig. 7.8 The procedure proceeds with gastrolysis along the greater curvature with preservation of the gastro-epiploic vessels (**a–d**). A sling is placed around the stomach for retraction. Lymphadenectomy of the celiac trunk can be now performed (**e–i**)

7. The Atlas Ligasure device is used to mobilize the greater curvature of the stomach by dividing the gastro-colic ligament from the pycorus, with preservation of the gastro-epiploic vessels Afterwards, the short gastric vessels are approached and divided up to the left crus of the hiatus (Fig. 7.8a–d).

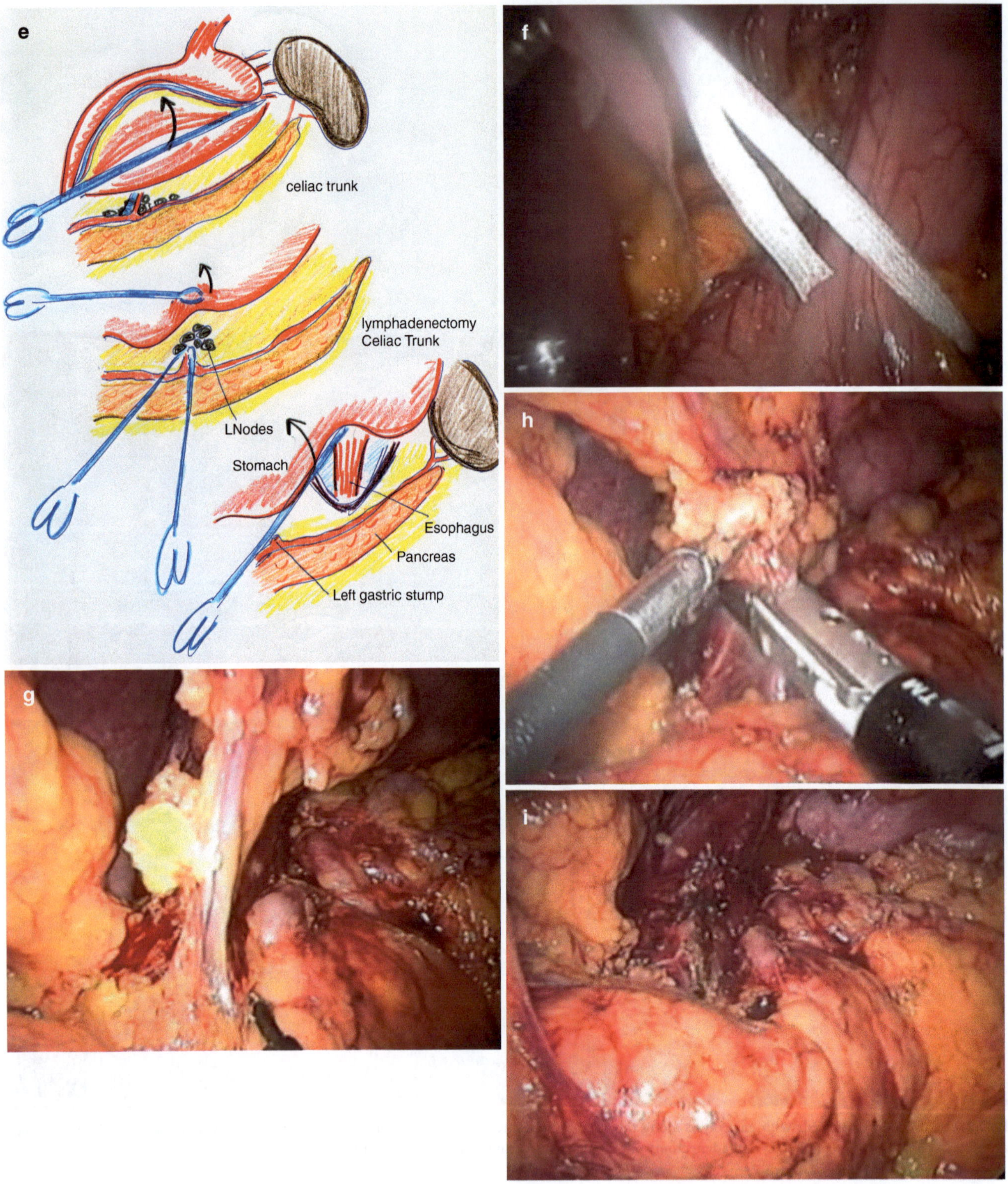

Fig. 7.8 (e–i)

8. By tilting the stomach or placing a sling around it (Fig. 7.8f) and dividing the adhesions present in the lesser sac, an extensive lymphadenectomy of the celiac trunk is performed (Fig. 7.8g, i), to be followed by division of the left gastric artery and vein by means of a vascular stapler or the Atlas Ligasure device (Fig. 7.8h). From there, the dissection is completed up to the hiatus.

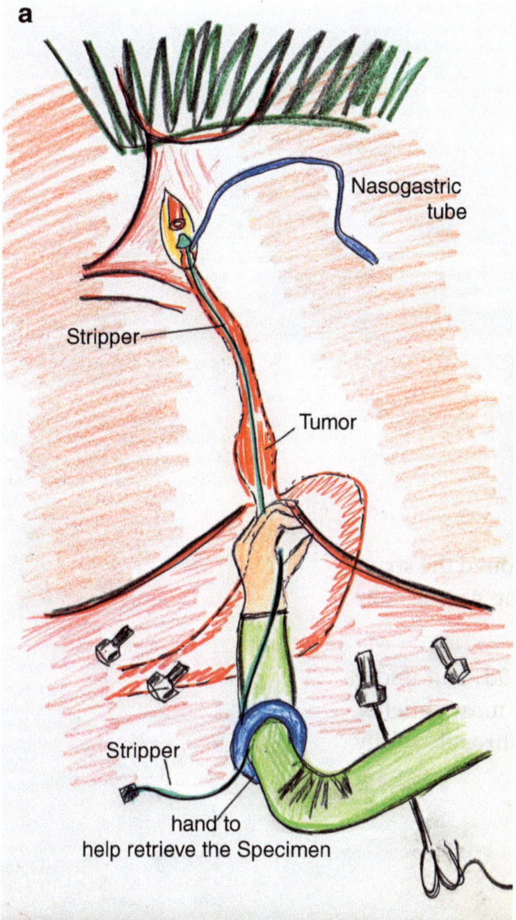

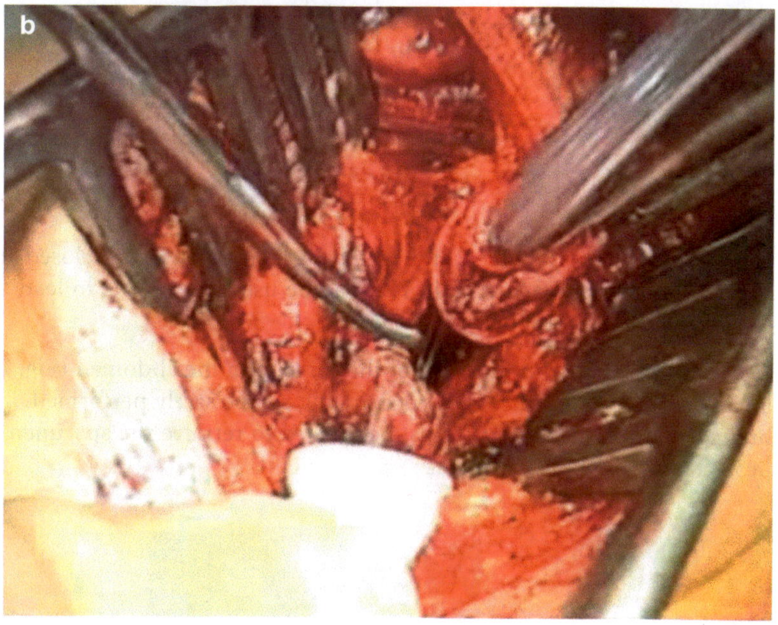

Fig. 7.9 (a–g) A cervical incision is performed and the eophagus is divided. The specimen can be retrieved by means of a stripper and exteriorized through the small and well protected (hand assisted) abdominal wound

9. The next step is dissection of the cervical esophagus by means of a right-side cervical incision (Fig. 7.9a, b).

10. At the same time, another surgeon introduces the HandPort system (Smith & Nephew, Inc., Andover, MA) through a 7-cm longitudinal periumbilical incision. Through the lateral left trocar, a venous stripper is introduced into the gastric lumen by a small incision in the lesser gastric curvature and then pushed up to the cervical dissected esophagus. If the stripper cannot be pushed because of the obstruction caused by the tumor, the feeding tube can be withdrawn via the small opening in the stomach and then exteriorized. The stripper can be attached to the nasopactric tube and pushed up. The

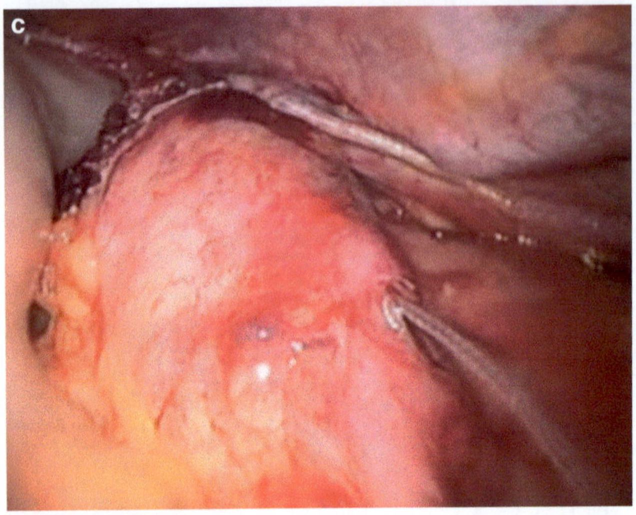

Fig. 7.9 (c)

cervical esophagus is divided, after which the most distal part is closed around the stripper. A NG tube is attached to it. This can be used afterwards to lead the gastric tube upwards to the cervical incision. (Fig. 7.9a–c).

11. In this way, with the hand of the surgeon in the abdomen (Fig. 7.9d) and under laparoscopic vision, the controlled stripping can be safely performed. In most patients, branches of the vagal nerves must be divided to retrieve the specimen through a fully protected periumbilical incision.

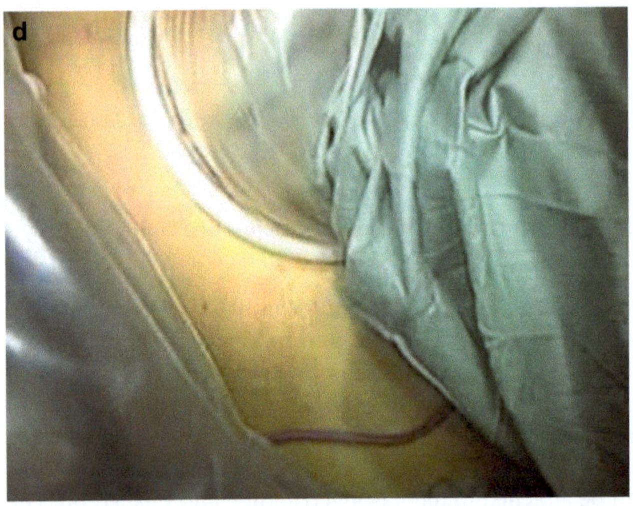

Fig. 7.9 (d)

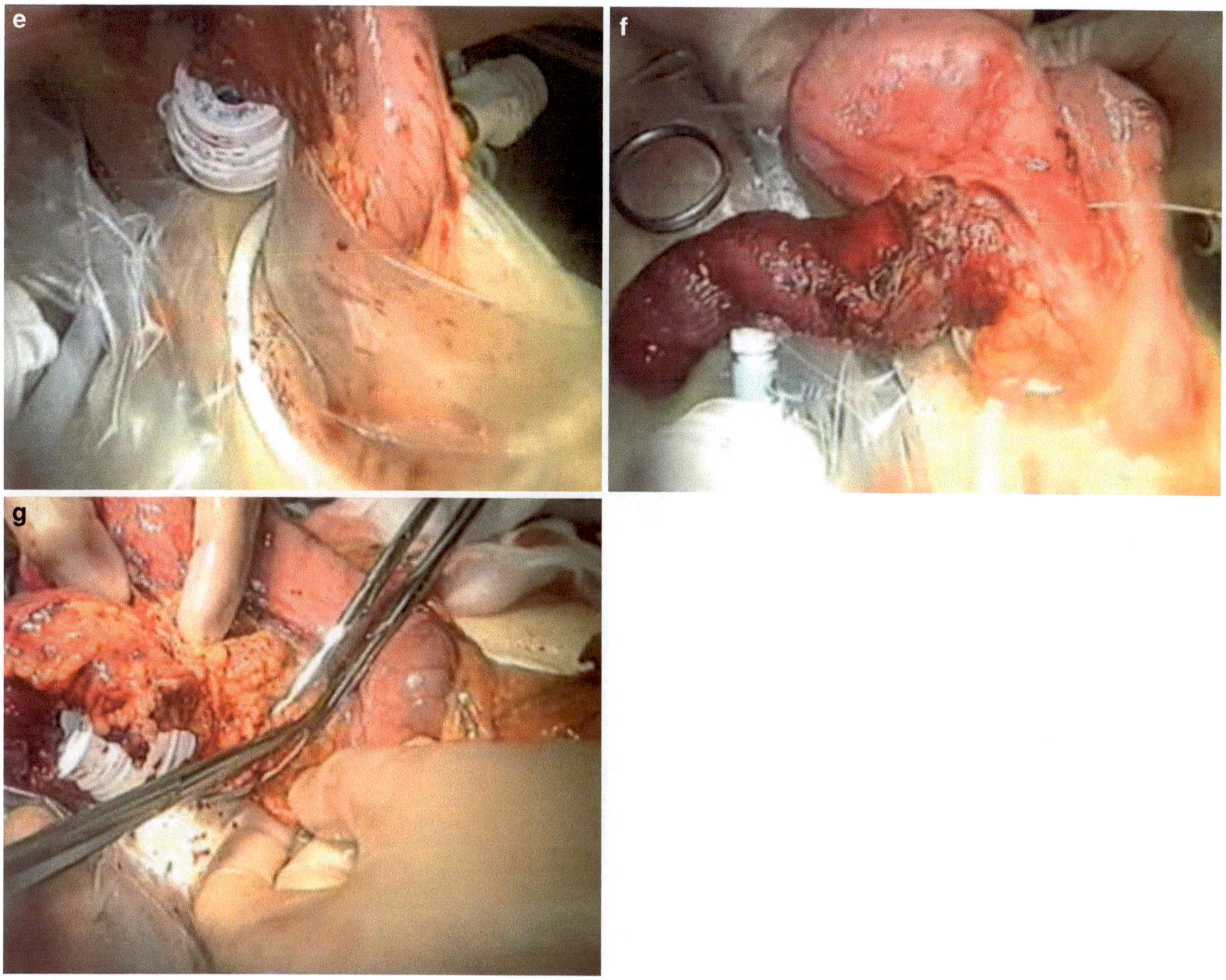

Fig. 7.9 (e–g)

12. Once the specimen is retrieved outside the abdomen (Fig. 7.9e–g), the mobilization of the stomach is completed, and the gastric tube is created, 4 cm wide, by using the

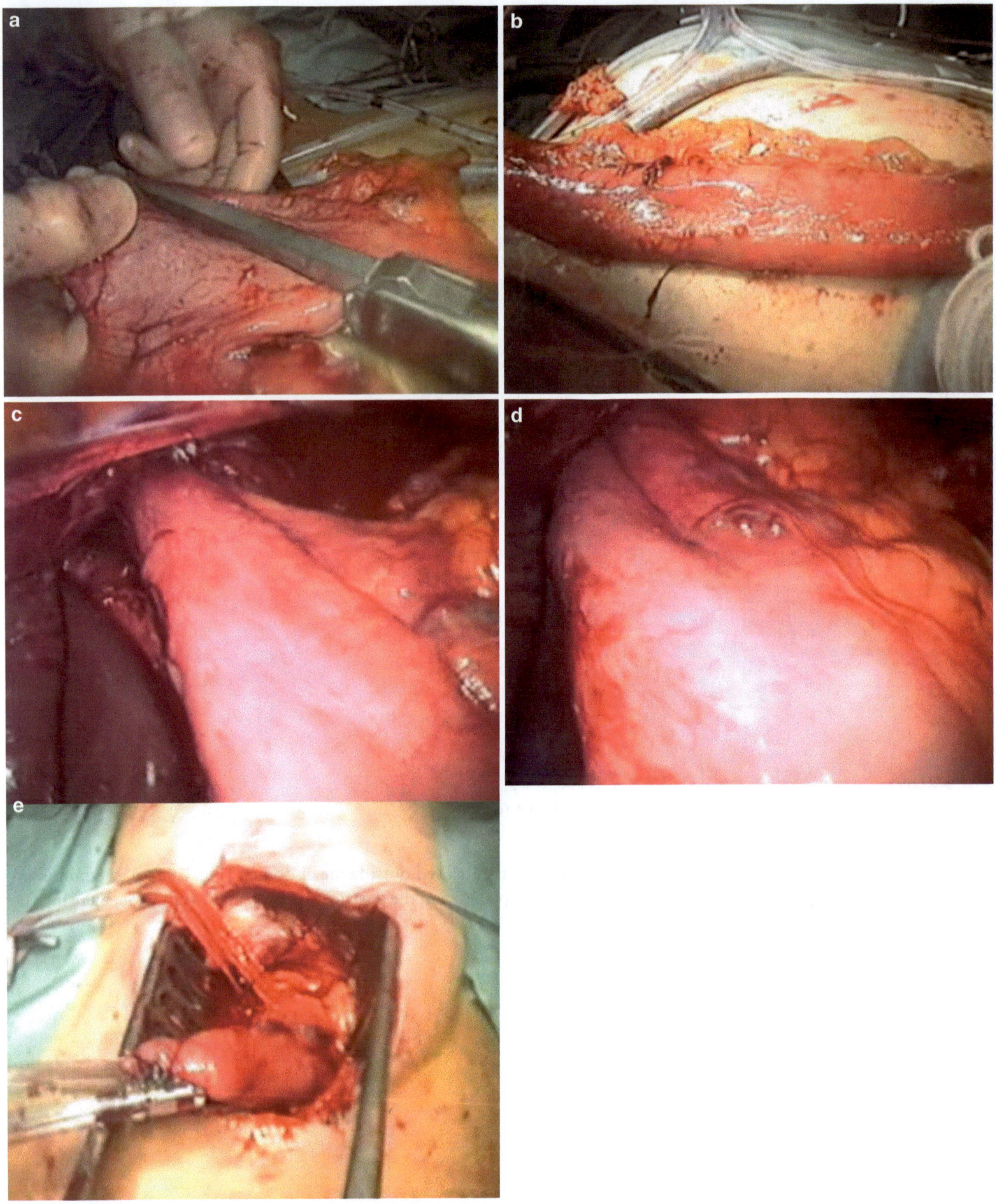

Fig. 7.10 (a–e) Once the specimen is exteriorized, a gastric tube (4 cm) is created by means of 100 mm GIA device along the greater curvature. The good vascularized gastric tube is oversewn, attached to a NG tube and pulled up into the cervical wound and anastomosed. Through the small laparotomy a jejunostomy catheter is introduced and both thoracic cavities are drained by means of drains introduced through the abdominal trocars ports (f)

100-mm GIA stapling device (Fig. 7.10a, b). The gastric tube then is oversewn and attached to the nasogastric tube and replaced in the abdomen. Next, the pneumoperitoneum is reestablished, and the gastric tube is placed under vision into the cervical esophagus by traction of the nasogastric tube (Fig. 7.10c–e). A laparoscopic end-to-side cervical anastomosis is created by using a one-layer suture technique.

Fig. 7.10 (f)

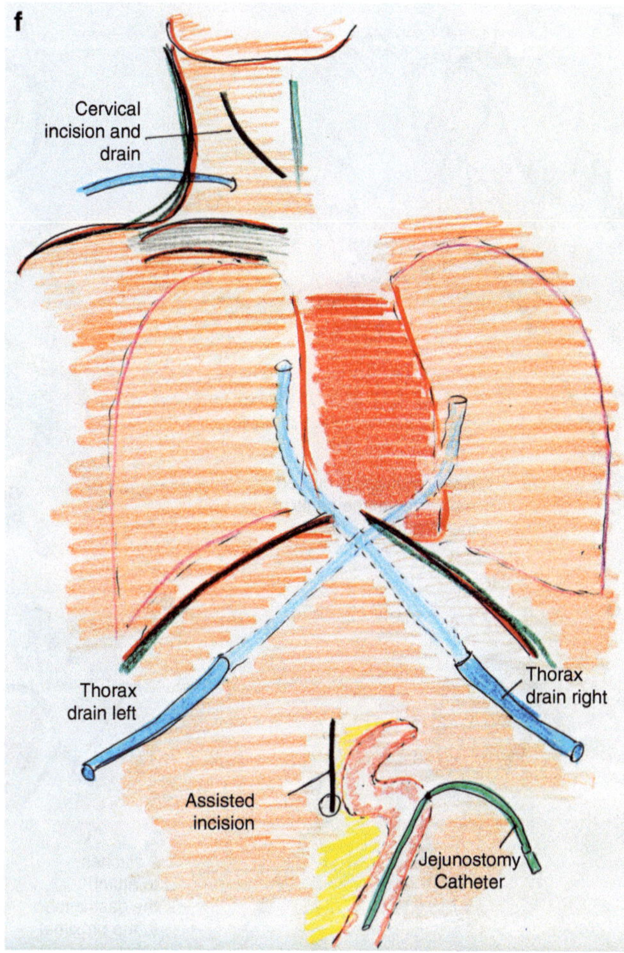

13. Through the transumbilical incision, a jejunostomy feeding tube was placed for feeding, and the two thoracic cavities were drained by two thoracic drains placed through the trocar openings (Fig. 7.10f). In none of the patients in this series was a Kocher maneuver, a pyloromyotomy, or a pyloroplasty performed.

14. An alternative method is to prepare the gastric tube intraabdominally. Once the gastric mobilization has been accomplished, by means of an blue endostapler 6 cm the stomach is divided to create a gastric tube along the greater curvature (4 cm width). Once

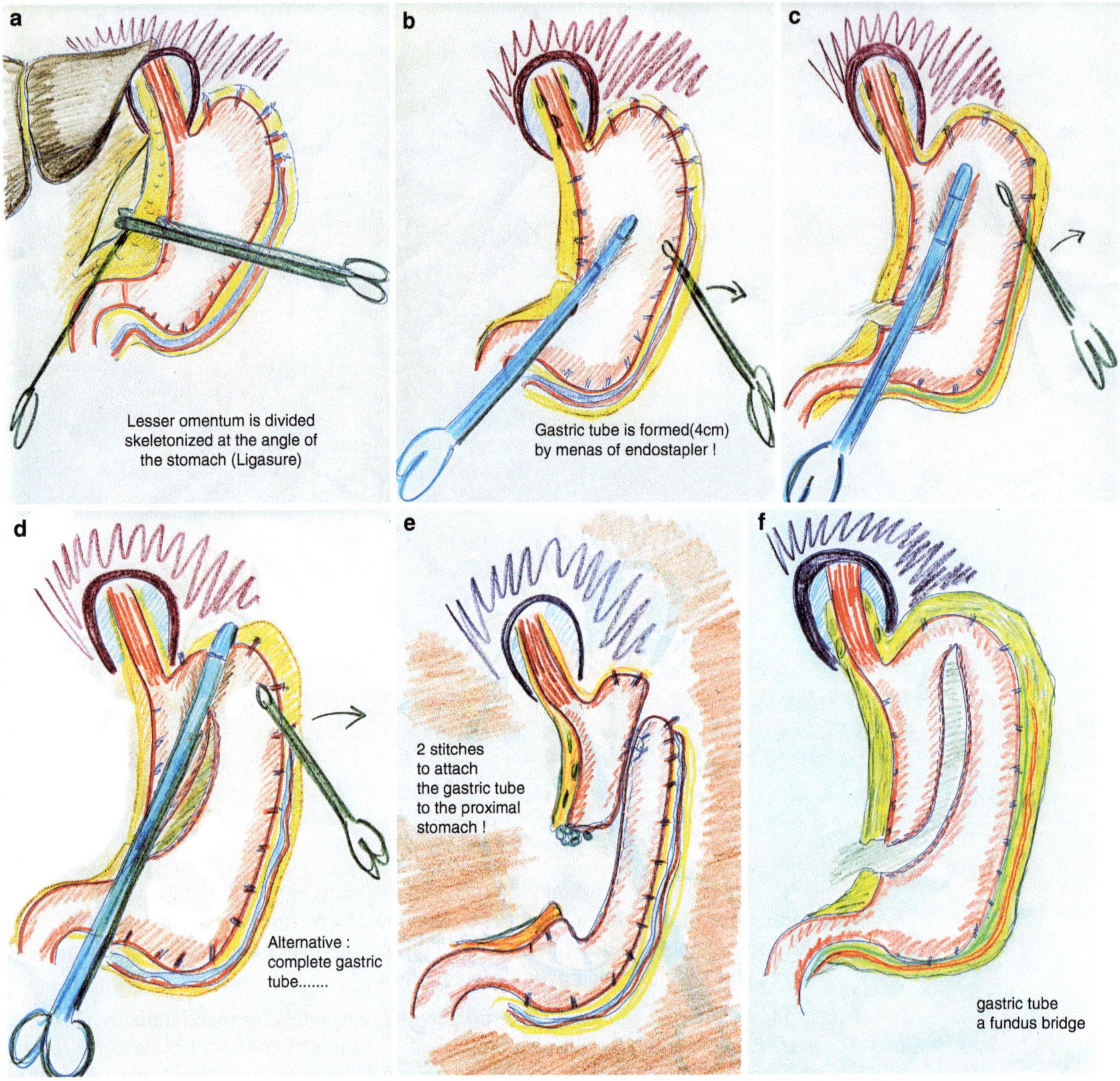

Fig. 7.11 (a–f) An alternative method is to prepare the gastric tube intracorporeally by means of the endo-stapler. Once divided, the fundus is attached to the gastric tube by means of two strong stitches. Other option is to leave a small bridge at the fundus instead of 2 stiches!

this is done, the gastric tube is attached to the gastric fundus by two strong stitches (Fig. 7.11a–e). From the neck, the specimen can be retrieved and in this way the complete

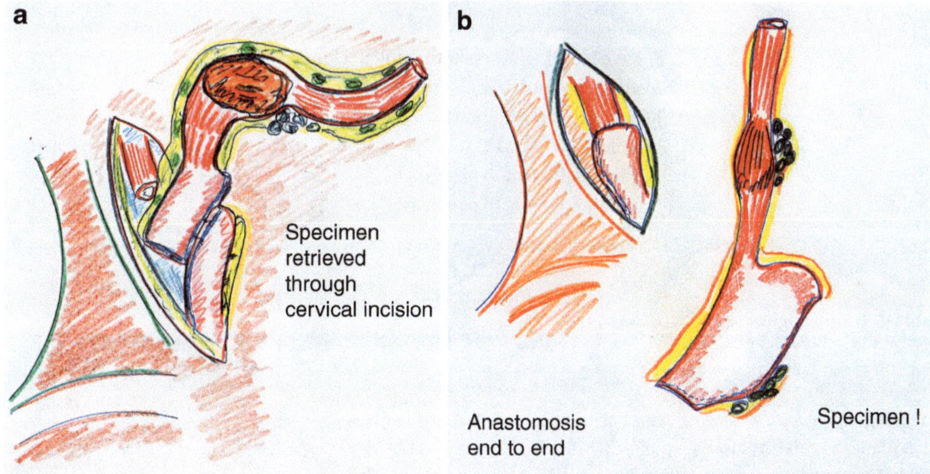

Fig. 7.12 (a, b) After retrieval of the specimen through the cervical incision, anastomosis between the esophagus and the gastric tube is manually performed

specimen and the gastric tube are exteriorized into the neck (Fig. 7.12a). After resection, esophago-gastric tube anastomosis will be performed (Fig. 7.12b).

This second option, without assisted abdominal incision is more difficult to perform, because in most of the cases, the esophagus above the carina and for a distance of a couple of centimeters is not dissected free during the mediastinal dissection. Therefore, it is difficult to retrieve it easily through the neck incision. My advice is to use the first option and to exteriorize the specimen after stripping through a small assisted abdominal incision.

Postoperatively, patients are ventilated mechanically at the ICU and extubated when their hemodynamic and respiratory conditions are stable. Extubated patients are admitted to the medium care ward and from there to the regular ward.

Patients are fed through the jejunostomy feeding tube from the first day after their operation, until the oral feeding can be completely resumed.

On postoperative day 5, a swallow X-ray examination is performed to assess the anastomotic and gastric tube passage. When no leakage and a good passage are seen, the nasogastric tube is removed and oral feeding is started. Patients are discharged when they are completely mobile and able to feed themselves orally.

Own Experience

Results

Between January 2001 and January 2005, 57 consecutive patients with a squamous cell carcinoma or an adenocarcinoma of the low distal esophagus or G–E junction were included for laparoscopic transhiatal esophageal resection [9].

Fifty-seven patients were approached laparoscopically to undergo a transhiatal resection. From them, 7 patients were found not resectable (12%), because of the presence of liver metastases; the presence of portal hypertension, or ingrowth in the pericardial sac or in the pulmonary vein. Finally, 50 patients underwent laparoscopically assisted transhiatal esophageal resection.

Nine patients (18%) were converted to open procedure; however, laparoscopic mediastinal dissection of the esophagus could be accomplished in 45 patients (90%). The reasons for conversion are listed in Table 7.1.

Tumor characteristics are given in Table 7.2. Tumor-free margins (R0) were obtained in 41 (82%) of the 50 patients, whereas in the other 9 patients, circumferential margins were microscopically affected (R1, 18%). The median number of harvested lymph nodes was of 14 in the whole group. The median operation time was 300 min (265–320 min) and a median blood loss of 500 mL (400–650 mL). Median postoperative ICU stay was 1 day (1, 0–2, 0 days) and the median hospital stay was 13 days (11–16 days).

Table 7.1 Reasons for conversion

Reason for conversion	Number of patients
Splenic bleeding necessitating splenectomy	2
Insufficient visualization due to liver	3
Evaluation of resectability	
Solid celiac trunk	2
Tumor adherent to pleura	1
Tumor adherent to pancreas	1
Total	9 (18%)

Table 7.2 Oncological characteristics of patients

Characteristics	Laparoscopic transhiatal esophageal resections ($n = 50$)
Histologic type	
Squamous-cell carcinoma	12 (24%)
Undifferentiated	1 (2%)
Adenocarcinoma	37 (74%)
TNM stage	
I	3 (6%)
IIa	10 (20%)
IIb	6 (12%)
III	31 (62%)
Tumor differentiation	
Good	3 (6%)
Moderate	10 (20%)
Moderate/poor	8 (16%)
Poor	29 (58%)
Location of the tumor	
Median	35 cm (33–41)
Radicality of surgery	
R0	41 (82%)
R1	9 (18%)
Number of harvested lymph nodes – median (interquartiler ange)	14 (10–19)

Morbidity and Mortality

One of the patients considered nonresectable because of the presence of a portal hypertension died during the postoperative period. Thus mortality of the whole group was 1.7%. No hospital mortality was recorded in the series of 50 patients resected.

Postoperative complications occurred in 21 patients (42%). Pulmonary and cardiac complications were observed in 9 (18%) and 3 (6%) patients respectively. Two patients (4%) had to be reoperated. Details of postoperative morbidity are depicted in Table 7.3.

Comments

In the randomized study by Hulscher et al., transthoracic esophageal resection with abdominal and mediastinal lymph node dissection (two field lymphadenectomy) were compared with the classical transhiatal approach [4]. The transhiatal approach had lower morbidity than the transthoracic approach. Even if a trend was observed with the advantage for the transthoracic approach in tumors located in the mid-esophagus, the median survival and disease-free survival for the most common very low esophageal and junction cancers were not statistically significant.

Compared with the right thoracoscopic approach, the transhiatal approach seems more suitable for junctional tumors because it approaches the tumor directly on both sides in relation to both thoracic cavities and its possible extension into the cardia. Also, the value of initial diagnostic laparoscopy for the assessment of resectability is

Table 7.3 Morbidity after laparoscopic transhiatal esophageal resection

Variable	Laparoscopic transhiatal esophageal Resections ($n = 50$)
In-hospital mortality	1 (1.7%)
Short term morbidity	
Patients with complications	21 (42%)
Pulmonary complications	9 (18%)
Cardiac complications	3 (6%)
Recurrence nerve palsy	3 (6%)
Chylus leakage	1 (2%)
Cervical fistula	4 (8%)
Evisceration	1 (2%)
Long term morbidity	
Stenosis requiring endoscopic dillatation	4 (8%)
Reoperation	2 (4%)
Inspection cervical anastomosis	1 (2%)
Correction of evisceration	1 (2%)

given in this series in which 12% of patients initially approached for resection were considered unresectable because of diverse reasons. Moreover, the thoracoscopic approach of these distal tumors can be hampered by the localization of the tumor at the costal-phrenic space. Furthermore, laparoscopic transhiatal approach will permit perfect visualization of the mediastinal structures in relation to the tumor up to carina, making this operation no longer a blind procedure, in addition to avoiding the hemodynamic instability during the conventional dissection by the use of the retractor and manual dissection.

Retrieval of the tumor through a small well-protected transumbilical incision instead of through a cervical incision may avoid the appearance of port-site metastases as in the case of laparoscopic colonic surgery for cancer. Moreover, once the specimen is retrieved, dissection around pylorus and the origin of the gastroepiploic vessels can be accomplished followed by formation of the gastric tube, using the conventional GIA-100. In this fashion, the operation is time sparing and cost-effective.

Current use of pyloroplasty remains controversial as well [10]. Many authors still include the drainage of the pylorus in the operative procedure. In the current study, the avoidance of this pyloroplasty has not lead to any gastric tube emptying problems during the postoperative period. Therefore, we do not recommend a routine pyloroplasty as part of the gastric tube formation.

References

1. Lewis I. The surgical treatment of carcinoma of the oesophagus with special reference to a new operation for growths of the middle third. Br J Surg 1946;34:18–31
2. Orringer MB, Sloan H. Esophagectomy without thoracotomy. J Thorac Cardiovasc Surg 1978;76:643–654
3. Law S, Wong KH, Kwok KF, et al Predictive factors for postoperative pulmonary complications and mortalitry after esophagectomy for cancer. Ann Surg 2004;240:791–800
4. Hulscher JB, van Sandick JW, de Boer AG, Wijnhoven BP, Tijssen JG, Fockens P, et al Extended transthoracic resection compared with limited transhiatal resection for adenocarcinoma of the esophagus. New Engl J Med 2002;347:1662–1669
5. De Paula AL, Hashiba K, Ferreira EAB, et al Laparoscopic transhiatal esophagectomy with esophagogastroplasty. Surg Endosc 1995;5:1–5
6. Dallemagne B, Weerts JM, Jehaes C, et al Subtotal esophagectomy by thoracoscopy and laparoscopy. Minim Invasive Ther Allied Technol 1992;1:183–185
7. Pinotti HW, Zilberstein B, Pollara W, Raia A. Esophagectomy without thoracotomy. Surg Gynecol Obstet 1981;152:345–347
8. Makay O, van den Broek WT, Yuan JZ, et al Anaesthesiological hazards during laparoscopic transhiatal esophageal resection: a case control study of the laparoscopic assisted versus the conventional approach. Surg Endosc 2004;18:1263–1267
9. Scheepers JJG, Veenhof AAFA, van der Peet DL, van Groeningen C, Mulder Ch, Meijer S, Cuesta MA. Laparoscopic transhiatal resection for malignancies of the distal esophagus: outcome of the first 50 resected patients. Surgery 2008;143:278–285
10. Mannell A, Mcknight A, Esser JD. Role of pyloroplasty in the retrosternal stomach. Results of A prospective, randomized, controlled trial. Br J Surg 1990;77:57–59

8

Robot-Assisted Thoracolaparoscopic Esophagectomy

Richard van Hillegersberg and Judith Boone

Introduction

As the esophagus has a unique longitudinal lymphatic drainage system in the submucosal layer, lymph node metastases of esophageal cancer can occur along the entire esophagus from the cervical to the abdominal part. The optimal treatment for esophageal cancer, therefore, consists of transthoracic en bloc esophagectomy (TTE) with an extensive mediastinal and abdominal lymph node dissection (LND). This approach through thoracotomy is accompanied by significant morbidity, which is predominantly due to cardiopulmonary complications.

To reduce the surgical trauma and thus the morbidity of open TTE, less-invasive surgical techniques such as transhiatal esophagectomy (THE) were introduced. A randomized controlled trial on TTE vs. THE has shown the latter to carry a lower complication rate.[1,2] However, since with THE the esophagus is stripped out of the mediastinum, only a limited LND can be carried out without dissection of the upper mediastinal lymph nodes. Consequently, a trend toward a better survival for TTE over THE was detected.[1,2] Statistical significance was not reached, but this was most probably a result of the fact that the study was underpowered.

Minimally invasive esophagectomy (MIE) was introduced to further reduce morbidity. With regard to MIE, the world's largest series on thoracolaparoscopic esophagectomy has shown a significantly lower blood loss and morbidity compared to open TTE. However, the survival after this procedure was worse than after open TTE (3-year overall survival rate for Stage II patients of 20 vs. 50%, respectively). This could be explained by the fact that a less extensive en bloc resection was preformed due to the disadvantages of "conventional" scopic surgery, such as a 2D vision, disturbed eye-hand coordination, and fewer degrees of freedom.

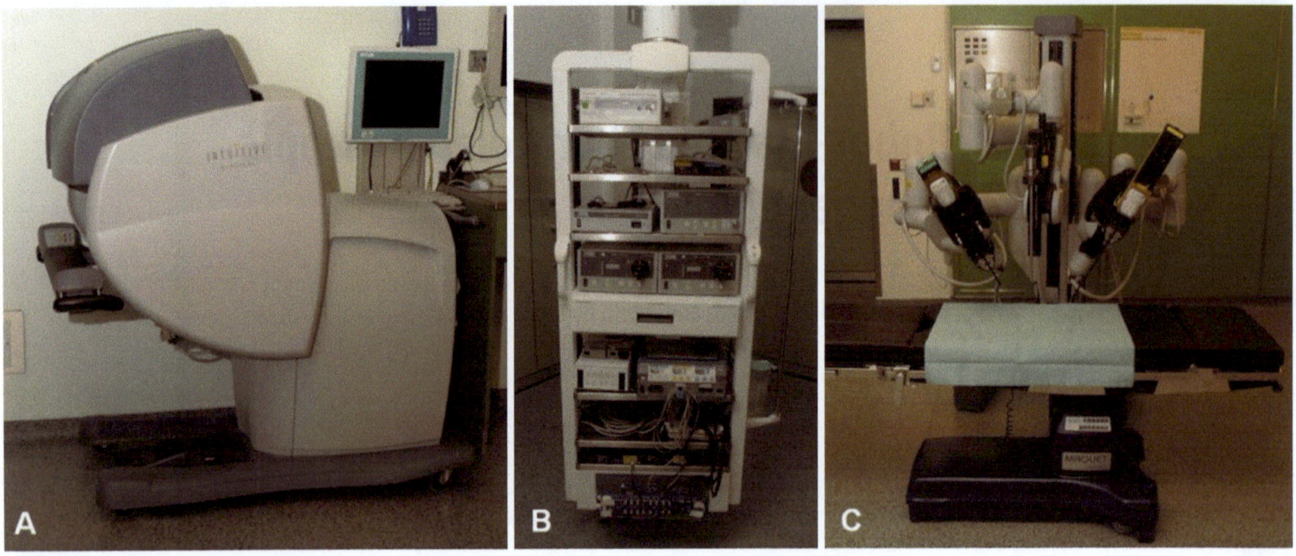

Fig. 8.1 (a-c) The Da Vinci® surgical system consisting of the surgeon's console (A), the accessory cart, (B) and the robotic surgical system (C)

Robotic systems have been developed to overcome the limitations of conventional scopic surgery. The Da Vinci® robotic system consists of three parts (Fig. 8.1): (a) the 3-armed robotic system which is positioned next to the operating table; (b) the console of the robotic system with joystick-like hand controls and with foot pedals through which the surgeon can control the arms of the robotic system and (c) the accessories cart which holds, e.g., the light sources and focus control. The Da Vinci® robotic system offers the surgeon a tenfold magnified, 3D view on the surgical field. The surgeon's tremor is filtered and the articulated surgical instruments allow for more degrees of freedom. These advantages facilitate a precise dissection in a confined operating space.

Robotic surgical systems have successfully been applied in various specialties such as urology, gynecology, cardiothoracic surgery, and general surgery. For radical prostatectomy, the robot-assisted approach has shown to be superior to the conventional laparoscopic approach and has therefore become the treatment of choice in many centers. Robotic systems may also be of added value in thoracoscopic esophagectomy, by facilitating a more accurate mediastinal dissection of the esophagus with the surrounding lymph nodes when compared to conventional thoracoscopic esophagectomy.

The first case description of thoracoscopic esophagectomy aided by the Da Vinci robotic system was published in 2004 by Kernstine et al. Simultaneously, a robot-assisted thoracoscopic esophagectomy (RTE) technique was developed in the University Medical Center Utrecht and clinically used since 2003, as the standard surgical approach to esophagectomy for esophageal cancer patients.

Surgical Technique

Before we introduced RTE into clinical practice, we have tested the optimal thoracic port positions and optimal position of the robotic system in a laboratory setting on living pigs and human cadavers. To reach the entire mediastinum from diaphragm to thoracic aperture, a dorsocranial position of the robot was found to be optimal, with ports in triangular formation (Fig. 8.2).

The newly developed thoracoscopic procedure was initially combined with laparotomy for creating the gastric conduit and for performing an upper abdominal LND. After the first 16 cases, the learning curve for this procedure had stabilized, and a complete minimally invasive procedure was introduced. The laparoscopy was performed without

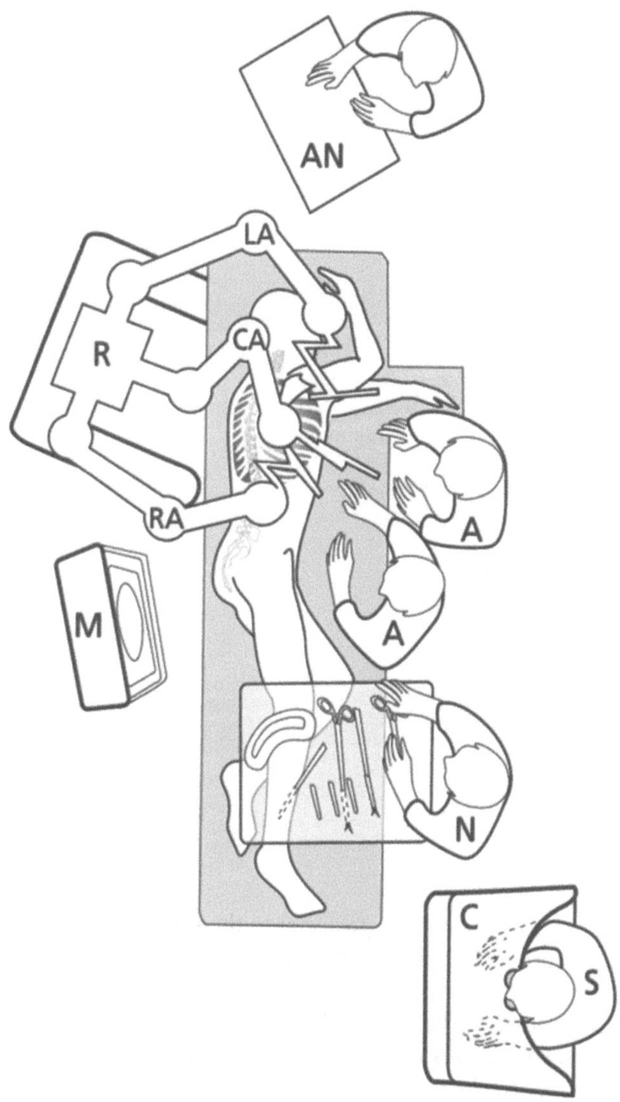

Fig. 8.2 Setup on the operating room during the thoracoscopic phase of RTE. The robotic system (R) is placed on the dorsocranial side of the patient. From behind the console (C), the surgeon (S) controls the left robotic arm (LA), right robotic arm (RA), and the camera arm (CA). The surgeon is assisted by a surgical assistant (A) and a scrubnurse (N). *M* monitor; *AN* anaesthesiologist. (Figure has previously been published: Boone et al. [1])

robotic assistance as our experimental studies revealed that large ranges of the robotic arms would limit the use of the robotic system in this part of the procedure.

During the thoracoscopic phase, the patient is intubated with a left-sided double-lumen tube and positioned in the left lateral decubitus position, 45° tilted toward prone position. In this position, the right lung is out of the operating field without retraction following desufflation. The robot was positioned on the dorsocranial side of the patient. A surgical assistant and a scrubnurse were on the anterior side of the patient. Three robotic ports were placed identically in all patients. A 10-mm camera port was placed at the 6th intercostal space, posterior to the posterior axillary line. Two 8-mm ports were placed just anteriorly to the scapular rim in the 4th intercostal space and more posteriorly in the 8th intercostal space. Two thoracoscopic ports were used in the 5th and 7th

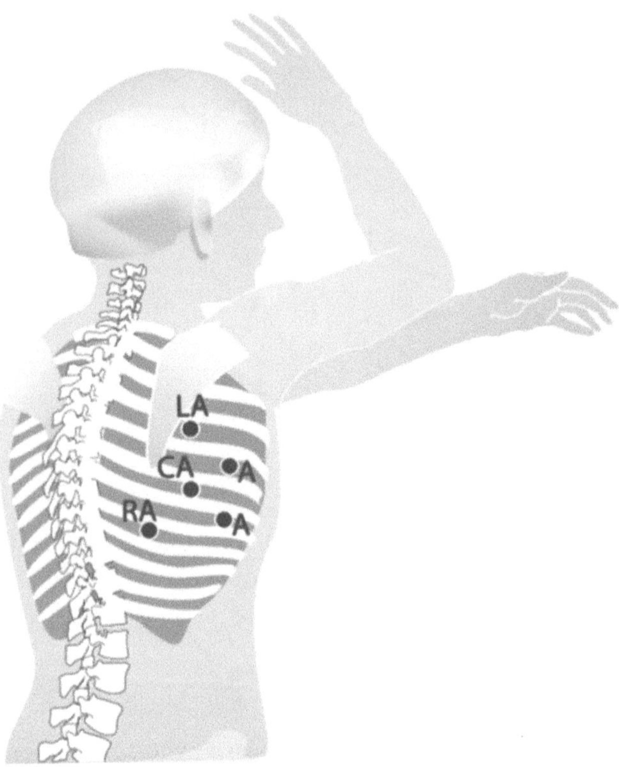

Fig. 8.3 Trocar position during RTE. Triangular position of the robotic trocar ports (*LA* left robotic arm; *RA* right robotic arm; *CA* camera arm). Two ports (A) are used for conventional scopic assistance, such as suctioning and clipping. (Figure has previously been published: Boone et al. [1])

intercostal spaces, just posterior to the posterior axillary line. These ports were used for conventional thoracoscopic assistance, such as suction, traction and clipping (Fig. 8.3).

After division of the pulmonary ligament, the parietal pleura was divided at the anterior side up to the level of the azygos vein. The azygos vein was ligated with sutures and clips. The mediastinal pleura above the azygos vein is ligated up to the thoracic inlet and a proper tracheal LND is performed.

Then the parietal pleura was divided at the posterior side along the azygos vein and including the thoracic duct. The thoracic duct was clipped at the level of the diaphragm to prevent leakage. The tumor and adjacent lymph nodes were dissected en bloc, with clipping of the aortoesophageal vessels. The right vagal nerve was identified and dissected below the level of the carina. A penrose drain was placed around the esophagus to facilitate traction. In this way the entire thoracic esophagus was mobilized from the thoracic inlet to the diaphragmatic reflections. Finally, a subcarinal LND was performed. The specimen included the lower and middle mediastinal, subcarinal, aortopulmonary window nodes, and right-sided paratracheal nodes. A 24-F chest tube was placed and the lung insufflated under direct vision. The patient was then put in supine position.

Through a midline laparotomy, the greater and lesser curvatures were dissected and a 3- to 4-cm wide gastric tube was constructed with staplers. The left gastric artery and vein were then transected at its origin, with concomitant resection of local lymph nodes. A feeding jejunostomy was installed in first jejunal loop after Treitz ligament. The cervical esophagus was mobilized through a left-sided longitudinal neck incision. A hand sewn end-to-side esophagogastrostomy was performed in the neck using one layer PDS 3/0 running sutures.

In case of laparoscopy, five abdominal ports were used (Fig. 8.4). A 10-mm camera port was introduced at the left midclavicular line at the supra-umbilical level and, a 12-mm working port was placed at the contralateral side. Two 5-mm working ports were placed at the subcostal area on both sides. A 12-mm port was placed pararectal right for

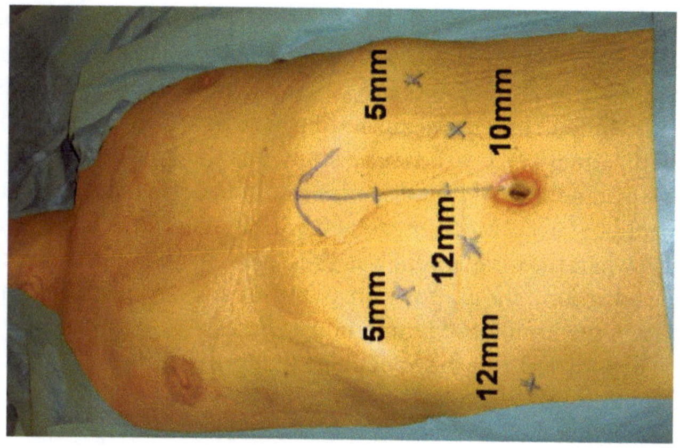

Fig. 8.4 Trocar positioning during the laparoscopic phase. 10-mm trocar: for camera. 5-mm trocars: working ports. 12-mm right pararectal trocar: for liver retractor. 12-mm paraumbilical port: ultracision device

the liver retractor. The abdomen was insufflated to a carbon dioxide pressure level of 15 mmHg. The greater and lesser curvatures were dissected with ultrasonic coagulating shears. The left gastric artery and vein were then transected at their origin, with resection of local lymph nodes. The hiatus was opened and the distal esophagus dissected from the right and left crus. Carbon dioxide pressure level was then reduced to 5 mmHg to avoid a high intrathoracic pressure. After cervical esophageal transection, the esophagus and surrounding lymph nodes were pulled into the abdomen under laparoscopic vision. A 7-cm transverse incision was made at the level of the left supra-umbilical port to extract the specimen and stomach using a wound protector. Outside the abdomen, a 3- to 4-cm wide gastric tube was then constructed with GIA staplers. The stapled line is routinely oversewn with PDS 3/0 to prevent local complications. In the neck, an end-to-side handsewn anastomosis was made between cervical remnant esophagus and the gastric conduit.

Results

Our first publication of 21 esophageal cancer patients, 15 male patients, and 6 female patients with a median age of 62 (7–78) years having undergone RTE has shown this technique to be feasible. Robotic set-up time was 7 (median, range 4–15) min. The median duration of the robot-assisted thoracoscopic phase was 180 (range 120–240) min and of the total procedure 450 (range 370–550) min. The robotic system facilitated a precise dissection along the vital mediastinal structures such as the pulmonary vein, the trachea, and the aorta. Blood loss was low: 400 mL for the thoracoscopic phase and 950 mL for the entire surgical procedure.

Patients were ventilated for 2 (median, range 0–126) days. Median ICU stay was 4 (1–129) days and total hospital stay was 18 (11–182) days.

Median pulmonary complication rate was 48%. A steep decrease in pulmonary complication rate was noticed from 60% in the first 10 patients to 32% in the last 11 patients. This represented the learning curve of both the surgical and anesthesiological team. In-hospital mortality was 5%.

Adenocarcinoma and squamous cell carcinoma were equally distributed (48 and 52%, respectively). Most patients had advanced stage disease (76% Stage III–IVa). R0-resection rate was 76% and no R2 resections were carried out. A mean amount of 20 lymph nodes were dissected.

Currently, we have treated approximately 100 esophageal cancer patients by RTE. The pulmonary complication rate has further decreased to 30%. Resected specimens are analyzed by one experienced pathologist in gastrointestinal oncology. The median amount of resected lymph nodes in our medical center is approximately 31.

An important difference between RTE and open TTE is the preservation of the azygos vein. In (robot-assisted) thoracoscopic esophagolymphadenectomy, the azygos vein is generally left in place, as the scopic ligation of the numerous intercostal veins is technically difficult and time-consuming. One may postulate that this could affect the extent of mediastinal LND. A cadaveric study was therefore initiated to determine which percentage of mediastinal lymph nodes would be left in situ when the trunk of the azygos vein would be preserved. A mean of 0.67 (95% Poisson CI 0.32–1.23) lymph nodes were left in situ when the azygos vein was preserved. In 60% of cadavers, no lymph nodes at all were found around the azygos vein. In those cadavers, additional azygos vein resection did not add to the number of lymph nodes dissected.

In addition, one may postulate that preserving the azygos vein may affect the circumferential radical resection (R0) rate. Yet, the results of our patient series on RTE have shown that the R0 resection rate is similar to that reported in open TTE. Thus, leaving the azygos vein in situ during (robot-assisted) thoracoscopic esophagectomy neither affects the extent of mediastinal lymphadenectomy, nor the R0 resection rate.

The gastric conduit is the most commonly used reconstruction for the digestive tract following esophagectomy. The linear stapled line is routinely oversewn to prevent leakage at this stapled line, and to avoid damage to the mediastinal structures by possible protruding staples (Fig. 8.5). Some surgeons performing MIE create the gastric conduit laparoscopically as well, in order to accomplish an entirely scopic surgical procedure. Because oversewing the stapled line by means of scopic instruments is technically difficult and time-consuming, this routine step is often abandoned. In our first 15 RTE patients, we did not oversew the stapled line. This resulted in leakage at the linear stapled line in 2 (13%) patients. Since then, we have reintroduced this routine practice, and no local complications at the stapled line have been encountered afterward. It should therefore be recommended to always oversew the gastric conduit linear stapled line, irrespective of the surgical approach.

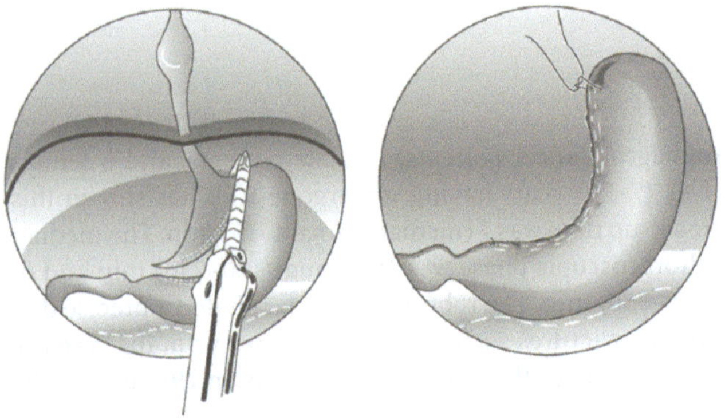

Fig. 8.5 The gastric conduit is created by means of several linear staplers (*left*). The gastric conduit stapled line is routinely oversewn with PDS 3-0 to prevent complications (*right*)

A second indication for RTE is giant esophageal submucosal tumors. In 2008, we have published the first case worldwide of RTE for a giant submucosal tumor of the upper esophagus in a young patient in whom a mesenchymal malignancy was highly suspected. Although histopathologic analysis of the resected specimen revealed the mesenchymal tumor to be benign, therapy would have been similar, as the enucleation of a large (>8 cm) esophageal leiomyoma would create muscular defects too large to achieve tension-free sutures.

Discussion

RTE is a safe, feasible technique, accompanied by significantly lower blood loss (median 650 mL) than open TTE (mean 1,900 mL). This is of particular clinical interest, as several studies have shown that esophageal cancer patients with major blood loss receiving allogenic blood transfusions have a significant worse prognosis than patients without transfusions.

The 3D, tenfold magnified view of the surgical field provides for an extensive en bloc dissection of the esophagus and the surrounding mediastinal lymph nodes. With a median number of 30 dissected lymph nodes, the extent of lymphadenectomy of RTE is similar to that of open TTE. When surgically treated by a THE, these tumor deposits would not have been resected.

The operation time of RTE is currently longer than open TTE. With increasing experience and consistency of the surgical team including the employment of a physician assistant specialized in robotic surgery, operation time may be expected to decrease further.

At present, the morbidity of RTE is comparable to that of open TTE. A steep decrease in pulmonary complication rate was noticed when comparing the last series of operated patients with the first. With 35%, the pulmonary complication rate of the last series was comparable to the open transhiatal approach. An additional reduction in pulmonary complications may be anticipated with increasing experience and consistency of both the surgical and anesthesiological team. Still, during RTE, similar to open TTE but in contrast to open THE, the right lung is deflated for 2–3 h to achieve optimal exposure of the mediastinal structures. Deflation with subsequent reinflation of the lung is accompanied by the release of various cytokines and chemokines. As these inflammatory mediators may cause pulmonary complications, effort should be undertaken to antagonize their production. This may be achieved by anesthesiological strategies (e.g., protective ventilation strategies for the deflated or the dependent lung, or systemic administration of anti-inflammatory or immunosuppressive drugs) and surgical strategies (e.g., less manipulation of the deflated lung with surgical instruments or optimal patient positioning so that gravity can aid in retracting the deflated lung).

To confirm our data and to assess if long-term oncologic outcome of RTE is comparable to open TTE, more prospective studies with a longer follow-up of larger study populations are warranted. We are, therefore, pleased to see that other institutions have commenced RTE. For the ultimate comparison of RTE, open TTE and conventional thoracoscopic esophagectomy, a randomized controlled trial is currently being conducted.

Reference

1. Boone J, Draaisma WA, Schipper MEI, Broeders IAMJ, Rinkes IHMB, van Hillegersberg R (2008) Robot-assisted thoracoscopic esophagectomy for a giant upper esophageal leiomyoma. Dis Esophagus 21:90–93

Index

MIX
Papier aus verantwortungsvollen Quellen
Paper from responsible sources
FSC® C105338

If you have any concerns about our products,
you can contact us on
ProductSafety@springernature.com

In case Publisher is established outside the EU,
the EU authorized representative is:
Springer Nature Customer Service Center GmbH
Europaplatz 3, 69115 Heidelberg, Germany

Printed by Libri Plureos GmbH
in Hamburg, Germany